Fat & Thin

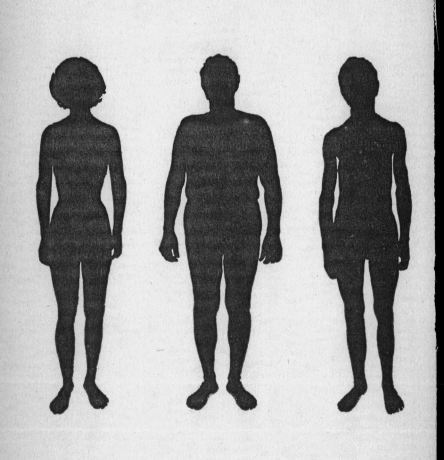

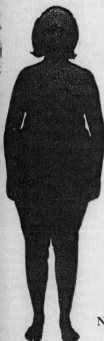

Fat & Thin

A Natural History of Obesity

Anne Scott Beller

McGraw-Hill Book Company

New York   St. Louis   San Francisco   Bogotá   Düsseldorf
Madrid   Mexico   Montreal   Panama   Paris
São Paulo   Tokyo   Toronto

Reprinted by arrangement with
Farrar, Straus & Giroux

First McGraw-Hill Paperback edition, 1978
Designed by Patricia Given Dunbar
1 2 3 4 5 6 7 8 9 0 FG FG 7 8 3 2 1 0 9 8

Library of Congress Cataloging in Publication Data

Beller, Anne Scott.
  Fat & thin: a natural history of obesity

  Reprint of the ed. published by Farrar, Straus and Giroux, New York.
  Bibliography: p.
  Includes index.
  1. Obesity. 2. Obesity—Social aspects. 3. Body, Human—Social aspects. I. Title.
RC628.B357   1978   616.3'98   78-6679
ISBN 0-07-004413-9

For A.

Acknowledgments

The author is indebted to Professors Francis Johnston of the University of Pennsylvania and Akkaraju Sarma of Temple University, and to Doctors Denis Abelson and Albert Stunkard, each of whom read and commented on all or parts of this book in manuscript.

Rosalind Layton, Michael Hoffacker, Marge Hebert, and Margaret Harvey gave tireless and invaluable bibliographic assistance, as did other members of the staff of the Ardmore Free Library and the library of the Philadelphia College of Physicians. Thanks are also owing to Marion Styer of the Montgomery County–Norristown Public Library for her unflagging help in tracking down books and other materials through inter-library loan, and to Jeannie Goodman and Ave Longley for moral, bibliographic, and editorial support.

Contents

Fat & Thin

Introduction

We live in a Malthusian universe, with population and food supply
leapfrogging each other toward what the demographers have daunt-
ingly described as the "limits of growth." World population passed
the four billion mark in 1976; and despite a recent dip in projections it is expected to pass the eight billion mark by the year 2020.
World grain reserves, meanwhile, have dwindled to the vanishing point and fluctuated between three weeks' and three months'
reserve rations since the famine year of 1974. With world food
backlogs at an all-time low, and world population figures at or
close to an all-time high, it may be timely to recall that obesity, the
dependable bugbear of cardiologists and fashion editors, may once
long ago have served nature's purpose, if not her grand design, by
outfitting the species with a built-in mechanism for storing its own
grain reserves in the form of fat.

   In the last forty years it has become fashionable among physicians, insurance underwriters, psychotherapists, and taste makers
to inveigh against overweight as the common enemy, and over the
years campaigns mustered in this cause have raised legions of col-
lateral specialists and specialties: The United States' diet industry
alone has been estimated to gross over $100 million a year, and the
figure rises annually. In terms of mounting scarcities and food

shortages, though, it may be profitable to remember man's humbler beginnings as a species struggling to survive and prosper in an environment that offered few options between feast and famine. Man's prehistory in Europe, Russia, and northern China is that of a species making its way at the edge of a glacier whose unpredictable stops and starts had direct and sometimes cataclysmic effects on the prevailing food supply.

Plants had relatively little place in the Paleolithic hunter's diet, and the romance of the hunter's life has been played up in the popular literature, its chanciness played down. Luck and accident have always been basic items in the hunter's tool kit, and like other great predators, our reindeer- and bison-hunting forebears lived from one windfall to the next. They might enjoy huge kills one day and then go hungry for days or weeks on end. Survival therefore dictated some metabolic compromise between feast and famine, and the emerging species must have "learned," anatomically, to store food under its own skin in times of glut, and to live off that stored subcutaneous surplus when the climate, the season, and the vagaries of the animal species it hunted resulted in scarcities and famine. With personal and population viability the reward for the so-called "thrifty" genotypes (people anatomically designed to store the greatest amount of fat in the least amount of time and to release it as parsimoniously as possible over the long run), it is not surprising that even present-day populations still contain large numbers of people whose genes dispose them to overweight.

Obesity has had a bad press in the medical journals and the fashion magazines; we eat more regularly now than our hunting ancestors did and the ability to store fat is thus no longer lifesaving. If anything, the actuarial tables suggest that it may be just the opposite. The present book acknowledges obesity as maladaptive in a time and culture in which the fluctuations of food supply are minimal and the physiological drawbacks of obesity are of more immediate medical concern than the ecological likelihood of famine. In doing so, though, it will attempt to retrace the ecological, genetic, and climatological history of obesity as a physiological response to environment, and in the process to suggest some morally and culturally neutral ways of dealing with the problem, even in the face of long genetic odds favoring the accumulation of fat in the fat-prone individual, and his or her possibly constitutional predisposition to chronic overweight.

Such odds entail the probability that a certain proportion of the general population will always have an uphill battle to fight against overweight. This genealogical probability is one of the better-kept secrets of medical history. Obesity has been identified as a "disease," with a stipulated cure (dieting) and an acknowledged etiology (gluttony). But to many of the afflicted the cure has always seemed at least as bad as the disease, and the medical profession has had its work cut out for it in putting its prescription into practice. To help it in this task it has enlisted an army of concerned family members, journalists, and other amateurs in the uphill effort to put fat people on a diet. The effort is a well-meant and generoushearted one and needs no apology. But meanwhile a considerable body of facts, figures, and general information seems to have gotten lost in the shuffle and, given the prevailing clinical view that obesity is a disease, and the pervasively moralistic tone of most popular writing on the subject, it has generally escaped notice that there exists a substantial body of medical and scientific literature pointing to the underlying constitutional (i.e., genetic) factors in overweight, and to possible ways of manipulating these factors in the patient's favor. A serious attempt to bridge the gap between the hortatory literature of the diet experts and the popular press, on the one hand, and the more culturally neutral but largely underreported message of medical, anthropological, biochemical, research, on the other, may therefore be seriously overdue.

Taste and fashion make strange bedfellows: In the current campaign against overweight the taste makers have found allies among the insurance underwriters. Aesthetics aside, actuarial studies linking overweight to increased mortality from various causes began to appear in print early in the century and received wide recognition and acceptance within decades of their appearance. Half a century later a generation of practicing physicians—and the public to whom they ministered—had mastered the official orthodoxy that fat is suicidal: a sin, that is, at best; and at worst a sort of felony.

The insurance studies that ushered in a brave new world in body images for American adults were first published in 1912, and the precepts they encapsulated have since taken on a cultural weight of their own and given rise to a folklore in their own right. We are taught that being fat increases our chances of dying of heart disease, diabetes, and nephritis; recently, asthma and even homicide have been added to the list. As if being fat were not enough in and of itself, the overweight are thus forced to carry around a burden of guilt and anxiety as excess psychological baggage in addition to the excess ponderal baggage of their own fat. And in terms of sheer numbers, we are speaking of no mean minority: The most recent figures published by the insurance companies in 1959 replaced the concept of average weights with the concept of ideal weights, and seemed to suggest that fully 40 per cent of the adult female population of the United States might thus be seriously overweight, with figures for adult males running them a close second. (If an obesity rate of 40 per cent seems high, Americans can nevertheless take some comfort from recent data released by the Baden-Württemburg State Medical Association, which estimates the German obesity rate for both sexes at close to 70 per cent.)

Like most revisionist dogmas, however, the 1959 *Build and Blood Pressure Study* upon which the American estimates are based, and the rhetoric that it gave rise to in medical and public health circles, may have overreached its mark and carried the swing of the pendulum too far in the other direction. For one thing, recent research has raised the question of what constitutes a proper definition of obesity and overweight in the first place.

While to date none of the published height-weight tables has made any really workable provision for estimating degree of general fatness apart from such closely related factors as over-all physical size and body build, it is known from more sophisticated measurement techniques that individuals can and do vary considerably, not only with respect to their subcutaneous fat deposits, but also with respect to their bone size and total amount of muscle tissue. Fat football players, for example, are rare; and yet football players are almost invariably above both the ideal and the average weights for men of their height and age.

The concept of average or mean figures is a useful one for scientific research, but the average person is an abstraction and for purposes of everyday life the abstraction itself is a meaningless one. At the level of the here and now we are all deviate, aberrant, and unique. Circumstances alter cases, and the genes or gene systems that control body size are at the mercy of environmental factors too numerous to calculate and of genetic factors too genealogically remote to retrieve and reconstruct. Moreover, in a country whose present citizenry and its gene pool have been recruited from virtually all corners of the populated globe, the concept of an "average" body shape or size, as of an "average" hair color, blood type, or cranial index, is even less conclusive and less binding on any given individual than it would be in most other regions of the inhabited world.

By the same token, research on the genetics of obesity, and recently published studies of individuals' feeding and activity patterns, have confirmed the informal observation that certain people do indeed seem to have a greater tendency to manufacture more fat, calorie for ingested calorie, than other people do, and that, in some cases, this tendency may rest on measurable individual differences in the underlying genetic equipment that each individual brings to the act of eating and metabolizing food. Well documented in certain strains of laboratory animals, such inherent differences in the way in which human beings process ingested foodstuffs are only now receiving the attention due to them both in professional journals and in clinical practice.

Thus, as medicine comes closer and closer to achieving the status of an exact science, and grows farther from its original status as a variously practiced art, further refinements in the data of individual differences will be sure to come to light, and patients at either end of the ideal weight spectrum can be expected to gain increased insight into, and better control over, the day-to-day management of fundamental metabolic problems they may be genetically programmed to contend with for the rest of their lives.

Further objections to the conclusions suggested by the actuarial tables can also be raised. A general criticism leveled by the anthropometricians against the ideal-weight tables is that the group of people whose measurements they represent may be socially, economically, and even ethnically nonrepresentative of the population as a whole. Because only a limited and self-selecting group of Americans buys life insurance to begin with, the people whose ideal weights are enshrined in the resulting tables are usually white, economically comfortable, and of predominantly northern European extraction; their diets may contain substantially more protein than the diets of less affluent groups, and they may come from an ancestral stock that is thinner, longer-legged, and more physically active and "outdoorsy" than that of the population at large.

Figures based on the ideal weights of such people may therefore be somewhat biased in favor of thinness and legginess. Body size, endocrinological systems, and soft-tissue components are inherited to some degree as a total package, and what may be conducive to longevity in one such package may not be conducive to longevity in another. Smaller-scale population studies, meanwhile, have found striking differences with regard to average weights and heights among various ethnic subgroups of Americans. In a recent Providence, Rhode Island, study, for example, middle-aged Italians of both sexes were found to be shorter and to have much higher obesity rates than other groups studied, while fully 72 per cent of Jewish women in the same area were found to be "overweight"— that is, between 16 and 35 pounds over their ideal weights as defined by the *Build and Blood Pressure Study* of 1959. On the other hand, it emerged from the same study that far fewer Jewish women than Italians were actually "obese"—i.e., more than 35 pounds above the "ideal" weight for similar women of the same age and height. From other studies we learn that black women, to cite a third case, tend to be fatter than white women of the same height at all ages once they are out of their teens, although they are generally comparable to, or even thinner than, whites as children. It would seem, therefore, on the basis of the data cited here, that there is indeed a strong ethnic component to patterns and degrees of overweight among given subgroups of Americans, and that this component shows up most strongly among the women—as opposed to the men—of the various ethnic groups reported upon.

Other objections to the life-insurance ideal-weight tables, finally, speak to the lack of uniformity with which the height-weight data on which they are based were originally collected; to their failure to distinguish between degrees of overweight and the specific effects of such differences on actual mortality figures; and to the fact that within each age group only the first 14 per cent of deaths are correlated to weight variables, leaving the remaining longer-lived 86 per cent of overweight subjects unaccounted for in terms of risk from overweight. In fact, if we read them closely, what the insurance tables actually show is that as the overweight population grows older, its risk of dying from the effects of obesity declines and continues to decline with increasing age. Overweight subjects who do not die in their late thirties, their forties, and their early fifties show much less discrepancy from the mortality figures for normal and underweight subjects than we would be led to expect if obesity were the sole causal agent of high death rates from overweight. In other words, if an overweight person manages to survive his fourth, fifth, and sixth decades, his chances of living to a ripe old age are not very different from those of the population at large.

Attempts to refine our ideas about what is and what is not "abnormal" with respect to body fat have accordingly come in for increasing attention in an effort to pin down the facts embedded in the figures. Definitions of obesity based on actuarial figures leave much to be desired: Depending on the investigator, obesity has been defined as starting anywhere from 10 to 25 per cent above actuarially "normal" weights for a given height. Considering that the norms themselves are somewhat suspect to begin with, it is clear that defining obesity in terms of departures from such norms is an even riskier undertaking than setting up norms in the first place. To answer objections of this sort, the newer height-weight tables have tried to make allowances for differing body builds by constructing special subtables for small-framed, medium-framed, and large-framed individuals—each with a range of some 10 to 15 pounds' leeway on either side of the norm. The idea is fine in theory but may bog down disappointingly in practice: Untrained people are simply not very good judges of their own "frame" size relative to other people's. Medium-sized people who have grown up surrounded by smaller siblings, friends, and peers will probably tend to rate themselves bigger than an experienced anthropometrician would, and small people who live in the midst of people as slender and diminutive as themselves will tend to visualize themselves differently than those who live surrounded by giants do.

Something less subject to the vagaries of ego and biographical accident is therefore obviously called for, and various attempts have been made to measure body fat in a more systematic fashion than this, ranging from skin-fold caliper readings to underwater weighing devices and other even more esoteric measures based on the biochemistry of lean tissue versus that of fat. The rationale for underwater weighing is that fatter individuals are more buoyant, or "floatable," than leaner ones and therefore weigh less than lean people when submerged; by comparing underwater weights with scale weights according to certain formulas, scientists can assess the fat content of bodies with a reasonable degree of accuracy. A less dramatic but equally accurate way to determine the thickness of a given individual's fat is to take skin-fold caliper measurements. A skin-fold caliper is a pincer-shaped device with a measuring dial that pinches up a section of skin and fat and measures the resulting double fold of flesh in millimeters.

Generally speaking, adult females have an upper reading of about 30 mm. on the back of the upper arm midway between the shoulder and the elbow; caliper readings for adult males are somewhat lower than this (23 mm.), and anything above that line for either sex constitutes statutory obesity. This determination seems as serviceable as any other now in use and correlates very highly with densitometry (underwater weighing) measurements; for purposes of the present survey it has therefore been adopted as a good working criterion of obesity. A very rough approximation of skin-fold caliper measurements can be had by pinching the appropriate site on the back of the upper arm between the thumb and finger; a double fold of over one inch for a man, and of over one and a quarter inches for a woman, puts the individual into the lower ranges of obesity by this criterion. And, if all else fails, there is always what certain clinicians have only half facetiously called "the eyeball test": in all probability a person who looks too fat actually is too fat—including, of course, the person everyone knows best from his or her own image in a full-length mirror.

Given these general cautions about what is and is not implied about obesity in the height-weight tables, and what is and is not commonly extrapolated from them in terms of concomitant mortality figures for the population as a whole, the time may well be ripe for a systematic detailing of the medical research of the last twenty years on the genetics, geography, physiology, and cellular anatomy of fat in this and other populations. While the evidence is still far from complete, enough information has accumulated recently to motivate a fresh look at what has been passing for common knowledge for the better part of three decades. And as for the 40 to 70 per cent of the American population to whom weight gain or loss is a more or less daily preoccupation (as estimated from the amount of inspirational literature that exists on overweight, and from the great numbers of proposed cures for it currently in circulation), it would seem that new light on this much-belabored subject could not come any too soon.

What passes for common knowledge in one generation is fortunately subject to revision in the next, and the widely accepted folk wisdom that gluttony is the sufficient cause of obesity has come under increasing suspicion of late on the part of scientifically sophisticated researchers in the fields of nutrition and endocrinology. It may be little consolation to someone with a weight problem to be told that even if he eats a supposedly normal number of calories for someone of his age, height, activity level, and general body build, his genes may still condemn him to go on accumulating excess fat at the predictable snail's pace; but it may be a relief to learn that it is his body and not his character that is primarily implicated in the process.

Such distinctions would be of less moment if it were not for the fact that overweight may have serious social consequences as well as physical ones. In a society that abhors overweight, the social repercussions of obesity are not insignificant. Fat army recruits can be dismissed or reassigned for cause; fat high-school seniors have been shown to have less chance of being admitted to the colleges of their choice than thinner schoolmates with identical College Board scores and grade-point averages. We are dealing here with the direct economic consequences of what is after all a physiological anomaly, and not a disabling one at that. The effect is nevertheless just as economically compelling as it would be if, like an actual physical disability, it directly affected the individual's labor market value and ability to perform a certain kind of job.

For women the economic repercussions of overweight can be even more serious than for men, a reflection of the strong element of economic market value involved in the happenstance of face and figure; by limiting her choice of college in late adolescence and thus significantly restricting her subsequent marital options in her early twenties, a woman's tendency to gain weight may have a substantial, if not a major, effect on her social and socioeconomic status as a married adult, feminist theory and practice notwithstanding.

Other, subtler forms of social bias against the overweight may add psychological insult to economic injury. Manifestly aberrant and different, the obese form a visible minority group of their own, and are thus open to all the special social and psychologically aversive effects of minority-group membership plain and simple. The fact that obesity is supposed to be reversible, while skin color and national origins are not, may make the stigma all the harder to deal with, for it adds a prescriptive and homiletic element to what is at heart not a social problem or even necessarily a psychological one, but a simple and often intractable problem in the physics and arithmetic of basic energy exchange.

Central to the question of fat storage in man and other mammals is an understanding of the energy exchange between warm-blooded animals and their environment, and the resulting thermal equilibrium that must be set up and maintained at all costs between them. The by-product of all metabolic operations is heat, and the integrity of an animal's physiological functions can only be supported within certain narrow limits of thermal tolerance. While people may vary from each other relatively little with respect to their basic thermal needs, there are, demonstrably, considerable variations between any two given individuals with respect to the amount and kind of food they must take in to maintain optimal deep-body temperatures and the proper equilibrium between their skin temperatures and the surrounding air. To some extent, at least, these differences are probably due to differences in the individual's internal metabolic engine—differences that may have their origins in the structural and anatomical design of the body and its fuel-burning machinery or, alternatively, in the chemistry of the smelting process itself—differences, for example, in the amounts of various enzymes individuals may have at their disposal for metabolizing foodstuffs, converting food to fat, and releasing the converted fat from its storage depots in the cells when called upon to do so.

Food is, of course, in the last analysis the only outright physical means there is toward the anatomical end of getting fat, and to say that people burn fuel and run their metabolic engines at different rates is not to quarrel with the basic economics of fat accretion and weight gain in the first place. Starving people do not gain weight no matter how sluggish their metabolisms may be; and fat people do lose weight when they are systematically underfed, no matter what kinds and amounts of enzymes they may be able to bring to bear on the nutrients in their systems. Within these limits, however, circumstances will probably always alter cases by however slight an amount, and the rates at which individuals gain or lose weight will never be quite the same for any two different people—even those living under identical conditions. Starvation for one individual may be no more than short rations for another; one man's feast may be another man's famine. Inside the body it takes food to generate heat, and how much food it takes to keep the individual furnace stoked is not a matter of taste but of metabolism.

Subcutaneous fat can be visualized as a depot for reserve fuel, a potential source of heat that is on tap to the animal at some crucial moment when food itself, in its primary and edible form, may not be immediately at hand. Understandably, then, the economics of metabolism are only one step removed from the ecology of climate and food supply and from the various local food chains that depend on climatological factors for their structure and their ongoing day-to-day checks and balances. Thus the history of human obesity, far from being a moral saga, is, in the last analysis, largely an ecological one.

In those parts of the world where the rigors of climate precluded dependence on a steady and infinitely renewable food supply, man's genes may have programmed him to accrue fat at a heightened rate and with special efficiency. It is little wonder, therefore, that the climates where food supplies are seasonal and chancy have also tended to be those that produced a disproportionate number of fat, or at least bulky, people. The fact that subcutaneous fat is also a good insulator from environmental cold can only have speeded up the process of genetic selection in favor of the fuel-economizing and fat-accumulating, or, as geneticist James Neel has called them, the "thrifty" genotypes. A good thick layer of fat between the viscera and the skin will tend to keep body heat where it is needed most—that is, in the heart, the lungs, the intestines, and other internal organs—and keep it from being freely lost and dissipated into the surrounding air, where it is of no immediate use or survival value to the animal itself.

Seen in historical perspective, then, and without the aesthetic and ethical cobwebs that may attach to the subject of overweight in the context of affluent, famine-proof, post-1930's America, the problem of human obesity proves to yield an interesting object lesson in the history and geography of the species as a whole. For while full-blown famine may never become a living reality for the average American or northern European of this generation, its existence on the Malthusian agenda of other less highly developed and less geographically favored countries is already inarguable and will demand increasing attention from all of us within the coming decade. Americans, both fat and thin, have already been requested by their less fortunate neighbors to pull in their belts as at least a nominal first step toward world-wide food redistribution programs; the ugly American of the fifties may in the process find himself being updated into the fat American of the eighties.

In the meantime, though, it may be well to remember that to the starving peoples of other nations most Americans look fat whether they conform to the ideal heights and weights of the United States actuarial tables or not. To the literally starving, the fine line between well fed and overfed may not be immediately apparent. Conversely, and in the not too distant future at that, the women's-magazine aesthetics of skin and bones may be due for a cultural overhaul in their own right. For while it may be true, as Cyril Connolly suggested, that within every fat man there is a thin one trying to escape, it is probably equally true, from another point of view, that buried not too deeply in the collective unconscious of the species as a whole is the memory of starvation, crop failure, herd extinction, and famine.

That this memory may have become encapsulated in the genes and the actual cytoplasm of the evolving species—with important repercussions for the obese, the chronically hungry, and the economic planners of the food-producing countries—will be the burden of the following chapters to point out. And in the meantime, whatever else the data to be reviewed here may prove, it is to be hoped that they may go at least some way toward defusing the guilt and anxiety that fat people in this culture learn to live with from their earliest social and medical encounters. For in the long Malthusian breadline we may all be queuing up for shortly, the fat can take comfort from the knowledge that they can afford to go to the end of the line, secure in the assurance that their genes and metabolisms can be counted on to give them the extra day's, week's, or month's worth of energy surplus that may be just what it takes to survive in a world with more and more people and less and less available food.

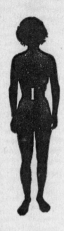

Geography:
Some Latitudes and
Longitudes of Human Size

The Ice Age has been called the Age of Man. The end of temperate weather more than a million years ago set the stage for the emergence of man as we know him from the bloodlines of less evolved hominids of the ancestral home range in Africa. The geographical and climatic background for this evolutionary drama was glacial. *Homo sapiens* came of age in an era that saw the rise of the woolly mammoth and the disappearance of the saber-toothed tiger, the ascendancy of the cave bear, and the demise of the tortoise in central and northern Europe. Before the onset of the last great glaciation, mean annual temperatures in central Europe stood some 20 degrees higher than they do now, and the Biblical metaphor of the Garden of Eden may therefore have firm empirical taproots in the unwritten history of the species and its collective genetic memory. When man first began to make the zoological transition from apelike to manlike *Homo erectus* forms, and the subsequent geographical transition from Africa to Europe, subtropical animals like rhinoceroses and elephants still grazed unconcernedly in England, and cercopithecoid monkeys and lions still roamed at large in northern Spain.

But this climatic Eden was short-lived, and the subsequent history of the period was marked by increasingly violent oscillations from hot to cold and resulting shifts in food supply, culminating in longer and longer periods of greater and greater cold. Cold became the limiting factor in subsistence, reproduction, and survival of many European mammals. Winter had come to the Garden of Eden, and cold, or relative degree of it, was therefore soon to be counted among the major modeling forces at work on the evolving species, especially in the more northerly reaches of its habitat.

The evolutionary pressures in this respect must have been at least as intense on man's developing brain as they were on his differentiating physique and soma: Man's adaptation to cold has always been cultural as well as physical. Without the use of fire, of shelter, and of hunting and trapping tools and clothing, it is doubtful whether our hairless and otherwise poorly insulated and vascularly rather unresourceful species could have survived its first mid-latitude winters, with or without a cave to shelter in.

But culture does not tell the whole story; adaptation to cold was also physical and morphological. It is an axiom of evolutionary theory that crisis conditions in an animal's ecozone will either put paid to the species in its extant form or stimulate finer adaptations and cleverer physiological accommodations to the environment. The glacial period that came to the end of its cycle and finally waned some 12,000 years ago in northern Europe saw the transition of man from a small-brained, stoop-kneed pebble hurler and flint collector to a fully erect biped, an artist, and a protoscientist. These changes in nature and human nature augured well for the reproductive exuberance of the species. One of *Homo sapiens'* first major population explosions in Europe occurred somewhere between 20,000 and 12,000 years ago, at which time it has been estimated that the total population of France alone increased from 15,000 to 50,000 human beings. While figures like these may sound trifling in the light of today's population problems, in its own time and place the increase was enormous and weighted with consequences for the future of the species.

Among the somatic changes entailed in this ancient population explosion and demographic shift northward into Europe and Siberia were changes in weight and stature. The earlier hominids had been small and slender animals; their descendants, especially in the colder climates to which they migrated, were bigger and heavier creatures than the ancestral prototypes. And, if current figures are an accurate reflection of past trends, we can also assume that men were getting stockier, fleshier, and muscularly sturdier as they got taller. In northern Europe and Asia, at least, the glacier that left so many of its geological marks on the hills and valleys exposed by its retreat left marks on the physiques of creatures living close to its edges before the end of the Ice Age too. It is in this sense that glacial ice may be said to have molded not only the land it covered but also the animals whose ecozones were bounded by it as well. Like other mammals, the evolving species of hominids who were our ancestors rose to the occasion by putting on weight, flesh, bone, and stature.

The point is not an unimportant one: If man's genetic and environmental response to cold involves a demand for extra stature, and extra weight to go with it, the response is one that he shares widely with other animals. This observation has become one of the capstones of modern zoological theory. Nineteenth-century naturalists cataloguing newly discovered animal species in their burgeoning collections began to formulate ground-breaking observations about the anatomical fit between the body morphology of an animal and the climate from which it hailed. Basic exploration of the human and animal hinterland had of course first begun in the sixteenth century, but it was left to later generations to fill out the picture, and the German biologist Carl Bergmann was among the first to draw the connection between size and climate in the animal kingdom. The various subspecies up for Linnaean classification among animals from the subarctic taiga and the hitherto unexplored Canadian and Siberian tundra were comparatively larger than those already classified, and Bergmann drew the conclusion that cold-dwelling subspecies tend to be considerably bulkier, heavier, and taller than their warm-dwelling conspecifics—an observation that has gone down in the annals of zoology as Bergmann's rule.

The rule rests on good empirical evidence. Many of the largest sea and land mammals in the world today are to be found in the northernmost reaches of the Northern Hemisphere. (The same rule applies in reverse to the Southern Hemisphere; but since most of the world's major land masses lie in the northern half of the globe, the zoological record is relatively richer and clearer in the north than in the south.) And the finding makes excellent anatomical sense as well: Size and general bulkiness give the animal a significant thermal advantage in a cold climate. This is because, as an animal gains in size, the increase in its accompanying skin surface is relatively much smaller than the simultaneous gain in its total bulk. Since every extra inch of skin is also a site for potential heat loss, gain in bulk (and weight) at the expense of the relatively minor gain in skin surface needed to cover it is, in the long run, an efficient and economical way to minimize heat loss. (This is one of the reasons, incidentally, that babies are so much less efficient at keeping themselves warm than adults are: Because of their thin, stick- like arms and legs, babies have proportionately greater total skin surface areas per unit of weight than adults do, and tend to lose heat faster than they can generate it.) By the same token, the large-boned and barrel-chested peoples who inhabit cold countries (and mountain areas in warmer ones) share with the polar bears, moose, and the now-extinct woolly mammoth the clever adaptive strategy—increasing bulk and weight at the expense of surface area—that is such a major thermal advantage to animals that live, reproduce, and winter in cold climates.

Bergmann's rule still stands as formulated; but the nineteenth-century anatomist J. A. Allen elaborated on it in a doctrine that has become known as Allen's rule and that is usually cited as a corollary to Bergmann's: The protruding parts of the body of most animal species tend to be shorter in the groups that inhabit the colder portions of the species' natural range, and longer in the groups that inhabit the warmer parts of that range. The principle is a simple one: Where rigors of climate place a strong premium on an animal's ability to maintain body heat, the shorter its legs and arms, the less difficulty the animal will have in maintaining them at optimal operating temperatures—and the less heat it will stand to lose from them in frigid weather.

Human beings are no exception to this widespread zoological imperative; like dogs, corn, and cattle, *Homo sapiens* comes in many different shapes and sizes, and the range of variation is so large and so predictable in terms of climate that it constitutes what amounts to a living object lesson in Bergmann's and Allen's rules. The Masai and other Africans of the upper Nile Valley are, for example, among the tallest people in the world, with an average male height of about six feet, and they live in one of the notable hot spots of the inhabited world. The Lapps of the Fennoscandian region—much of which is well within the Arctic Circle—are extremely short-legged; Lapp men average just a little over five feet in height, while the women's average height is a mere four feet six. Ecologically speaking, Lapps and Masai live at opposite ends of a bipolar climatic continuum; but there are national differences in shapes, sizes, and limb proportions even among groups of people living at roughly the same latitudes and longitudes of the globe—and even here the differences calibrate relatively neatly with temperature. Thus Greeks, Turks, and Italians share almost the same geographical latitudes and longitudes, but there are mean annual temperature differences among their various countries and these differences are reflected—at least to some extent—in average male heights. Turks are the shortest, and shortest-legged, of the three groups; not unexpectedly, Turkish annual mean temperatures are also the coldest of the three groups.

To account for the differences of physical types among whole populations of human beings living at some significant geographical distance from each other, anthropologists and human biologists have tried to accumulate height and weight statistics on large numbers of people throughout the world. The data are still far from complete, but when they are all in they will no doubt form a compendium that will be helpful in settling questions about the relative importance of genes and environment in governing body weight and stature for any given group, and may as a dividend give us valuable indirect evidence for the comings and goings of various tribal and ethnic groups over the course of the great uncharted migrations of human prehistory.

Meanwhile, individual studies of human weights and statures are in good basic accord with the theoretical implications of Bergmann's and Allen's rules. They show that not only are the northernmost subjects of world-wide human demographic studies absolutely heavier than the southernmost ones, but that they are also relatively heavier in terms of weight per unit of height. So far, however, data on Allen's rule are somewhat harder to come by than those on Bergmann's; but it is a fairly safe guess even so that the increased bulk of cold-climate animals and human beings is going to be greater in the torso than in the legs and arms; this is because there are general biological and even architectonic limits to the maximum height of animals, but fewer and less binding limits on maximum weight. The result is that—beyond a certain upper limit at least—weight can be concentrated only in the torso as it increases and not in the arms and legs.

Thermal factors as well as architectonic ones may also be operating here. The anthropologists Carleton Coon, S. Garn, and J. Birdsell explain the "globularity" of cold-dwelling members of a species in geometric terms: The mammalian torso is spherical, and its surface increases according to a geometric formula involving the cube of the total mass. Its limbs, on the other hand, are columnar rather than spherical and therefore answer to different geometrical laws. Arms and legs also present much more surface area to the world than the torso does, thereby exposing more skin per unit of length than the more dense, spherical, and massive torso does. Science seconds the popular stereotype of lanky, leggy individuals as being "all skin and bones." A classic illustration used in human biology texts to show the differing total skin-surface areas of long, lean individuals (human and otherwise) versus short round ones makes its macabre point by illustrating the two types in their "skinned" states, like animal hides sketched side by side on the printed page. The heat-adapted, linear "hide" takes up significantly more space on the page than the more compact, cold-adapted hide does—an object lesson, though fortunately only a graphic one, in the comparative geometry of human physique.

The result of such human and mammalian geometry is that short arms and legs form rounder, hence more spherical, "columns" than long ones do, and are therefore easier to keep warm at low temperatures than long ones are. According to this line of reasoning, the rounder and more spherical the arms and legs, the better it will go for the animal in a cold climate—especially in the middle of winter or in prolonged exposure to wind and snow.

To state the theory is one thing, but to go about proving it is of course another. Physical anthropologists have been trying to tease out the empirical connections between fact and theory for half a century. If it is true that people in cold climates tend to be heavier than those in warmer ones, the difference is one that ought to be demonstrable in terms of differing average or mean weights between the two kinds of populations on the basis of climate alone.

The fact that such differences do exist would certainly constitute strong supporting evidence for the hypothesis that ability to store fat, bone, and muscle may be a primary physiological response to life in a cold climate—or at the very least to some other, second-order environmental or economic factor associated with those climates. In this respect, broad-scale population studies that map the incidence of high weights, and high weights for height, of people living in (and presumably adapted to) cold climates bring us one step closer to validation of the well-known empirical finding that people, as well as animals, who live in cold climates tend to be larger and heavier than people who live in warmer ones, as predicted by Bergmann's rule.

Such studies do exist, and fortunately for the status of the theory, they do tend to bear out the assumptions implicit in it. Anthropologist D. F. Roberts studied some 220 groups of adult populations from all parts of the world, and his results, published in 1953, confirmed the impression that there is indeed "a very marked tendency for most 'very high' weights to occur in cold areas and for 'very low' weights to occur in hotter regions." Roberts plotted height-weight ratios relative to an isotherm of 50° F. mean annual temperatures. The 50° isotherms run just north and south of the equator, forming bands that connect all regions on the globe where mean January temperatures are roughly 50°. The areas bounded by it in the Northern Hemisphere lie slightly above the Tropic of Cancer and include parts of the southern tier of American states; the Atlantic coast of the Iberian Peninsula; the Mediterranean and Saharan sections of Morocco, Algeria, Libya, and Egypt; most of Jordan and Iraq and Iran; northern India, and southern China. The finding that people farther from this line tended to be heavier than those closer to it proved to hold good on a world-wide basis for both hemispheres, and even turned out to cut across racial and subracial categories as well. Mongoloids living twenty degrees of latitude north of the 50° isotherm, for example, tended to be heavier than Mongoloids living closer to it or south of it, and the degree of divergence from average weights actually turns out to follow the degree of geographical distance from the 50° isotherm with a remarkable degree of fidelity.

Fortunately for the status of Bergmann's rule, the same generalization was also found to hold true even when other factors were varied. The rule operated, in other words, regardless of extraneous variables like age and sex; twenty-year-olds in colder segments of the area tended to be heavier than their age mates in warmer latitudes, and females from colder climates outweighed males from warmer ones. Temperature, in short, seemed to have the final say in determining body weight and took precedence, in a sense, over such variables as age and sex, which are otherwise known to be important factors in human bulk.

Sample sizes of Roberts's populations varied from a low of 20 individuals to a high of about 3,000; and given the large number of discrete groups on which these data were based, the scientific validity of his findings is impressive. The subjects' ages ranged from twenty to forty. (One interesting corollary to emerge from the study, incidentally, was the finding that weight per height in both sexes seems to increase on the order of about 4 kilograms [8.8 pounds] between the ages of twenty and forty on a more-or-less world-wide basis, even in very primitive cultures where people continue to lead physically active existences until well into middle age.)

The possibility arises that the strong relationship found between weight and annual mean temperature might be a mere fact of increasing stature: Taller people, everything else being equal, will tend to have longer arms and legs than average, and longer bones will in turn tend to increase a person's weight, even in the absence of increased fat and muscle tissue to go with the longer bones. This problem was dealt with by means of appropriate statistical tests, and on the basis of these tests Roberts determined that height per se could not be held accountable for the increased weight of the cold-dwelling subjects. Even at the same height, cold-adapted people still outweighed heat-adapted ones. Furthermore, variations within each particular sample followed very much the same temperature gradient as variations between whole groups—so that even within highly localized areas the southernmost inhabitants of the area had the lowest weights per height, and the northernmost ones were heaviest for their stature. (Except below the equator, where, of course, these relationships were geographically reversed.)

Putting these findings in their proper historical perspective, Roberts found that, at least among tropical groups, the lowest weights occurred where the particular sample was thought to have occupied the area for the longest time. For example, wherever an equatorial group was known to be the aboriginal, or earliest, ethnic group to have populated that particular area, its weight proved to be lower than that of later comers from cooler parts of the region. This observation makes good anthropological and evolutionary sense, for the finding may be interpreted to mean that the earliest and longest settlers of any given locale will tend to be more thoroughly adapted to local conditions than recent immigrants; later arrivals, on the other hand, may still reflect genetic adaptations to the homelands from which they originally migrated.

Roberts's findings were among the first in a series that all pointed unmistakably in the same general direction. French anthropologist Eugène Schreider had earlier carried out a much smaller-scale study along the same lines, correlating heights, weights, and body surface areas for peoples of different geographical areas. Schreider's results were very similar to those later compiled by Roberts. Other investigators soon followed suit, with strikingly similar results. Among the most interesting of these studies were those of Russell Newman and Ella Munro, who set out to replicate Roberts's data in the United States, using a sample of U.S. Army recruits. Their study confirmed Roberts's data with regard to weight per height and the cold-warm temperature gradient. But in addition they made the interesting discovery, overlooked by Roberts, that the relationship between height and weight was strongest when it was tabulated not in terms of the mean annual temperature (as Roberts had assumed) but of the mean January temperature instead. It is where winter temperatures are coldest, in other words, and not necessarily where mean annual temperatures are most rigorous, that the biggest Americans are bred and raised. This means that even where summer temperatures are high, it is the coldness of the cold winters that counts—a discovery that suggests beyond doubt that the true significance of the correlation between weight and climate must lie not in the relevance of either height or weight to *heat* adaptation—as Roberts incidentally had tentatively proposed—but in its relevance to *cold* adaptation. The accumulating evidence thus began to point ineluctably to the conclusion that, in the matter of physique and body build at least, cold may turn out to be a more potent genetic selector than heat, especially in the temperate climates where such adaptations could be expected to go either way with almost equal probability.

But this is not to say that in more extreme climates heat does not exert its own not inconsiderable pressures on physique—pressures that may make themselves felt even within the relatively small-scale microgeographies of given land masses and continents, and Africa is a good case in point. In sub-Saharan Africa, for example, the tall, thin Masai live and farm in an environment that is for all intents and purposes significantly hotter and drier than that of their shorter and sturdier near neighbors the Kikuyu, who live barely a day's walk from them in the neighboring uplands. Both groups have inhabited their respective areas for centuries, and the difference of physique between them probably represents age-old genetic adaptations to their respective and very different econiches. The same distinction holds true for the long, lean Watusi and their fatter, shorter neighbors the Hutu. Cold or hot, man must, to keep alive and functioning, maintain his internal organs at a critical thermal set point of about 98.6° F. (Interestingly enough, man has a comparatively low thermostat setting compared to other warm-blooded animals; normal temperature for dogs is about 102.8°, while pigs have a normal temperature of 103° and chickens of 107°.)

The long-legged and narrow-headed Masai live and raise cattle in open savanna where daytime temperatures regularly rise to 110° at noon. To keep heart, lungs, brains, and innards at an optimal operating temperature of 98.6° or thereabouts at midday under the grueling open sun, the Masai must make shift to radiate a high percentage of their own body heat back into the surrounding air—and their long, lanky limbs and torsos are admirably designed to do just that. (Even the shape of their heads contributes to the proficiency with which Masai, and other lanky Nilotic African tribes, manage to minimize thermal overload and transfer heat away from their own bodies and back into the environment. Russian anthropologists have determined that when a heating lamp is held vertically at an established distance from a random series of human skulls, heat rises much more slowly inside the cranial box of the longer and narrower skulls than it does inside the rounder ones.)

Surprisingly, at least from the outlander's point of view, the African continent represents a true ecological melting pot; when it comes to physique and stature, African ethnic groups run the gamut from the shortest to the tallest of known human populations, from the towering Watusi, Dinka, and Shilluk herdsmen of the upper Nile marshes, on the one hand, to the Bushmen and diminutive Mbuti Pygmies of the Ituri Forest on the other. Heat may not be the only determining factor here, however; relative degrees of humidity and dryness in Africa apparently bolster and amplify the basic thermal factors operating on human physique. In the equatorial rain forest, where the air is so heavily saturated with moisture that sweat never has much of a chance to evaporate, the resulting clamminess may act as a sort of perpetual wet blanket—and, as it happens, a (relatively) cool one. Man happens to be the sweatiest animal on record, and this generalization applies to both cold- and heat-adapted groups of people. Eskimos, for example, are said to have the greatest number of sweat glands per inch of skin surface of any major ethnic group so far measured—a peculiarity that may be related to the extraordinarily high temperatures that may be reached inside a well-heated igloo, especially by a person dressed in furs from head to toe; and one which clearly has no effect one way or another on the average Eskimo's simultaneous adaptation to extreme environmental cold.

But whatever the relationship of sweatiness, humidity, and heat to body build, the effect is probably an important one: It is in areas where humidity is high, and not necessarily those where mean annual temperature is low, that the shortest and fattest Africans are to be found. And the anatomical consequences are not confined to body weight and stature alone: All measurements seem to broaden out where there is high year-round humidity, including the breadth of the nose and the width of the face and cranial box.

Where mean annual temperatures are lower than they are in Africa, however, the rule does not seem to apply or may even operate in reverse; for, interestingly enough, the major exceptions to the general cold-warm distribution of tall peoples are mostly noticed in the wet western coasts of continental and peninsular land masses. Some climatologists have pointed out that, given the prevailing world wind patterns from west to east, the western coasts of any given body of land tend to be warmer and wetter than eastern ones—a provocative finding when applied to such linear types as the Scandinavians and Montenegrins, among others.

A digression, or even some special pleading, may be in order here: Observations like the foregoing tend to rouse the bemusement—if not the downright disbelief—of nonanthropologists. We are all armchair geographers of sorts, and the exceptions to Bergmann's and Allen's rules and their corollaries are legion and come easily enough to mind. B. Rensch, a statistical-minded biologist working in this area, played devil's advocate by putting the respective rules to the test of the extant zoological cases, as they were then known. He found that of the total sample of known animal specimens, only about 70 per cent actually conformed to the so-called rules; the remaining 30 per cent of animals tested thumbed their noses at the theory and went their own way with respect to size, limb length, bulk, and skin-surface area.

Whether Rensch's conclusions constitute proof of the theory or disproof depends to some extent on the bias of the person assessing the results; a physicist, for example, might tend to be impatient with a "rule" that operates only 70 per cent of the time, while a social scientist, on the other hand, might be deeply impressed by such broad generalizability. This is because workers in the biological and social sciences have learned to be more tolerant of departures from "universal" values and norms than engineers, metallurgists, and atomic scientists can ever allow themselves to be; they have to be, because the world they are attempting to understand is a vastly richer and more complex one than the world addressed by the so-called hard sciences. No physical anthropologist would want to go on record as maintaining that tall, lanky Swedes got the way they are by spending appreciable parts of their lives working under the hot sun, or that warm, sunny Italy does not produce its fair share of short-legged, barrel-chested, and therefore presumably cold-adapted individuals. But, by the same token, no physical anthropologist would care to throw out Bergmann's and Allen's rules on this basis either; in anthropology, as in most of the social sciences, a statistical conformity rate of 70 per cent remains a respectable figure and one to be reckoned with.

The relative linearity of warm-dwelling peoples, and the relative globularity of cold-dwelling ones, goes back to the Paleolithic era at the very least, and is probably more closely related to climatic factors than to dietary ones—all evidence of plump Italian sopranos and thin Scandinavian fishermen notwithstanding. The beautiful and mysterious Venus figurines of Stone Age Europe, Russia, and Siberia date to the Upper Paleolithic, or in other words to a period roughly 18,000 to 25,000 years ago. Even making allowance for whatever poetic license the sculptors may have chosen to take with the basic form, the figurines probably bear some credible relation to the models who actually posed for them, for the Stone Age artists were working within a highly realistic convention, and the archaeological evidence can therefore be assumed to establish an empirical record as well as a merely aesthetic one.

The women immortalized in Stone Age sculpture were fat; there is no other word for it. But they certainly did not get that way eating pasta and bread, as modern orthodoxy explains such matters. Upper Paleolithic peoples were still hunter-gatherers and not peasants or agriculturists, and bread and pasta had yet to be invented for some several hundred centuries. Thus, the endomorphy which was undoubtedly already a prominent feature of the physiques of our European forebears, to judge by the evidence of the Venus figurines, cannot really have been a function of a high-carbohydrate, low-protein diet as postulated for later, farming peoples and for obese Americans today. On the contrary, the European hunters of glacial times lived almost exclusively on meat. Winters were long and severe, and the only vegetable foods available on a year-round basis (mosses, lichens, and some grasses) are not ones that man has ever been physiologically equipped to digest. Meanwhile, though, the evidence of the figurines is ungainsayable: Obesity was already a fact of life for Paleolithic man—or at least for Paleolithic woman.

It is hard to avoid the conclusion that genes for corpulence already existed to some degree in these resourceful but hard-pressed hunting groups carving out their difficult existence at the edge of the Swiss and Scandinavian glaciers in the Paleolithic hinterland. For life along the perimeters of the glacial moraines cannot have been an easy one, and in such rigorous climates obesity cannot by any stretch of the imagination have been the outcome of simple gluttony (as may or may not be the case in industrialized societies today). Europe in the last glacial period was far from being a land of milk and honey; the winters lasted for ten months at a stretch, and were considerably colder than they are now at the same latitudes. In such environments the ability to store surplus fat in useful amounts under the skin on the least possible total food intake may have made the difference between life and death, not only for the individual but—far more important in terms of the evolutionary history of the species—also for the family and tribal group as a whole.

In the meantime, armchair geographers and other disbelievers to the contrary, such studies as have already been done along these lines do indeed tend to confirm the relevant hypotheses. The rationale for these observed relationships rests on the assumption that, by and large, the predominant physical type within any given region will be one that over the years has proven to be well adapted to the ecological peculiarities of that region—or, at the very least, not ill adapted to it. The odds against blond hair in a sunny tropical climate are long; fair-skinned people do not do well in hot, open savanna unless they spend most of their working hours indoors, sheltered from the sun. The local gene pool in such a climate will therefore contain few genes for blondness, and many for dark skin and hair. Conversely, in cloudy countries, children with light skin and hair are able to extract more Vitamin D from sunlight than their darker-haired brothers and sisters can, and it is therefore the blonds who thrive. Over the centuries, therefore, cloudy countries will tend to accumulate genes for blondness in their local populations, and genes for dark hair will gradually tend to get scarce.

As with skin and hair color, so with height and weight. Both heat and cold are stressful to the organism, but different climates put different thermal loads on the populations indigenous to them, and in northern Europe, at least, temperature extremes have usually run to cold, not heat. Body size is not the only piece of anatomical evidence on hand to prove the point; other factors, like fat and body hair, can be called upon to bolster the case. Presence or absence of body hair or fur is a well-known concomitant of thermal adaptation in other species of animals besides our own; zoologists can gauge an animal's place of origin from the thickness of its pelt, and, in a recent and rather startling object lesson in animal thermodynamics, scientists at the University of Maryland who bred featherless chickens in an attempt to cut processing costs in the commercial poultry industry found that the nude chickens tended to weigh some

6 per cent more than their feathered conspecifics. This finding suggests, perhaps more graphically than zoologists had any right to expect, that increased body weight may be one of the first physiological responses a warm-blooded animal can make to cold stress, and we are probably safe in betting that man follows suit in this respect too, however hairless and featherless he may be relative to most other animals.

A large proportion of the increased weight of nude Maryland chickens was due to bone and muscle; but in man there is evidence that body hair and fat may have a similar connection. Swedish anthropologist Bengt Lindegård studied a group of 320 twenty-year-old Swedish Army recruits and, in the process of correlating various indices of masculine body traits, found that while the recruit's body hair itself bore no particular relationship to other signposts of masculinity, it did correlate positively with the amount of fat on the subject's trunk. In other words, the more body hair any given individual recruit had, the more subcutaneous body fat he was likely to have as well. Both fat deposition and body-hair growth are under the control of roughly the same adrenal hormones, and it may very well be that both of these traits are thus being mediated by cold-adaptive responses of the adrenal glands of these particular young men. Whether the response is a genetic one or an environmental one is a question that has tantalized anthropologists for decades.

The case for the genetic underpinnings of body composition in various populations is a strong one; but to state the case for genetics is not to deny the importance of environmental factors as input either. The two things can be irritatingly difficult to factor out unless we look at children in their growing periods, transplant them from their normal "habitats," and see what happens to them as adults. Phyllis Eveleth's study of American children raised in Brazil is a case in point. Eveleth compared growth records of American children against growth records of ethnically and socioeconomically similar children raised in Iowa, and found that the Brazil-raised children weighed less, and had smaller calf widths and smaller yearly weight increments, than the home-grown group in Iowa. J. Millis investigated the same question in Malaysia with similar results, and E. E. Hunt compared body weight and height data from groups of English and American children raised in the tropics and noted a definite tendency for higher weights and higher weights-for-height to be found in colder-dwelling children by the age of five and a half years. These differences persist into adulthood, and studies like these therefore make it obvious that environment has an important part to play in human weight and stature; they also confirm that genetic endowment is never the only factor, although in the long run it may turn out to be the limiting one.

But although our genes may prescribe how tall or how heavy we are ever eventually likely to get under one set of environmental extremes as opposed to another, they do not constitute an absolute stranglehold on development or possibility; physique is in some respects plastic and, especially during the growing period, responsive to change both for the better and for the worse, however these may be defined. Evolution can only operate where environment has already done its basic modeling, for even when the environment has altered the rules of the game by raising or lowering the limits of weight and stature, natural selection still goes to work on what's left—the, finished product is always a joint effort of genes and habitat. The subtle interplay of constitution and environment is one that is still ongoing, for the species as a whole, and can be assessed for the asking in the fascinating phenomenon of the so-called secular trend. The secular trend documents the curious fact that since about the middle of the last century, the average stature of people all over the world has been increasing significantly, raising the possibility that if things continue as they have been going we will end up a species of giants and thereby outrun our natural resources and food supplies even if we manage to put the lid on population in the interim.

The usual explanation offered to account for the secular trend is a change for the better in overall nutrition, particularly in the nutrition of growing children. But other, more bizarre hypotheses have been offered to explain the trend. These include the artificial extension of daylight brought about by world-wide use of electricity and kerosene to light homes well beyond the normal hours of natural daylight. Increased light exposure can affect stature by acting as a retardant on the pineal gland (a small, light-sensitive organ in the brain that is involved in activating the various hormonal systems that turn on maturation and puberty), thereby delaying the onset of puberty, prolonging total length of adolescence, and thus in the long run postponing the date of full maturation well past its expected deadline. All these factors would tend to increase the growing time of the long bones and could thus, ultimately, eventuate in a longer-legged and hence taller population at large.

In much the same vein, though perhaps even more exotic in conception, is the speculation that the secular trend toward increased height may be due to the increased use of central heating in homes and schools, which would in effect create artificially tropical mini-environments for growing children, leading to delayed puberty, increased bone growth, and postponed maturation—all of these factors resulting, again, in longer limbs and hence in increased adult stature over the long term.

From an empirical and scientific viewpoint all these theories leave much to be desired. The only thing that can safely be said at present is that, for any given individual, adult body size and stature must depend on a multiplicity of interlocking constitutional and environmental factors, not all of them measurable or even dimly understood. At the present state of our knowledge about these matters, the safest guess seems to be that the relative contribution of genes and environment is probably about fifty-fifty, with environment providing the empirical, day-by-day checks and balances to basic programs legislated in utero—or even earlier—by the genes themselves.

Studies like Eveleth's, Roberts's, and Newman and Munro's document the world-wide phenomenon of above-average weight for height, and general bulkiness (including in all probability a certain degree of corpulence as well), for colder-dwelling members of a species relative to warmer-dwelling ones. They do not, in and of themselves, tell us anything about nature's means of bringing such differences about; and while the details of some of the investigations described here seem to suggest a strong genetic component at work, we are still in the dark as to how the causal connections may actually be operating on a day-to-day, gene-to-gene, and enzyme-to-enzyme basis.

One guess is that the intervening genetic variables may be hormonal. Cold stress stimulates the adrenal glands, which respond by increasing their secretion of the adrenal hormones. These act in tandem with the sex hormones estrogen and testosterone to govern fat storage, muscle building, and the rate at which the growing ends of the long bones are programmed to close. If these hormones are oversecreted in a given individual, or if cold stress affects their timing by speeding up the endocrinological master plan, the growing ends of the long bones may complete calcification well ahead of schedule, and the resulting physical type (short-legged, muscular, and inclined to be frontally stout) ends up conforming almost exactly to the physical model demanded by Bergmann's and Allen's rules for cold-dwelling individuals. The so-called Alpine physical type so regularly described by early anthropologists is almost a caricature of this hormonal master plan. Short-legged, barrel-chested, and snub-nosed, the Alpine type is one that is well represented in all the mountainous areas of Europe and South America today, and seems to constitute a living embodiment of the morphological principles spelled out in Bergmann's and Allen's rules.

Recent investigations into the biochemistry of the obese support this rationale, and ring a minor but interesting change on the basic thermodynamic givens of height, weight, and climate. It has been reported, for example, that endomorphs (i.e., plump, relatively short-legged people) tend to have higher excretion rates for the metabolites of the major adrenal hormones than other physical types do. When given ACTH, the pituitary hormone that stimulates the adrenal gland to produce its own hormones, the endomorph's output of adrenal hormones is often two to three times greater than that of any other body type's. Among the hormones involved is hydrocortisone, or cortisol, which has a reputation for greatly stimulating appetite. The anatomical consequences of this hormonal peculiarity speak for themselves in the rounded body configurations of endomorphs. On the other hand, under the same dose of ACTH, ectomorphs (thin, long-legged, and relatively unmuscular people) have the least increase of adrenal hormones of any of the major body types.

The terms "endomorphy" and "ectomorphy" have their origin in William Herbert Sheldon's well-known and much-discussed typology of body build. Sheldon's contribution to the study of physique was to describe it in terms of three major components present in varying degrees in individuals of every size and shape. These are the soft roundedness of "endomorphy," the squared-off muscularity of "mesomorphy," and the lean legginess of "ectomorphy."

The principles that underlie Sheldon's somatotyping are not totally at variance with those that appear to be operating on height and weight in response to climates. Looked at from the standpoint of Bergmann's and Allen's rules, for example, one would not hesitate to predict that typical warm-dwelling populations ought to be leggier, leaner, and hence more "ectomorphic" than cold-dwelling ones; and with some exceptions here and there in northern Europe (notably Scandinavians and highland Scots) this prediction is largely borne out by the observable facts. By and large, most ectomorphs are to be found in the warmer latitudes, with mesomorphs and endomorphs overrepresented in the cooler ones.

This sort of somatic adaptation to the environment is the stuff of which evolution is made, and probably comes about through minuscule and unremarkable shifts in gene frequencies between one generation and the next, unheralded and unnoticed by anthropometrists and ordinary citizens alike. The glacier's advance some 1,600,000 years ago put strong adaptive pressures on emergent local populations of all animal species living close to it, but the pressures must have been particularly intense when it came to *Homo erectus,* our immediate hominid forebear, whose northerly dispersal and proliferation into Europe and Siberia was destined to proceed on a makeshift, hit-or-miss fashion more or less in time with the glacier's own inexorable advance.

In our own time and place and at our own moment in history we would expect such adaptations to be minimal. Modern technology takes the sting out of many environmental extremes and provides a thermally protected environment for most human beings—especially those born and raised in the industrialized countries of the Northern Hemisphere. Modern housing, central heating and air conditioning, ready transportation facilities, and the mass production of warm clothing all serve to homogenize existing disparities between climatic and economic extremes, and to minimize the individual's actual exposure to cold stress even in the dead of winter. Culture insulates us from the environment more pervasively and more dependably than physiology does, and this is even truer in the twentieth century than it has ever been in the past.

This being so, it is all the more interesting to see studies like Roberts's, Newman and Munro's, and Eveleth's, all of which document the extraordinary degree to which modern man still seems actively programmed to conform to the anatomical blueprints laid down by Bergmann's and Allen's rules. For in spite of the nicely insulated thermal cocoons in which most of us are raised and cosseted from the cradle to the grave, we continue to be larger in the colder reaches of our habitat and smaller in the warmer ones. Adaptation for thermal efficiency in man appears still to be going on, with important species-wide ramifications not only for stature and weight but also for the closely related propensity of cold-adapted peoples to manufacture (and store) undue amounts of subcutaneous fat when food supply and economics give them the ecological leeway—and impetus—to do so.

In this sense perhaps it may be fairly said that our bodies and our genes have far longer memories than our minds and archives do. Imprinted somewhere in the code of our basic cytoplasm is the long, varying, and harsh prehistory of the species—a record that our written histories will never reach far enough back into the past to bowdlerize. And meanwhile, in a world where ecological reversals may not be as unthinkable as we have been educated to suppose, we may find this unwritten blueprint a richer resource for survival than we have recently tended to give it credit for. In diet-conscious twentieth-century America, fat may never become beautiful, but under certain not altogether unforeseeable circumstances it may turn out to be a very useful commodity even so.

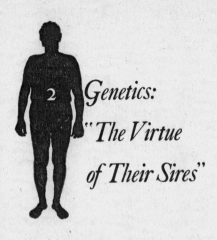

2 Genetics: "The Virtue of Their Sires"

For centuries farmers and livestock breeders have made a living from the common knowledge that certain strains of domestic animals are easier to fatten up than others. Sizable fortunes have been made on the propensity of the Aberdeen Angus to mature earlier and fatten more evenly than other breeds of cattle; sheep growers have learned to capitalize on the known likelihood of the Southdown breed to fatten too early for mutton, the Blackface too late for lamb. Even in the wild some animals can and do fatten on differing food intakes and caloric regimes from that of related others: A recent report from the World Wildlife Leadership Foundation says that the oryx, a North African antelope species, yields the same amount of meat on only half the daily food ration of cattle living in the same environment. The tendencies of the Middle White pig to develop well-turned hams, and of the later-maturing Large White to yield the best bacon, of the Berkshire hog to run to fat, and of the Razorback swine to muscle, form the taxonomical working capital of the British and American pork-breeding industries among others. Specialized knowledge about the growth rates and body morphologies of genetically different strains of domestic animals is the cornerstone of multimillion-dollar industries in all the major meat-eating countries of the world. "There is in cattle, there is in horses," Horace wrote, "the virtue of their sires."

Economic realities like these reflect the zoological fact that different breeds of the same species have widely differing abilities to store fat, even when all other factors (amount and kind of feed, grazing habits, range size, climate, etc.) are held constant. There are fat and lean breeds of dogs, poultry, sheep, pigs, mice, rats, and cattle. The differences are visible; they can be exploited for profit, aesthetics, genetic engineering, and laboratory experimentation. And yet, when it comes to human beings, a stubborn folklore resists the insight that, like most other mammalian species, we harbor subgroups in our midst who run to fat and others that can't be fattened up to win a bet.

Much of the incoming evidence runs counter to the received idea that we are what we eat, and challenges the simplistic medical and moral assumptions on which this popular shibboleth is based. In 1966 researchers at the Vermont State Prison set out to test the notion that there are innate variations in the ability of different people to store fat; sixteen volunteers were drafted for an experiment in the systematic overfeeding of adult human males. (The merits of using prisoners for research purposes may be open to argument, but as such things go, it is easy to imagine less humane experiments.) The volunteers were put on a high-calorie regimen for a period of about seven months. For the duration of the experiment, bouts of high caloric intake and *high* daily activity cycles alternated with periods of high caloric intake and *low* activity cycles. Body composition changes, weight gains, and changes in the size and number of adipose tissue cells were measured at various junctures during the seven-month period.

The results were various and provocative. Although not a single subject failed to gain weight on this program (there was an average weight gain of 24.8 per cent for the group as a whole), one subject never did gain more than 18 per cent of his original weight, in spite of food intakes ranging from 4,000 to 7,000 calories a day. For the entire group, weight gains ranged from this minimum of 18 per cent to an unenviable maximum of 31 per cent of the original body weight. In all cases the number of fat cells remained constant; only the size of the cells themselves changed to accommodate the growing increment of fat.

Even so, there were interesting changes in the post-experimental body composition of various volunteers over the seven-month period; in some subjects, for example, the weight gain consisted almost entirely of fat, while in others there was an increase in lean tissue too—presumably in the form of muscle added during the periods of high activity. Since all subjects ate the same amount of food and took the same amount of exercise for exactly equivalent numbers of hours, differences in the gains of fat and muscle can only be explained by innate differences in the ways in which these individuals were converting their food to tissue as time went by. What these variations involve physiologically can only be guessed at. The Vermont experiment establishes once and for all, however, that such differences do exist, and that they play no small part in the propensity of one individual to run to fat, and of another to resist fattening, against long caloric and bio-energetic odds. Dieting back down to pre-experimental weights wound up this groundbreaking experiment. To nobody's great surprise, this part of the venture was much less agreeable—and took longer—than Phase I.

The variability of the "caloric cost of the kilo" has been argued on and off for years in European medical circles; M. J. Demole calculates that according to the constitution of a given individual, it may take anywhere from 6,000 calories for a constitutionally lean person to gain one kilo, to 2,500 for a metabolically obese person to gain the same amount of weight. Estimates based on a random sample of patients seen in a normal medical practice do not of course have the scientific validity of measurements taken on a group of sequestered prison inmates whose comings and goings can be monitored around the clock for a seven-month period, and whose activities and food intake can be metered by instruments for months at a time. All the more convincing, then, that the two sets of figures should agree so closely, and despite the enormous differences in life-style and geography of the populations concerned.

But the caloric cost of the kilo can have its upside limits even among the obese. A club in France for men weighing over 100 kilos not long ago accidentally brought light to bear on the fact that, even for grossly overweight individuals (100 kilos equals 220 pounds) there may be a hitherto unexpected upward limit on the amount of weight that can actually be stored as fat. To their own and their colleagues' surprise, some applicants in the 95- to 99-kilo range, who were probably already obese by any ordinary clinical standards, simply never could gain the extra pound or pounds needed to qualify for membership in this unusual fraternity. Fat as they were, they could never get beyond a certain ceiling on their own overweight, no matter how hard, faithfully, and pleasurably they tried.

This finding may be cold comfort for people on their way to the last of the 100 stipulated kilos against their own will and inclination, but it is still food for thought. And the other side of this dubious coin, for those of the obese who have often had cause to wonder where it would all end, is the fact that there are also certain people who never do gain much weight or store many surplus calories in the form of fat no matter how much they force themselves—or are forced by well-meaning bystanders—to eat. In other words, the immutability of the equation between excess calories ingested and the weight that is automatically supposed to accrue from them may prove on second thought to be subject to a wide range of empirical ifs, ands, and buts. Human metabolism, commonly assumed to be an absolutely unvarying example of the laws of thermodynamics in action, has proved upon closer examination to be subject to a wide range of variation among individuals and even whole populations. One researcher, for example, has estimated that a certain subpopulation of urban Indian beggars he studied probably lives, reproduces, and raises its children more or less successfully on a total intake of something just over 700 calories per person per day. And while one hesitates to raise questions about the quality of a life lived on 700 calories a day, the point is that these people can and do subsist, bear children, and even have grandchildren on this regime. They survive and endure, in other words, even if they can hardly be said to prosper.

Just the opposite can happen too. Other investigators doing closely controlled clinical studies have found that, depending on metabolic factors that vary at random from one subject to the next, it can take anywhere from a low of 1,250 to a high of 3,000 calories to add a pound of fat to the patient's own pre-experimental weight. In 1967 D. S. Miller and P. Mumford published their report of an experiment with two American college students, a man and a woman, who were systematically overstuffed (to the tune of 37,300 surplus calories above normal for him and 20,100 for her) during a six-week period. Their caloric intake was metered by the experimenters; both subjects wore pedometers throughout the period to measure their caloric output in terms of activity; their urine and feces were measured every three days and analyzed for residual caloric contents. Pre- and post-experimental body composition factors were measured by sophisticated biochemical assay and skin-fold caliper readings. At the end of the six-week period, the expected weight gains (without water) should have been 4.1 kilos for him and 2.2 kilos for her; with water these sums should have risen to 6.2 and 3.3 kilos respectively. Instead, the two subjects showed total weight gains of 1.3 kilos for him, and 1.2 kilos for her— amounts which, the authors note, fall easily within the range of simple day-to-day variations that are normal for any given individual, overfed or not.

Intrigued by their own results, the researchers went on to test their findings with a group of fourteen nonobese college students— and, somewhat to their own surprise, managed to replicate their own earlier results almost exactly. And the conclusion does not seem to be limited to people with normal body weights and metabolisms; the medical literature is full of findings like these: E. M. Widdowson and his colleagues showed that in a California high-school population, for example, obese adolescents' daily food intakes ranged anywhere from 1,950 to 2,540 calories per day; while in the Obesity Clinic of Guy's Hospital in London, T. Hanley found that intakes of newly admitted severely obese patients ranged all the way from 750 to 3,200 calories a day, with no immediately discernible relationship between the recorded intakes on the one hand and the measured body weights on the other.

It seems fair to conclude, then, that like farm animals and laboratory mice, different genetic strains of human beings metabolize their food in individually idiosyncratic ways and may therefore for all intents and purposes be as variable in their ability to store fat (or avoid storing it, as the case may be) as any two specimens of domestic pigs or fowl.

Such an assertion flies in the face of much current physiological theory and practice, which assumes a sort of one-man, one-vote (1 calorie, 1 erg) model for weight gain, as if the human body were a mass-produced internal combustion machine made to certain stan-

dardized zoological specifications to which we or at least our medical practitioners and diet brokers were magically privy. The fact is
of course that the production of human beings is still in this sense a
cottage industry, and the offspring of human matings are therefore
as various and metabolically unpredictable as the parents themselves. It is, on closer analysis, no more revolutionary to say that
genes govern fat than to assert that long-legged parents tend to
produce long-legged children, or to predict that the offspring of two
blue-eyed parents will be blue-eyed too. Everything else being
equal, tall parents do tend to have tall children; conversely, no
amount of orange juice, fortified milk, or treadmill running will
ever produce a seven-foot basketball player from a long line of
short-legged, barrel-chested Alpine ancestors, unless somewhere
along the line there has been genetic admixture with considerably
more long-legged ectomorphic forebears.

The assertion that we are what we eat must therefore be modified
in view of what we now know about patterns of assortative mating
and the probabilities of gene frequencies, gene recombinations, and
heredity. We are what we eat only insofar as our basic heredity permits us to assimilate our own food and maximize our own growth
within certain limits laid down for each of us at the moment of conception by the random but irrevocable throw of the genetic dice.

At the moment of conception we receive as our genetic capital
exactly one half of each parent's full complement of genes and
chromosomes. The physical traits which we will go on to exhibit as
children and adults therefore represent various, probably not entirely random, permutations and recombinations of each of a pair of
possible simple traits inherited from each of our two parents: a father's nasal cartilage, a mother's nostril, father's father's jawbone
and chin, mother's father's skull cap, etc.

In theory these traits should combine quite randomly; in fact their
combinations are probably governed by structural matches and mis-
matches along the length of certain chromosomes (the long rib-
bonlike structures in each human cell upon which the genes are
strung side by side like beads) and also perhaps by certain innate
compatibilities and incompatibilities between newly combining
traits. For example, genes for a certain height of nose bridge may
be less compatible than others with genes for a certain width of
nasal septum; genes for hemophilia may be more compatible than

others with genes for color blindness, etc. These phenomena are relatively easy to study and identify in fruit flies and domestic plants, and they are not impossible to document in human beings too.

Apart from the purely structural restraints on the expression of any one of a pair of two genetic traits (restraints which may come about because the two genes in question are too far apart on their respective chromosomes to match up successfully in the new genetic individual, or because one of them may code for enzymes which do not make good chemical or molecular sense in the context of the individual about to be born) there may be some innate dynamic restraints on gene recombinations too: Complementary traits inherited in good faith from paired parental chromosomes may simply not work together in the new individual. The result is a damaged, or perhaps even an aborted, fetus.

By studying the actual frequency with which certain genetic traits show up in certain special groups of people, and comparing them to the expected and normal frequency for the same trait in the population at large, geneticists can draw reasoned conclusions about what combinations of genes may or may not be harmful, dysfunctional, or even downright lethal in a given population. Variations in the expected frequencies of fat children born to fat and thin parents are one of the many kinds of genetic probabilities that can be calculated in this way. Where there are shortfalls, we can assume that this particular combination of traits in the parents was lethal for a certain kind of body composition in the child. Where there are surpluses, we can assume that the same parental traits were lethal for just the opposite kind of build. These relationships are enormously complicated to figure out and it may take a team of highly trained geneticists and biostatisticians to do so. But for fat people at least the game would seem to be worth the candle.

Sex is the key to this complicated Mendelian maze. Traits that are in some way genetically linked to the sex of an individual are probably the easiest to deal with in genetic research; we know from long experience, statistical and otherwise, that during any significant period of time an almost equal number of children of each sex is born. (Actually, slightly more boys than girls are born, but the difference is not statistically important.) J. Lawrence Angel's study of the abnormal frequencies of male and female children among the offspring of different combinations of parental body types (e.g., fat mother/thin father; thin mother/thin father, etc.) resulted in the interesting finding that something other than the normal fifty-fifty boy-girl sex ratio seems to be involved when we look at parental pairs from the point of view of obesity and thinness.

Angel found that in two kinds of such parental combinations—fat fathers married to average mothers on the one hand, and average fathers married to average mothers on the other—there were fewer male offspring and larger families than there were, for example, among fat fathers married to fat mothers and average fathers married to fat mothers. Anomalies like this in the sex ratios of offspring of a given kind of union are generally considered by geneticists to point toward serious underlying constraints on the excluded gene combinations, operating imperceptibly at some point in early intrauterine life. From the resulting shortfalls of boy or girl babies in the particular group being scanned, geneticists can deduce that the missing—or, as more often happens, the underrepresented—sex has been the early precocious prenatal victim of an unlucky gene or new gene combination located somewhere along the length of one of the sex chromosomes. Reanalyzing data from the 1920's, E. E. Hunt found strikingly similar patterns, and concluded that "the evidence of sex ratios indicates that boys are least likely to be born of slender mothers, or from two fleshy parents, or parents of dissimilar build."

If we are reading these statistical omens correctly, it would seem that some gene close to or dependent upon the gene locus for fat in males tends to put the genetic damper on the number of male children a fat father could normally be expected to have. At the same time, though, this very gene or gene sequence seems paradoxically to be operating so as to increase the total number of children the fat father is actually likely to sire over the long haul, at least when he is mated to an average, nonfat female for the length of their child-bearing years.

Exactly what this finding portends is difficult to say. Statistical anomalies of this sort may or may not point to the underlying existence of strong causal relationships (what Borges has called the "divine labyrinth" of cause and effect) between two sets of factors, but they do nothing to explain the relationships themselves or to map their physiological antecedents and interconnections upon the

complex somatic terrain where they are destined to work themselves out.

Angel's study has been widely questioned; it has also, however,
been at least partially supported by evidence from other, unrelated
research. Work along these lines was particularly popular in the
twenties and thirties and inspired a rich mix of studies almost too
numerous to mention. Studies carried out by R. F. Withers on an
English population tend to confirm Angel's data in some particulars, and recent American research, more anthropometrically and
less genetically oriented than Angel's, has affirmed the general
finding that fat fathers do indeed tend to have larger families than
thin or average fathers do. Whether the unusual fertility of fat men
as opposed to thin ones has a direct biological basis, or whether it
is grounded in some more general second-order effect of fleshiness
in males (sensuality? impetuousness? fatherliness above and beyond
the usual cultural norm?) remains a question that can only be decided by further research. The phenomenon is there; it remains to
be explained.

The fertility rate of any given group of people is the result of a
blend of factors, by no means all of which need necessarily be
physical. For example, in a study of United States Army men,
Newman found that significantly more of the fat soldiers were
married than the thin ones; the same trend for obese males to be
married, and to be married at an earlier age than most other males
in this population, may be all that is needed to account for their
high fertility rates. Obviously, the over-all length of time that a
couple has been married will have an important bearing on that
couple's over-all fertility; people marry early or late, but regardless
of when they marry they all tend to complete their families and stop
having children at more or less the same age. Couples who marry
young, therefore, have a running start on those who put off marriage till a later date, and their fertility rates reflect their marital
precocity. The precocity itself of course remains to be explained.

Additional evidence for the genetic influence on obesity and
various lesser degrees of overweight comes from indirect observation of the link between obesity, on the one hand, and other physical traits already known to be under strict genetic control on the
other. Trunk hair in males is a case in point. Trunk hair and body
fat seem to be closely linked genetically. Per Bjürulf took anthropo-

metric measurements of Swedish Army recruits and found that the thickness of an individual recruit's subcutaneous fat depot was positively correlated both with the girth of his biceps muscle and with the amount of hair on his trunk. While muscle size can be increased to some extent by exercise, on an over-all, population-wide basis, hereditary factors are probably much more crucial to muscle size than other factors are (Richard H. Osborne and Frances De George, for example, give biceps measurements a heritability quotient of 68 per cent, which is lower than that for stature but higher than that for head circumference and body weight). Elsewhere, body-hair growth has been proven by S. Garn and E. L. Reynolds in very different kinds of studies to be one anthropometric feature that seems to be under fairly strict genetic control; and the fact that subcutaneous fat is so closely correlated to anatomical features (like body hair) which are already known to be controlled by genes would therefore seem to argue for a similar genetic influence on body fat itself.

Bjürulf's additional observation that men with large biceps measurements tended to be fatter than average reflects the interesting discovery that muscle and fat seem to have some kind of natural anatomical affinity for each other—a finding emphasized by Jean Mayer's studies of obese adolescent girls in the northeastern United States. In Mayer's study, girls who were above the average weight for their age also tended to have larger muscles and bigger bones than girls of average or below-average weights; like Bjürulf's Swedish Army men, from whom they are separated by the width of an ocean and a certain breadth of age and sex, subjects who were high in one tended to be high in the other too. Contrary to popular preconception, in other words, muscle seems destined to call to fat; the two tissues have an affinity for each other that is not easily explained away.

Intrigued by the finding that fat men seem to be hairier than others, Bjürulf went on to test the genetic component in the correlation by distinguishing between two basic elements of body fat. The assumption implicit in this distinction is that there are two major limiting factors on the amount of fat that any one individual can store in a lifetime; one (presumably inherited) is the number of fat cells the individual is born with or acquires at the very latest within the first few months or years of life, and the second (presumably environmental) is the size of each individual adipose tissue cell in and of itself. Overfeeding in adults results in a sort of over-all inflation or ballooning of each fat cell to several times its original size; but the actual number of fat cells in an individual's adipose tissue reserve depot remains the same throughout most of life, and seems to be determined at or slightly after birth: Once past the first few months of life, fat cells probably do not divide, and any additional volume in the over-all subcutaneous fat depot can only be managed by increasing the actual size of the cells already assigned to the individual by genetic birthright at conception.

Assuming the existence of these two basic components of body fat, there is therefore good reason to suspect that trunk hair, insofar as it *is* related to fat cells in an individual's body, should be much more directly connected to the total *number* of fat cells than to the particular *size* of any individual cell. Not surprisingly, Bjürulf's data tended to confirm this hunch: In men with identical skin-fold caliper readings (i.e., identical amounts of body fat) body hair was much more profuse in those whose fat measurements depended on a higher total number of adipose tissue cells than it was in those whose fat was mostly due to increased cell size.

The finding is a puzzling one, especially since we tend to think of body fat as a feminine secondary sex characteristic, and of body hair as a masculine one. One possible explanation may be that both body hair and subcutaneous fat are normal adaptive responses to the stress of environmental cold in both sexes. If so, anything that favors the development of the one should theoretically favor the development of the other as well. In women estrogen normally suppresses the growth of body hair; even so, however, women in cold climates tend to be hairier than women in warmer ones—a phenomenon with a long and interesting ethnic pedigree. (As a general rule, Europeans, Asian Indians, and the Ainu people of Japan have substantially more body hair among both sexes than Africans, Mongoloids, and Amerindians do; and although the exceptions to this generalization are too numerous and too unaccountable to prove the rule, the possibility that body hair has something to do with adaptation to cold remains an acceptable working hypothesis until a better one comes along.)

Like differences between species of animals, differences between groups of people sharing the same econiche at given moments of time and space seem to have come about as a result of adaptations to stressful local conditions, through processes working and re-working the basic genetic material over time. Evolutionary theory suggests that ethnic differences are the result of local geographical imperatives: The light skin and eye color of northwestern Euro-peans probably evolved in response to the prevailing cloudiness of their ancestral habitats, while the epicanthic fold of the Mongoloid eye may have been adaptive in climates that were both sunny and cold, etc.

The classical view of evolution as survival of the fittest is better applied to whole populations than to the individual alone; within species, evolution is expressed in terms of gene frequencies, not in terms of the absolute presence or absence of any one particular gene. The test of evolutionary success is proliferation. "Never forget," wrote Charles Darwin, "that every single organic being may be said to be striving to the utmost to increase its numbers." In the long run it is quantity, not quality, that counts. But survival of the fittest means survival to breeding age, and can only be measured in terms of the numbers of the survivors' offspring left alive to compete in the sexual sweepstakes of the next generation. For all intents and purposes selection is never absolute; there is no totally blond population of human beings—no population, that is, where blonds comprise 100 per cent of those born into the group; by the same token, there is no totally "black" population either, since albinos are born at a predictable rate even in the blackest of black African populations. Nothing in nature, and especially not in the richly mongrelized and biologically venturesome segment of it that amounts to human nature, is ever 100 per cent. As a species we have had the good fortune to stay labile and polymorphic, and thus have always had a genetic fallback position or contingency plan to resort to in the face of sudden ecological reverses.

Skin color seems to be a particularly sensitive trait with respect to evolution, probably because its effect on the skeletal develop-ment of women brings it to bear directly on the width of the female pelvis, and thus on the success of childbearing itself. For example, in countries that don't receive much sunlight dark-skinned people may not receive enough Vitamin D to build healthy bones, and the pelvic bones may become stunted during the growing period. When this happens in girls it may have disastrous consequences for future childbearing. But other physical and genetically governed traits are subject to environmental selection too. Like degrees of cloud cover and sunshine, though perhaps less directly, degrees of cold and heat in a prevailing habitat can have an effect on the body build of child-bearing females and hence on the group's over-all fertility rate as well. "What is bred in the bone," as the saying has it, "will never come out of the flesh." This aphorism may have been intended fig-uratively, but it contains the kernel of an unimpeachable anatomical reality; looked at from the cool clinical viewpoint of environmental adaptation, subcutaneous fat can be visualized as a sort of insula-tion worn under, instead of over, the skin; and the ability of fat people to maintain optimum operating temperatures for their inter-nal organs under thermal conditions in which thinner people tend to freeze is probably no small measure of their over-all reproductive success in cold climates.

Although the amounts and kinds of clothing and housing that are generally available, and people's economic and/or geographical access to them, may undercut the importance of actual physiolog-ical adaptations to climate in this day and age in most parts of the world, modern populations as a whole stubbornly continue to ex-hibit significant adaptive differences with respect to heat and cold. These differences have been mapped even within the geographical perimeters of the continental United States where, presumably, most people can avail themselves of warm clothes in cold weather, cool clothes in warm weather, and, for a price, fuel of some sort to keep their indoor temperatures at a relatively stable 60° to 70° on a year-round basis no matter where they live.

Even so, American-born white children are fatter than American-born black children, even when both groups are evenly matched for city of origin, social class, and presumably therefore also for diet, housing, kinds and amounts of physical activity, and various other sorts of environmental stresses and strains. Ethnic differences of this kind are already discernible in infancy, though there is some evidence that they tend to disappear after adolescence.

Earnest A. Hooton, assessing somatotypes of various American ethnic subgroups, came up with the finding that among white

Americans as a whole, obesity is lowest in people of British, Irish, or "old American" origins (i.e., families of many generations' residence in the U.S.), and slightly higher in people of Scandinavian and Germanic ancestry. According to Hooton's analysis, the fattest Americans of all tend to be people of Balto-Ugraic (i.e., Latvian, Estonian, Lithuanian), Central Slav, and Soviet Russian ancestry.

In attempting to get at the ethnic origins of his subjects from an even closer angle of view, Hooton analyzed his data according to his subjects' religious preferences as well as their ancestral geographic origins. Eastern European Jews had originally been classified with Slavic subjects on the basis of their geographic provenience; but differences emerged: In Eastern Jews, for example, the degree of endomorphy, or soft roundedness, was often accompanied by a low level of muscular development—in contrast to findings from other studies (such as Mayer's, mentioned earlier) in which muscle and fat seemed to be closely correlated and mutually self-entailing. Taken as a group, Protestants proved to be generally lean but unmuscular, while of all groups represented in Hooton's study, Roman Catholics proved to be the most muscular. (It should go without saying that data like these reflect geographic origins, social status, and job options of the people supplying them, rather than anything especially effortful or easy or fattening in the nature of their theological beliefs.)

While Hooton analyzed body build as a function of ethnic roots and ancestral geographic origins, other researchers have shown that there is a striking correlation between body build and an individual's city or state of origin within the United States. The leanest Americans come from the southeastern United States, while the fattest ones come from the mid-Atlantic states and the Midwest. On a cross-country basis, white Americans show a high degree of correlation between the mean annual temperatures of their birthplaces and their amount of body fat; black Americans show no such correlations—a finding that suggests that whatever is operating to calibrate degree of body fat to climate inside the somatic package must be a genetic rather than an environmental force, and one that is moreover more highly developed in whites than in blacks. Historically, this sort of interpretation makes good ecological sense, because the prehistory of the species in Europe has been much more thermally stressful than its prehistory in Africa ever was, and thermal adaptability in Paleolithic Europeans may well have gone hand in hand with the gradual bleaching or lightening that attended man's transition from the cloudless latitudes of his original African homeland to the sunless latitudes of glacial Europe to which he migrated in the Ice Age.

Findings like these run counter to so much of the regularly promulgated literature of the diet industry and the medical-advice-to-the-layman columns that a clarification seems to be in order, if not an out-and-out apology. There are, clearly, strong environmental forces involved in ethnic differences in overweight. Different ethnic groups have different cultures, and different cultures have different convictions about what, when, where, and how to eat. Food is of course in the last analysis the only outright physical means there is toward the end of getting fat. Starving people do not gain weight, no matter what ethnic group they hail from. Fat people do lose weight when they are systematically underfed, no matter what kinds and degrees of climates their ancestors were raised in. And at any given moment in history some societies will be richer and therefore more apt to have food surpluses on hand than others, and will therefore offer greater opportunities to overfeed their citizens than those without. These are inescapable inferences from observable facts, and no sensible person would want to take issue with them.

But to enumerate the cultural and environmental determinants of overweight is not to erase the notion that there are potent inborn physiological factors in this equation too; food surpluses may have to exist before significant members of a group can become obese, but they alone are not enough to bring about the overfeeding in the first place or the obesity in the second. To produce a substantial number of overweight people in a given population both constitutional and environmental factors have to coincide, and ferreting out the ways in which they do so has placed the epidemiology of obesity squarely upon the testing ground of the time-honored nature-nurture controversy once and for all. Do we get fat because we eat too much? Or do we eat too much because we are constitutionally programmed to run to fat? Arguments are still being heard on both sides of the case; the case itself is one that has been argued for centuries.

As early as the 1920's scientists were addressing themselves to the question of the incidence of fat children in families with overweight parents; various studies, both here and abroad, went on to document the unusually high number of fat children in families where either or both parents were overweight. The criticisms leveled against such studies on a theoretical basis were not unjustified; from statistics that simply enumerate the number of fat children born to normal and obese parents there is no easy way to determine on the face of it whether the children are fat because their parents are feeding them too much, or because their genes incline them to gain weight no matter how well or how sparingly they are fed in the first place.

But the investigators persisted, and as the data began to accumulate the picture that emerged seemed to be more and more suggestive of an underlying constitutional factor in overweight. Studies along these lines proliferated in the second quarter of the century; they include the work done by Bauer in Vienna, Dunlop and Lyons's studies in Edinburgh, and research done by Davenport, Rony, Gurney, Iverson, Fellows, and Ellis and Tallermann in various cities throughout Great Britain and the United States. Given the wide geographical range and the different methodologies brought to bear on each separate body of data, all these studies were in surprising general agreement as to the incidence of obesity in the children of fat parents, and vice versa: The cumulative weight of their findings was enough to suggest that when a child is overweight, there is fully a 70 to 80 per cent chance that at least one of his parents will turn out to be overweight too.

But the relationship is not a symmetrical one. Turning the question around the other way, it transpires that overweight parents have only about a 25 per cent chance of producing overweight children, which suggests that diet, mealtime rituals, food habits and other cultural factors are not enough in and of themselves to produce fat children 100 per cent of the time, even when both parents are overweight and, presumably, setting a hearty table not only for themselves but for everyone else in the family as well. On the contrary, it appears that an underlying genetic disposition has got to be there too; otherwise, *all* the children in the family would eventually turn out to be fat, rather than the mere 25 per cent who actually do. Results like these, replicated fairly extensively as they are by many independent investigators in many independent studies, are suggestive of a classical Mendelian segregation pattern and would seem at the very least to point to the existence of an underlying biological design in the heritability of overweight.

But ferreting out underlying patterns is only a beginning; scientific understanding demands details, testable hypotheses, measurable deviations from established norms. Singleton births do little to prove a genetic point, but twins provide a natural laboratory for testing genetic connections out. Identical twins are, genetically speaking, almost exact replicas of each other, and if their weights proved to be more alike than the weights of either fraternal twins or of any two random brothers and sisters in the same family, the assumption would be that it is the genes that are responsible for creating the difference. Closing in on the problem from this new angle, Horatio H. Newman, Frank N. Freeman, and Karl J. Holzinger studied the weights of identical twins and compared them with the weights of fraternal twins and same-sexed siblings in the same families.

In the case of body weight, their work established the usefulness of twin studies for basic obesity research beyond question once and for all. Newman, Freeman, and Holzinger's results showed that the difference in adult weight between identical twins amounted to an average of 4.1 pounds, while the difference between weights of fraternal twins was an impressive 10.1 pounds, and that between same-sexed siblings a still greater 10.4 pounds.

The high correlation between the weights of identical twins, and the much lower correlations between those of fraternal twins and same-sexed siblings, confirmed the hunch that there is a definite genetic basis for a given individual's body weight as an adult. Environmental factors may play a part in the picture, to the point of confounding the underlying constitutional patterns in ways too complicated to decipher—but they never operate in a genetic vacuum; an individual who is genetically prone to obesity will therefore have an altogether different "weight problem" from one whose excess weight is an accident of time, place, and the groaning board.

Parents have lately taken their blows for the appearance of obesity in their children, and certain theorists have gone so far as to trace the whole syndrome of adult obesity to thoughtless overfeeding in the first three years of life. But statistical evidence favors a more relaxed point of view. One way to come at the problem is to compare children's weights to the weights of their natural parents, on the one hand, and to the weights of their adoptive parents on the other. If there are greater similarities to the first than there are to the second, it is a safe guess that we are in the presence of constitutional factors rather than environmental ones. In a new assault on the age-old nature-nurture problem, Withers undertook this sort of comparison in 1964 with results that struck another blow for the constitutionalists over and against the moralists: Withers's research proved that the correlation between the body weights of natural children and their parents was significantly higher than the correlation between weights of adoptive children and *their* parents. Since both natural and adoptive parents probably over- and underfeed their children at about the same rate, it is probably fair to conclude that the child's receptivity in this situation counts for at least as much as the parents' generosity does. A similar study has recently been completed in Greater Montreal by Pierre Biron, who reported at a 1975 meeting of the American Heart Association on the relationship between weight and heredity in a total sample of 274 families, with results very similar to those of Withers. Biron concluded that the amount of food that is offered to a child may have relatively little to do with whether that child is ever likely to become overweight. Rightly or wrongly, some children are destined to be fat, whether they are overfed or not.

Genes have been called the raw materials of evolution. It is through the agonizingly slow and piecemeal weeding out of harmful genes, and the ongoing snail's-pace accretion of good or "fit" ones in a given population, that evolution from one form of life to another (at the species level) and from one set of physical attributes to another (at the population level) manages to take place. The process may take eons; even the fastest rates of evolution, as evolutionary biologist George Gaylord Simpson says, seem very slow to human beings—including paleontologists. But if genes are the raw materials of evolution, adaptation is the refinery in which these raw materials are duly processed. New gene sequences or mutations may appear at random, but they can only be incorporated into the total gene pool—or rejected from it—by the effect of ecological factors administering their presence or absence from the next generation's gene pool through natural selection.

Our success as a species has been put down to our history as biological generalists; like the rat and the cockroach, man is genetically prepared to turn on a biological dime in the face of new challenges to his livelihood, his fitness, and his over-all somatic ingenuity. As archaeologist Carl Sauer has pointed out, man is just as unspecialized with respect to his gut as he is with respect to his taxonomically famous and unspecialized hand. Our ability to use our hands for tool making as well as for grasping, climbing, and throwing is mirrored and amplified by our ability to convert a whole range of natural growing things into things that are good—or at least possible—to eat and digest. It is as omnivores that we have made our way as a species into literally every corner of the habitable world—and some that are well-nigh uninhabitable as well.

The trick of evolution is to adapt, but never to overadapt. Specialization is always a risky undertaking: Adaptation to cloudy climates may disqualify you for life in the hot sun; adaptation to cold climates on the other hand may carry vascular, social, and occupational risks later in life. Nevertheless, it is a safe bet, from the available evidence, that at some moment in man's climatic prehistory, such risks must have been acceptable ones; the genetic load implicit in the tendency to accrue fat must have been offset biologically by the generally better fitness of fat people in a cold environment than that of thin ones.

Man's arrival in Europe from his ancestral African and Middle Eastern homelands took place at a time of incipient and eventually cataclysmic change for the earth as a whole and for northern Europe in particular. And it was probably at that time that the new species exercised its biological option in favor of genes for overweight, writing off the long-term disadvantages of reduced speed and maneuverability, and perhaps a reduced life-span too, against the short-term advantage of survival from one bitter winter's day to the next. But without this biological option in the meantime—and without the genes that it eventually indemnified—some of us might well not be alive today to tell the tale.

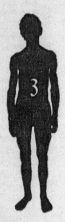

3 *Women:*
Venus as Endomorph

"I am resolved to grow fat, and look young till forty," said John Dryden's Maiden Queen, reflecting the seventeenth-century wisdom that being young entails a certain degree of fleshiness—or endomorphy, as anthropometrists would probably call it now. Revised over the course of several centuries, this orthodoxy has come full circle to its own antithesis: Nowadays it is assumed that fat is unlovely and, worse still, makes you look older than your years.

There are fashions in human beauty as there are in clothes and architecture, and the ideal of female fleshiness did not survive the turn of the present century. Of the many changes in public taste and standards that have meanwhile taken place, perhaps none is as thoroughgoing as the change in the publicly canonized version of what constitutes a desirable female body shape. Till early in this century, Venus was almost always drawn in the guise of an endomorph: moon-faced, pear-shaped, and well fleshed out. And the aesthetic ideal was not far removed from the living reality: Pound for pound and millimeter for millimeter, women have always been fatter than men.

The difference is already present in infancy. This fact would be less remarkable in and of itself if it were not for the corollary that

a) newborn girls in all ethnic groups, although they are fatter, weigh less at birth than newborn boys; and b) fat is only deposited in the fetus of either sex quite late in the last trimester of pregnancy, so that whatever differences there may be between the fat measurements of boys and girls at the moment of birth must have been achieved pretty much within the last two or three weeks of life inside the womb, and must therefore reflect strong physiological forces at work on the baby about to be born. Since mothers in the normal course of events cannot be expected to know the sex of the fetus they are carrying (and probably would not change their eating habits much accordingly, even if they did) the presumption is strong that the differences in body fat between girl and boy newborn babies is largely the outcome of built-in factors (like genes and hormones) rather than extraneous, environmental factors (like what and how much the mother eats during the last few months or even weeks of pregnancy).

The difference in fat between male and female babies at birth is measured by skin-fold calipers, usually applied at two sites: the skin over the triceps area on the back of the arm, midway between the shoulder and the elbow, and the skin on the fleshy part of the back just below the scapular bone, or shoulder blade. The male-female difference in skin-fold measurements is most noticeable at the latter site, and it is still apparent, though less so, at the site on the back of the arm. The consistent difference in amount of body fat between the two sexes is one that cuts across geographical and ethnic categories. In other words, within any given local or ethnic population, girls in the group will tend to be fatter than boys; furthermore, the relationship is one that holds good throughout the entire life-span when, as in later middle age, males begin to lose much of their muscle tissue and start to run to fat instead.

The fact that females are, from birth onward, fatter than their male counterparts may seem on the face of it a biological injustice as undeserved as any social or economic injustice exercised upon women by a male-dominated social system—especially to women who tend to run to more than their fair share of fat in the first place. We live in a culture that values leanness in both sexes; if there is any particular lesson for feminists in this preference it may be that the ideal of feminine beauty has thus come increasingly, within the span of the past half century, to reflect a male ideal model in preference to a typically female one. The status assumptions implicit in this choice are interesting. People tend to ape their betters, and women's aspirations to the unmodulated physiques of men express unvoiced, and until recently probably largely unconscious, judgments about the nature of male status and privilege as compared to their own. But from an anthropometric point of view the trend is a dubious one: Female fleshiness is a fact of biological life and one that has every appearance of having been programmed into the species long ago by nature.

This is not to assert that all women are born to be fat and might as well resign themselves to it, any more than it is to say that all men are born to be thin. Statistical averages for sizes and shapes are not binding on individuals; they are only extrapolations from measurements of large numbers of people within a given population. They tell us what the odds are that we will be of one size or shape rather than another, but not what particular body build any one of us as an individual is fated to be born with or to have assigned to him in perpetual care as an adult.

What has to be taken into account, anthropometrically speaking, though, is that the derived image of the twentieth-century Venus is that of a creature who is on the whole typologically unfeminine. The hipless and flat-chested mid-twentieth-century version of the familiar feminine cult figure is one who comes closer in actuality to the real-life model of an adolescent boy still deep in his growing period than to that of a historically "normal" adult female; the lanky Seventh Avenue epigone with her narrow pelvis and unremarkable behind conforms in many ways much more closely to a male skeletal—and adipose—model than to a typically female one. The role of the homosexual fashion designer in all this has probably been somewhat overdrawn by the exasperated (heterosexual) males who pay their bills; women have always known how to pick and choose among the competing images offered them by the fashion designers, and have certainly played a much more active, discriminating, and downright hedonistic role in the process than their husbands and fathers seem to want to credit them with. In the context of the new feminism, therefore, it may be well to remember that, for whatever reasons, the present model is one that has by and large been imposed on women by women: Men's calendar art and pinup magazines have usually dealt in somewhat more biometrically realistic images and ideals.

While naturally thin women and naturally fat men are far from uncommon, especially in the rich ethnic and anthropometric melting pot of twentieth-century America, there are nevertheless normative shapes and sizes for men and women, and normative sites and distribution patterns for body fat, and such norms vary quite predictably as a function of the subject's sex.

Men, for example, although leaner than women on the whole to begin with, do tend to deposit their fat more frontally than women do (that is, on the chest and abdomen) and may thus give the appearance—at least from the front—of being fatter than women with the same total amount of body adipose tissue. Women, on the other hand (disallowing for the moment the frontal fat represented by adipose tissue in the breasts), tend to deposit their fat more dorsally than men: Inch for inch, a woman may thus expect more of her excess poundage to migrate to the back of her body than to the front. This is true not only for that percentage of fat that accumulates in her buttocks, but also for the leaner part of her back as well. Thus, given two individuals, male and female, with an equal amount of total body fat, as determined by some nonmetrical test like creatinine excretion assay, or densitometry (underwater weighing) measurement, one can predict with a fair degree of safety that a skin-fold reading at any site on the back of the woman (except at the nape of the neck) will be fatter than an identical site on the back of the man; and conversely, that waistline skin-fold and upper abdominal measurements will tend to be higher for the man than for the woman.

Another sex difference in fat distribution between men and women is that men tend to deposit more of their total body fat on the trunk, as opposed to the arms and legs, than women do. Male fat therefore tends to be truncal fat, as well as frontal. And by the same token, fat men will exhibit a characteristic pad of flesh at the nape of the neck; when it is seen in women this phenomenon is known as a dowager's hump, in recognition of the age factor involved. The phenomenon is rarely present in women before menopause, at which time female hormone production is sharply reduced and women are more apt to manifest masculine traits (for example, hirsuteness and voice changes) than they are during their childbearing years.

Another typically masculine feature involves the vertical distribution of frontal fat in men. Much of the adipose tissue that a man accumulates on his front will be concentrated in the area above the navel; the low-slung Falstaffian paunch or beer belly is actually a gynoid (feminine) departure from the prevailing android (masculine) norm. More typically masculine on the whole is the barrel-chested pouter-pigeon shape, even though it involves some degree of adipose tissue build-up in the chest, thus mimicking mammary development and a misleading feminine body configuration. Fat women, on the other hand, contrary to the barracks-room ideal of pinup girls whose only visible frontal fat is limited strictly to their chests, will tend on the whole to concentrate their truncal fat below the navel and over the hips, leaving the waistline and chest relatively less well padded in comparison to the belly and haunches.

This brings us to the subject of breasts, a distinctively human biological invention whose evolutionary *raison d'être* has yet to be pinned down in the biological literature, and whose aesthetic and erotic fascination for a large percentage of the postpubertal male population in most cultures has never really been satisfactorily explained in the psychological literature either. The fatty female breast is a uniquely human phenomenon, and as such it is a zoological mystery of the first order. We are the only primates of record to have opted for permanently fatty breasts as a normal infant-feeding device: other nonhuman primate females, even though their nipples are placed similarly to those of human females and they feed their infants frontally in much the same nursing positions as we do, tend to have their chest fat much more evenly distributed over the entire chest wall than human mothers do.

Adipose tissue in the human breast expands with age and the number of children a woman has borne; it is liberally seeded throughout the basic glandular tissue of the breast and tends to displace it with increasing age. The popular assumption that big breasts guarantee a big milk supply in the lactating mother is false: Actually, according to some anatomists, the size of the areola is much more closely related to the size of the gland behind it (in much the same way that the root system of a tree is proportional to the size of its branches) than is the size of the whole breast itself.

Fat makes the difference; and the amount of fat present in the breasts is probably governed less by the size of the mammary gland itself than by the individual woman's own distinctive adipose tissue economy and her genetic predisposition to deposit what fat she has in one part of her anatomy rather than another. So, even though there may be relatively little difference in the size of the mammary glands from one woman to another, the propensity to put on fat has never guaranteed that the fat-prone woman will develop a bigger bosom than her leaner sister, and the best prescription for a big bust still remains to pick your ancestors accordingly; a big-chested grandmother is a better predictor of a big chest in any of her female descendants than the amount of food they eat or the weight they may happen to gain in the course of their post-adolescent lives.

The phenomenon of the fat human breast remains to be explained; in the meantime various speculative arrows have been aimed at it, without any of them having quite made their mark. Desmond Morris considers the human female breast to be a sexual signaling device. Normally among primates—as among most other mammals—male entry in coitus is from the rear, and that is where most female sex-signaling displays are located. But in human beings, according to Morris, the strong monogamous impulse programmed into the species depends on constant face-to-face contact not only during coitus but for all other social intercourse as well, with the result that during the long course of evolution from ape to man-ape to man, sexual signaling devices in human females have migrated from the back of the body to the front.

This argument may owe something to the reasoning of turn-of-the-century anatomist and zoologist Hermann Klaatsch, who linked sexual selection for chestiness with the heightened fertility that must once upon a time have seemed to be implicated in it. Sexual selection in favor of lactating women may therefore have come to focus on the size and shape of the engorged lactating breast itself. Because human babies may nurse for years at a time, their mothers' breasts remain "fat" much longer than the breasts of other lactating primates, and the man in the family might draw the somewhat erroneous conclusion that fat breasts equaled superfertility. (The facts of the matter are almost just the opposite: Nursing usually interferes with normal ovulation and thus acts as a sort of built-in contraceptive and child-spacing device.)

Other explanations for the fat human breast have been more down-to-earth and have sought to rephrase the question in terms of the distinctively human mother-child relationship. It has been suggested, for example, that the fatty female breast is a means of keeping breast milk at a kind of pediatrically optimal temperature, as a sort of anatomical homologue to a bottle warmer. (On the face of it, though, this explanation leaves something to be desired, since the best way of keeping breast milk warm would surely be to keep it closer to the chest wall in the first place, and thus closer to the original source of internal body heat.)

A fourth possibility is that in a hairless but upright species like man, a pendulous breast gives infants something to hang on to while the mother carries them around from place to place. Certain rodents simply hang on to their mothers' nipples for dear life when danger looms; and ape and monkey nurslings commonly anchor themselves to their mothers by clutching fistfuls of chest or shoulder hair. But this solution is not available to human infants, and the closest thing to it is the compressible, graspable adipose tissue of the human mother's breast.

Whatever the merits of each or any of these arguments may be, zoological evidence seems to favor the existence of a strong sexual component in the picture: Man is the only animal of record who focuses any particular erotic attention on the female breast; human females are by the same token the only animal of record to enjoy or solicit such attention to their breasts. The resulting consensus may conceivably have left its mark on demographic history. From the point of view of the aroused woman, eroticization of her breasts may act to increase her chances of mating and motherhood; as for the man who is inspired to arouse her, his continuing interest in her breasts may well have something to do with the fact that human females are the only known animals whose mammary structures are just as prominent between pregnancies as they are when bearing or suckling their young. It is adipose tissue that makes the zoological (and histological) difference between the engorged breast of the pregnant or nursing mother and the merely seemingly engorged breast of the normal adult human female.

Quite possibly the answer to the biological riddle presented by the human female breast includes elements of all of these explanations and theories: Evolution itself is rarely as single-minded and reductionist as the average ethologist's pet theory is. But however the case may finally be resolved, it is clear from the anthropological literature that latter-day American pinup collectors are not the only ethnic group, past or present, to have favored women with big breasts: of the Sirione of the Amazon River basin, Holmberg observed: "Besides being young, a desirable sex partner should also be fat. She should have big hips, good-sized but firm breasts, and a deposit of fat on her sexual organs." And the Sirione are not an isolated case: According to ethnographic reports in the Human Relations Area Files, the Alorese, Apache, Hopi, Kurtatchi, Lesu, Thongo, Trukese, and Wogeo all like their women on the bosomy side, if not downright obese. This anthropological cross section seems to cut a wide swathe across geographical and ethnic lines, and while it is by no means universal it is widespread enough to offer some consolation, however abstract, to fat women whose constitutions seem to offer them little choice in the matter, regardless of what the culture they were raised in wants of them.

Sex differences in body dimensions and contour appear at adolescence and tend to become more and more marked as time goes on. And because fat is such a characteristic component of female body tissue at all ages, but especially from adolescence on, adult feminine body shapes tend to be much more variable than those of men. Fat is an almost infinitely expandable and plastic tissue, as those who have too much of it are first to realize—whereas there seem to be distinct upper limits on the size of bone and muscle, the major components of body tissues in men. The plasticity of women's shapes and sizes as opposed to men's is reflected in the various sizing calculations used in the clothing industries that cater to men and women respectively: The women's clothing industry in the United States uses a total of sixteen different sets of measurement sites to standardize the full spectrum of women's sizes and shapes; while most manufacturers of men's clothing in the United States grade their patterns on the basis of two or at most six simple measurements alone, chest girth and sitting height being the crucial—and sometimes the only—ones. These disparities mirror the complex modulation and relief of the female figure, as opposed to that of the male's: While actual measurements at a given point of the body may be the same (or less) for women as for men, the distance between any two such points on a woman's figure is apt to be much larger than the same distance on a man's.

Other differences in the gross body morphology of men and women include differences in over-all stature, total body weight, and limb circumferences—to the point where some observers would list body size as a secondary sex characteristic in and of itself, along with beards and voice differences. "Sexual dimorphism" is the name given by zoologists to describe the total number and degree of gross anatomical differences that are normally found between males and females of the same species—excluding differences in the genital apparatus of the two sexes. In a majority of mammal species males are larger than females (exceptions like the European rabbit, the hamster, and the bat, where the female is significantly larger than the male, comprise only about one quarter of known groups), but in some species the difference is much more marked than it is in others—probably as a result of the ways different species have of making a living within a given ecozone, as determined by local food supply, water resources, and various other environmental stresses and strains, and the basic genetic equipment that is any particular animal's species-specific stock in trade.

Different environments impose different demands for defense and aggression on the animals inhabiting them, and defense of the territory is something that normally falls to the males of the species, leaving females free to deal with bearing and raising the young. Ethologists have theorized that in certain ground-dwelling primates, where the aggressiveness and physical robustness of males is in sharp contrast to the passivity and daintiness of females, certain features of the group's characteristic social structure seem to favor selection for exaggerated size differences between the two sexes too. According to Sherwood Washburn and Irven de Vore, for example, the average male savanna-dwelling baboon weighs 75 pounds, while the average female weighs 30 pounds—or, in other words, less than half the weight of the average male. Life in the open savanna where these animals make their home can be a dangerous one for ground-dwelling primates like baboons, as it must have been for man's earliest hominid precursors, who ranged much the same area as that now inhabited by the baboons. Large carnivores (particularly lions, but there are others too) share the baboon's habitat, and some kind of defense preparedness must therefore be built into the species' somatic equipment and into its social and behavioral repertoire as well.

The species has accordingly solved its defense problems in several ways. Baboons live and travel in bands which vary between about forty and eighty individuals; social groups within the band are organized in a sort of concentric pattern according to age and sex, with females and infants grouped with dominant "alpha" males at the center of the band, and young males deployed around the perimeter of the group for defense and lookout purposes. Mating couples are more or less permanently bonded, but the group leaders (the so-called alpha males, who are usually the largest mature males in the group) tend to form harems. This gives them sexual access to a larger number of the fertile females than other males have, and they therefore mate more often than other males do, with the not surprising result that they end up fathering more than their fair genetic share of the infants born within a given band.

Under these circumstances a large proportion of infants born in any given year will prove to have inherited these particular baboons' unique genetic traits (including male robustness and large body size) and these traits will therefore come to be liberally seeded throughout subsequent generations of baboons. Meanwhile, though, the greater number and genetic variability of the mothers giving birth to the alpha males' offspring in a given season will dilute any concomitant trend toward robustness in female newborns; in this way the males of the troop will tend to get bigger and bigger over the years, while the females remain more variable. The human model for social organization which this harem system most closely resembles is polygyny, a fairly common marital system among primitive (and some not so primitive) peoples all over the world, in which one man—usually a well-to-do and powerful one—takes several wives and thus ends up impregnating several women at a time, thereby managing to disseminate his genes much more widely and in a much shorter period of time than men with fewer wives.

Where this system prevails, so will its biological heritage: Polygyny promotes the genetic idiosyncrasies of alpha males, whether these consist of large noses or robust shoulders—or whatever else the anatomical and/or physiological factors are that are involved in the acquisition of social power, including male-female sex differences in species where males are the power wielders, females the housekeepers. This is not to say that it is the only possible or major system either in man or in other mammals. Among arboreal primates like gibbons, for example, who feed and nest in trees and whose natural predators are few and far between (or can at least almost always be outmaneuvered by climbing high or higher into the nearest tree) there is very little over-all difference between the lifestyles of male and female members of the species, and the difference between male and female body size is correspondingly unremarkable. Gibbons live in permanently bonded pairs and form small nuclear families of father, mother, and immature offspring not unlike the nuclear families of human beings today. Interestingly enough, gibbons turn out to be among the most monogamous of mammalian species. And ethological studies of other animals confirm the observation that lack of size and build differences between the sexes is a frequent characteristic of animals who live monogamously. It would be interesting to know what inferences, if any, could be drawn from this insight for the institution of human marriage in the twentieth century, and for the future of sexual egalitarianism in labor, education, and family life. The "little woman" of American folklore is a patent anachronism—both anatomically and psychologically—in a world that no longer has any particular reason to value the defensive prowess or sheer brawn of "big men." And yet, by all accounts, women still place a certain premium on height in the men they marry; taller is still better when it comes to choosing a husband in twentieth-century America, and most women will still "marry up" in a strictly postural, if not necessarily a social, sense.

Such genetic shibboleths die as hard as social ones, and there are still differences in degrees of sexual dimorphism between men and women in human groups just as there are in primate ones. If we accept the working hypothesis that sexual dimorphism stems at least to some degree from differences in social organization and economic life-style, the fact that there are body size and tissue differences between the sexes in human groups constitutes strong suggestive evidence for certain kinds of socioeconomic arrangements operating long ago in the past, even though we may never be able to prove the point definitively.

Human beings all belong to the same species, of course, but over the years geographical isolation from each other at certain moments in history may have produced gross visible differences between large groups of human beings living at some significant geographical remove from each other around the world. These differences are the ones that we now recognize as criteria for ethnic or racial distinctiveness. The flat face of the Mongoloids, the fair skin of northern Europeans, the red hair and freckles of some Irish groups, and the snub nose and slanted eyes of the Lapps, were probably originally all features of adaptation to environment worked out at one time or another in prehistory when the group (and its genes) was isolated from other groups for fairly long stretches of time due to some insurmountable ecological or social happenstance. Over time, populations living at some distance from each other and working out distinctive adaptations to prevailing local conditions will tend to come up with all kinds of virtually custom-made accommodations to a given set of environmental circumstances; and sexual dimorphism itself may long ago have been one of them—along with the distinctive hair forms and colors, nose shapes, limb lengths, and eyelid folds that distinguish one ethnic group from another even today.

Broadly speaking, the racial group with the least number of gross body differences between men and women are the Mongoloids. This is a category that would include most Chinese, Japanese, Indochinese, and Amerindians both north and south of the border. At the other end of this continuum are the Caucasoids (including white Americans, Europeans, Transcaucasian and Asian Indians, and most North Africans and Middle Easterners), who tend on the whole to show the largest degree of sexual dimorphism and male-female body-size differences of any of the three major racial groups. And with respect to sexual dimorphism, Africans and black Americans form a third group somewhere between Caucasoid and Mongoloid extremes.

Unlike baboons, however, selection for sexual dimorphism in human groups seems not to have favored exaggerated maleness in the male prototype so much as it has favored exaggerated femininity in the female. There is some evidence, for example, that Caucasoids produce women with the largest breasts and the widest pelvic flare, as well as the highest subcutaneous fat readings, of any of the three major racial groups.

Such differences between populations with respect to sexual differences in body size and shape must of course have many causes. Men are not baboons, and among the important determinants of sexual dimorphism in our own species, past and present, we have to number aesthetic factors as well as ecological ones. Men marry women for their looks, among other things, and aesthetic decisions about what constitutes feminine beauty in any given culture will no doubt eventually have to have some effect on that culture's gene pool too. The operating principle is a simple one. As much as any other factor, aesthetic choices govern the rate at which certain women get married—and bear children—as opposed to others, and thus have a direct effect on the over-all fertility of the woman in question. For there is a certain time factor involved in fertility: Women who marry, and especially those who marry young, will in the normal course of events produce more children and have higher fertility rates than those who marry late or not at all.

Of course sexual selection by face and figure is not the sole or even, perhaps, the major determinant of what genes get replicated from one generation to the next: Women in most cultures are valued not only as romantic and sexual objects but also as cooks, basket weavers, hide chewers, and clothing manufacturers—not to mention as housekeepers, conversationalists, and party givers. Women in various cultures often specialize in one or another of these skills, and if the husband's survival or social status depends on warm clothing, surplus baskets to trade, or well-patronized dinner parties, he will do well to look for a bride who is accomplished along these lines, whether or not she has a pretty face or an interesting figure to match it. Local ecological and economic considerations therefore can and do have at least as strong an effect as looks do on the emergence of certain physical types among women; in nomadic cultures where women, like camels, must walk and carry things great distances, a certain degree of skeletal sturdiness will always be attractive in a wife—and of course men looking for brides have always had an eye toward their aptness for childbearing. Wide hips and generous figures were therefore once in fashion, and rightly so.

The point has not been lost on primitive groups, nomadic or otherwise; among the Wogeo, according to a reporter in the Human Relations Area Files, "the petite has less aesthetic appeal than the massive, for girls pointed out to me for commendation were all somewhat large . . . with broad hips and powerful limbs." The same author was led to conclude that "as far as general body build is concerned, the majority of societies whose preferences in this matter are recorded feel that a plump woman is more attractive than a thin one"—obese North American and European women please take note.

There is no accounting in the long run for the aesthetic assumptions about what passes for feminine beauty in one culture as over and against another, but ecological factors undoubtedly impose their own strictures on the local labor pool—and hence on the local gene pool as well. And these strictures may get incorporated into the local aesthetic ideal as time goes by. Archaic subsistence patterns can be tentatively reconstructed by analogizing from the living patterns of primitive peoples alive today, and on this basis we can speculate more or less intelligently about the living patterns of extinct populations too. For example, where men and women perform just about the same kind of subsistence tasks, day in and day out, and eat more or less the same kinds and amounts of food while doing so, selection in favor of one body size and shape for men and another one for women would not make good evolutionary sense and would therefore probably be kept to a minimum. In point of fact, successful subsistence in this kind of economically egalitarian economy would probably depend on the easy interchangeability between workers of either sex, thus effectively doubling the labor pool whenever and wherever extra hands happened to be needed—as for example during harvesting or sowing.

The latter-day Indochinese can be taken as a case in point. There are relatively few size and shape differences between men and women on the Indochinese peninsula, and historically, the economic record bears the anthropometric record out; the economics of rice cultivation have a long local history and prehistory in Indochina. Thus the logic of Indochinese agriculture supports the view that when men and women do basically the same kind of work in the same kind of habitat, their bodies will come to resemble each other fairly closely in size and shape too.

The strong sexual dimorphism of European populations (especially northern Europeans), on the other hand, may reflect an almost diametrically opposite set of circumstances, and one in which a long history of cultural, ecological, and economic separatism between the sexes (perhaps even one with a strongly institutionalized sexist component) grew out of the unequivocal ecological realities of man's glacial prehistory in that part of the world, molding a social-sexual dimorphism just as compelling as the primary physical one.

This kind of sexual separatism—ecologically determined, anatomically built in—may have sprung from environmental conditions peculiar to man's Paleolithic life-style in the cold Pleistocene hinterland. In the absence of texts and records it is hard to test the theory out; on the other hand, though, Ice Age man in Europe was an artist as well as a hunter, and the mysterious Venus figurines, the tiny statuettes of opulently fleshy and probably pregnant female nudes, add up to a sample of some sixty or seventy more or less naturalistic icons of human females of the era. Assuming that figurative art establishes a historical record as well as a merely aesthetic one, we can deduce certain things about the living realities of the sculptors from the shapes and contours of the women who may once have sat for their portraits in limestone and mammoth ivory to them.

The famous Venus of Willendorf is probably the most admired and best known of the group. Seen from the front, Willendorf is almost perfectly globular: If one were to draw a line around her picture on a piece of paper her head and torso would fit into the circumference of an almost geometrically perfect circle.

What cultural and/or aesthetic role Willendorf and other figurines may have been meant to play in the societies that produced them is still not provable. By analogy to certain traditions in latter-day Western art, the first theory to be advanced was that the figurines were pornographic—erotic fetishes of sex-obsessed big-game hunters—or in other words, a species of Ice Age barracks-room art. Others believed that, like the reindeer, bison, and woolly mammoths he hunted, human females were objects of the hunter's sympathetic cult magic, and that these miniature icons of women in limestone and ivory represented wishful projections of the caveman's desire to conjure them up whenever they were absent or in short supply.

Anthropologically speaking, this idea is not as farfetched as it may sound at first blush. Scarcity confers value on an object, and women in Paleolithic hunting groups may at certain times and places have been at an enormous economic premium. In many primitive societies women are still traded in marriage like commodities and domestic livestock; and the practice was not uncommon in pre-Enlightenment Europe among the higher nobility for that matter either. By extension, the possibility that in certain political situations females were apt to be "hunted" almost as systematically as animals, and on much the same basis, has been seriously advanced by some anthropologists. In primitive subsistence economies where most of the food-getting activity depends on big-game hunting and is consequently restricted to men and older boys, little girls are an economic luxury item, and in lean years female infanticide is not an uncommon practice. The practice does not have to be formalized: Benign neglect of female babies can be counted on to thin out the populations of weanlings when food is scarce and the mother is hard pressed with other (male) mouths to feed. The predictable result, however, is that ten to fifteen years later there may suddenly prove to be a dearth of marriageable females in the group in question, thus setting off predatory raids against neighboring tribes for females. ("We marry our enemies" is the common ethnographic refrain from all corners of the inhabited globe.) In the process women, as a scarcity item, may easily become deified. The rags-to-riches metamorphosis, from despised muchness to prized minority, is not an unusual one; we have seen the same thing happen within our own lifetimes with respect to certain kinds of big-game animals, real estate, and fish.

The how and why of the Venus figurines and their corpulence may never be definitively spelled out, but from the anthropometric viewpoint one of the most interesting lessons to be learned from them is that, just as in similar populations in Europe of the present day, the fattest or at least the most globular of the figurines were usually found at sites which must have been the coldest for the periods in which they were sculpted, while the more linear of the figurines have generally been dug up from the more southerly, or at any rate the warmer, sites.

This being so, it would seem that the Paleolithic women who served as models for the Venus figurines, like the nonhuman fauna all around them at the time, were living under the ungainsayable anatomical imperatives of Bergmann's and Allen's rules. In part, therefore, their globularity may have represented not just a cold winter night's reflection of some erotic gleam in the art-ist's eye—or even a magical act to summon fertility and good luck in the (bridal) hunt—but also a predictable adaptation to cold by means of increased body fat. And if Paleolithic man in Europe val-ued fat breasts and haunches in his women, he had natural selection on his side: In a hairless species like man, fat had come to have a survival value of its own, especially thirty to twenty thousand years ago at the height of the Würm glaciation.

For life on the glacial tundra of northern Europe and Siberia was not an easy one—especially not for the female of the species—and endomorphy may have been one of the cleverest somatic strategies available to women making their homes as big-game hunters' wives at the edge of an advancing glacier. Henri Vallois estimates that less than 50 per cent of a given Paleolithic population could have been expected to live long enough to reach the age of 21; of these, only 12 per cent would finally make it past 40, and among this last handful of hardy survivors there would not be a single female. In Vallois's study of skeletons of Ice Age bands, not one woman in any of the groups he studied had ever made it past the age of 30.

Women in Ice Age Europe did not join in the hunt; the human mother-child relationship is a demanding and time-consuming one, and stalking and ambushing the huge herds of large hooved animals on which the hunters depended for the bulk of their food supply was a job for cooperative male hunting groups, not for women and children. Paleolithic women may have trapped small game and fowl, but many of the smaller rodents and burrowing animals which could be caught locally around the home camp during the glacial winters were hibernators, and in the protracted winters of the Ice Age it is unlikely that such animals formed any sizable proportion of the regular diet.

In a subsistence economy in which virtually all the food is there-fore contributed directly by males—with females having little if any control over their own immediate food supply—genetic selection would have to favor those women best able to accumulate the most fat, on the least caloric input, and in the shortest possible period of time. In this way, in the event of prolonged fasting between meals—lapses which might be all too common if hunters were ab-sent from camp on game forays for more than a few days at a time—the women left behind would have some dependable reserve food supply of their own to provision themselves and their nursing children. And while it is no doubt possible that meat could be and was frozen for storage against a rainy (or, more appropriately, a snowy) day, and against periods of prolonged sexual disfavor, widowhood, or any other unforeseeable social or physical disaster—it is clear that in the long run a woman's own stored fat must have been a safer, longer-lasting, and more dependable form of reserve food supply than frozen meat: an eminently moveable feast, and in the most literal sense of the term at that.

In short, it was clearly an advantage to a woman to be fat prone if she lived in a cold climate where her winter food supply was always at the mercy of someone else's economic efforts and social or sexual favor. During the long winter months, women in Paleolithic hunting cultures were in just such a position, and the same set of circumstances is not totally unknown even today. Customs and traditions in some subarctic cultures still bear witness to the extraordinary degree to which males in a hunting society may dominate the prevailing food supply, both at the source and even at the endpoint too: Among the Fennoscandian Lapps, for example, all food was once not only provided by men but was ultimately even prepared and cooked by men, and thereby controlled at the distribution point as well as at the source. This tradition was still in effect as recently as a hundred years ago, according to Björn Collinder, although it has since broken down, especially among the more assimilated Lapps of Norway and Finland. Even so, and regardless of who does the killing and cooking, it is clear that to be physiologically self-sufficient in a big-game-hunting society (or even a more evolved but equally sexist one, where big money may have taken over that section of the economy where big game leaves off) would always tend to be an advantage for a woman and her children—especially during the coldest months of the year.

In this connection, it should be remembered that Paleolithic winters were longer than they are at the same latitudes today. Adaptation to cold was therefore an almost all-year-round requirement at the height of the Würm glaciation, and while there were no doubt good years and bad years for the hunters, and seasonal ups and downs in the success of the hunt, the social organization of the Ice Age hunting peoples was probably always such that women and female children would normally be last in line at the end of the local food distribution chain. Under the circumstances, it paid women to be fat and stay that way as long as they could. But this wisdom had to become automatic and self-regulating before it could appear on a population-wide basis as part of the group's permanent adaptive armamentarium; and although the means for internalizing it may have been genetic, the feedback circuits perpetuating it must have been social and sexual as well.

The social connections are easy to imagine. Some of them may still be with us today in the institution of European monogamy, where the woman stays home and raises children while the man migrates out to some watering spot of the corporate wilderness every day and brings home his share of the corporate kill at weekly, biweekly, or monthly intervals. The sexual connections in this system are somewhat less easily reconstructed. Staying home with varying numbers of small children, wild or tame, is not generally considered the most erotically stimulating option available to women nowadays. But fat women may have the edge over their thinner sisters in this respect; researchers at Michael Reese Hospital in Chicago a few years ago came up with the startling finding that fat women are more sexually appetitive than thinner women are. The finding was unexpected because the investigators had started out with almost exactly the opposite hypothesis: Psychoanalytic theory had advanced the notion that fat women become fat and stay that way largely as a means of insulating themselves from the give and take of mature heterosexual relationships, however such things may be defined. Fat was seen in other words as a kind of somatic metaphor for the psychic armor fat people are supposed to have elaborated as a defense against sex and love. We live in a culture that pays extensive lip service to the notion that fat is morally and sexually repulsive, and it seemed a not unlikely hypothesis that the fatter a woman was the less likely she would be to have an active and satisfactory sex life—on the one hand because her partners could be expected to find her unappetizing to begin with, and on the other hand because the same defense mechanisms that were supposed to have led her to get fat in the first place should by the same token have operated to make her frigid in the second.

But the assumption did not test out. On the contrary, the fatter women in the Chicago survey were significantly "sexier" than the thinner subjects in the same experiment. In terms of erotic readiness and general sexual excitability, fat women outscored their thin sisters by a factor of almost two to one. Matched pairs of thirty fat and thin married women all reported roughly the same frequency of intercourse (about nine times a month); but a statistically over-whelming majority of the fat women stated that they would have preferred a higher coital frequency, while a significant number of the thinner subjects were perfectly contented with their sexual lots. The authors concluded that "these women obviously weren't overeating *instead* of having sex; their craving for both food and sex exists almost simultaneously." And by way of explanation, one of the coinvestigators offers the predictable psychoanalytic rationale that an underlying psychic hunger must be what lies behind the otherwise merely symbolically related appetites for (sexual) love and food.

In an intellectual climate—by now almost a reigning canon—that has tended to endorse psychoanalytic explanations for most human behaviors at the expense of more physiological ones, it is some-times useful to remember that man has a soma as well as a psyche and that the traffic between them is not all one-way. The fat woman's sexual readiness may be part and parcel of a generalized nervous-system syndrome in which appetite, once triggered—whether for food, sex, "love," housework, poetry, or anything else under the sun for that matter—may be much more difficult to turn off than it is in thin or normal women.

And men. For the explanation may be a psychobiological one. Research on the obese has shown them to be far more "persevera-tive" in their behavior than the nonobese. This means that once they have committed themselves to a given activity, no matter how dull or intrinsically unrewarding the activity itself may be, fat peo-ple will tend to persevere at it far more doggedly and for signifi-cantly longer periods of time than controls. This finding was a puz-zle to researchers studying the psychological correlatives of obesity; by no stretch of the psychoanalytic imagination can this particular twist of fat people's behavior be explained away as a defense mechanism, an infantilism, or a recognizable neurotic strategy. As a last resort, investigators in the field have therefore had to turn to a central-nervous-system rationale to explain the phenome-non; and here they seem to be on somewhat more convincing ground.

Arousal levels in human beings are known to vary widely; cues and sensory input from the environment that may catapult one person to his feet and halfway across the room may not even move his more phlegmatic brother to get up out of his armchair and see what is going on. In the classical layman's view of the characterology of the obese, the happy fat man is an imperturbable fellow, pacific and hard to arouse except when there is food on the table. This image of the phlegmatic fat man may have firm roots in the unedited phenomenology of everyday life, but it has a corollary that has received much less attention—to wit that, once aroused, the originally unexcitable fat person may be much more difficult to turn off than his initially more easily excited brothers and sisters. Inertia works both for starting and stopping, in other words.

In a series of experiments with obese subjects, psychologist Devandra Singh of the University of Texas reported that fat people seem to lack the ability to attain closure—or to put the psychological and behavioral brakes on—that other people have. "Situations that require the abandonment of one response and the development of a new response put obese subjects at a particular disadvantage," observes Singh. This difficulty extends from eating behavior—where the obese have a hard time knowing when to stop at the end of a calorically adequate or even superadequate feed— all the way to cognitive operations like doing arithmetic problems, forming and revising opinions, and forming and breaking daily habits.

Given the "perseverative" behavior of the obese in experimental situations, we can speculate that this kind of doggedness, when it is translated into emotional or appetitive situations, might very well turn into the erotic gluttony or unquenchability noted by William Shipman and L. Schwartz in the obese Chicago wives. An arousal system which is slow to fire but equally slow and difficult to damp down may be at the root of much biological and emotional "hunger" in the obese; and if this cerebral mechanism projects on the emotional level as a hunger for love and affection, it should not come as much of a surprise.

In evolutionary terms, meanwhile, the constant nagging state of affective arousal and hunger, with its concomitant and perhaps simultaneous hunger for food, affection, and erotic satiety or closure, might well produce a genetic master plan for a woman who is always more or less sexually ready and arousable (though probably, if we carry the hypothesis to its logical conclusion, correspondingly difficult to turn off). Just such a woman, however, will probably be more sexually receptive much more of the time than her less excitable sisters, and therefore—everything else being equal—will be more apt to conceive and bear children too, at least in eras and cultures where the means to ensure birth control do not come easily to hand.

Sexual readiness in the females of most primate and other mammalian species is usually seasonal and limited; the human female is unusual in her almost continuous sexual availability. Female orgasm is, as far as is certifiably known to date, a largely if not uniquely human phenomenon; man is, in Desmond Morris's words, "the sexiest primate alive." Human social organization and the hunter's peculiar biogram—his biologically programmed lifestyle—must thus long ago have combined to place a strong premium on any adaptive maneuver that would bind a woman over strongly to one particular man: The prolonged dependency of human children, and the inability of women in cold climates to provide for themselves and their children during their most fertile years without a man to hunt for them, must have fostered high dividends from the sexual capital of a woman's fidelity to the man who fathered her children and provisioned her (and them) with food. Under the circumstances anything that intensified her bond to the man in her life was bound to become an adaptive plus—and might thus get programmed into her and her daughters' genes. And while social reenforcement as represented by tradition, community pressure, and enlightened self-interest has probably always played a major part in keeping women monogamously contracted to the men whose children they bear, sexual loyalty is a potent reenforcer too—perhaps a stronger one for women than it is for men.

If we are right in postulating heightened sexual readiness in fat women, we are probably equally justified in going one step further and hypothesizing that fat women may thus also have a particular penchant for pair formation and for the monogamous impulse that has been one of the salient characteristics of our species since earliest recorded time. Research relevant to this issue is William Herbert Sheldon's classical assessment of physical types, and his remarks about the possible psychological and appetitive correlates of various kinds of body builds.

Fat, thin, or in-between, women are born endomorphs. Normal somatotypes for women, according to Sheldon, always lean more toward the endomorphic side of the spectrum than do those for men; this is in keeping with the higher fat content of women's bodies relative to men's—a distinction which starts in the womb. And endomorphy itself may dispose toward cuddliness in either sex: It is Sheldon's contention that, given their love of comfort, of company, of warmth and satiety, endomorphs may be the most sensual, and certainly the most affectionate and contact-oriented, of any of the three major body types. On the other hand, again according to Sheldon's logic, the long, thin, and "cerebrotonic" ectomorphs, whose linear builds and long arm, legs, and necks tend to give them more total skin surface and therefore probably more nerve endings per unit of weight than other somatotypes have, should prove to be the most sexually passionate and (in Sheldon's own words) "ecstatic" of the three major groups.

Are fat women sexier? Perhaps the last word on this subject will have to come from men; judgments about erotic desirability are, like most other matters of taste, largely in the eye of the beholder. Meanwhile, a strong presumptive case for the general desirability of fat women can be made from the ethnographic evidence: Of a total of twenty-six tribes from all over the inhabited globe who have ever been put on record as expressing any preference in the matter, only five preferred their women slender. To this meager roster should now be added, presumably, the vote of twentieth-century Americans and western Europeans; but even so, the naysayers are resoundingly outnumbered by those who like their women fat. And, from the distaff side of evolution, it should be added in all fairness that under the ecological and social circumstances in which fat women were evolving throughout Ice Age Europe, Russia, and Siberia, it paid a woman to be fat and to stay that way, at least throughout the span of her childbearing years. For this strategy was obviously a self-rewarding one wherever women were destined to be last served at a commissary run and provisioned by men. The evidence of the Venus figurines makes it clear that nature had got the message; and Ice Age man agreed. The resplendent endomorphy of the Venus figurines bears witness to an ecological lesson well learned.

But the same lesson may in the meantime have become inscribed all too indelibly on the genes of the hunters' daughters, an adaptive gamble that paid off handsomely in the hard times our species has been heir to but which, at 300 centuries' and several continents' remove, ended up creating far more problems than it solved. Modern woman in the Western world is still paying the price in terms of body fat—and, what is probably even more onerous in the long run, in terms of will power, self-approbation, and the almost chronic hunger of fat people in a thin culture.

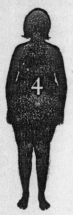

4 Pregnancy: Is Motherhood Fattening?

Testimonials and case histories record a familiar complaint, well known to readers of the dietmongers' ads: Mrs. X confides that as a bride she wore a size 7 wedding dress and her husband carried her across the threshold of their honeymoon cottage without missing a step. But after the first baby was born the idyl paled. Mrs. X's weight never got back down to normal and now, some two, three, or four babies later, the young mother weighs in at 197 pounds and suspects (rightly perhaps) that she has bartered away her waistline and her self-esteem for the sake of motherhood and multiparity.

In a culture that exalts leanness Mrs. X will do well to ask herself whether she has made a fair exchange in the process. Her written testimonial includes the token *mea culpa* of the chronically obese (I nibble all day; too much soda and potato chips watching TV at night) but her eyes in the diet-candy photograph tell a different story: In them we read the doubt—virtuously suppressed but still more or less ascendant—as to whether any normal human being can really go from 107 to 197 pounds in eight years' time, and from a size 7 dress to a size 20, just by drinking eight ounces of Pepsi every night after dinner and demolishing the odd box of Mallomars. And all this while leading a life that is as active as most in mid-century industrialized America—hoisting babies, chasing toddlers, going up and down stairs at least fifteen times a day and usually with a baby, a laundry basket, or a heavy vacuum cleaner in tow at that.

"My womb undoes me," cried Falstaff, unmanned by the womanish belly that precedes him wherever he goes; Mrs. X does have a serviceable womb in good working order inside that belly of hers, however, and she is right to have her doubts. Before marriage and motherhood she sat safely behind a typewriter all day and had doughnuts every morning at coffee break, but rarely gained a pound. What happened between then and now to throw up this wall of flesh between the real Mrs. X and her fat postnatal alter ego? Her obstetrician may be sympathetic and will probably put her on a calorie-restricted diet to stem the tide, but will have neither the heart nor the office hours available for lengthy clinical explanations. Briefly, what happened to Mrs. X is that she got pregnant, not just once but two, three, or four times, and carried two, three, or four healthy children to term. Pregnancy, as it happens, is for most women a lipogenic (that is, a fattening) state, and Mrs. X has multiplied her original risk factor by the number of times she has undergone it and the number of babies she has borne while doing so.

The importance of fat-tissue economy in successful childbearing has been largely overlooked in twentieth-century American obstetrical practice; American gynecologists were notorious not so long ago for trying to keep weight gain during pregnancy artificially low through diet and sometimes even medication—including hormone therapy. In fact it used to be normal prenatal medical procedure in this country to keep a woman's total weight gain during pregnancy at 15 to 18 pounds, or in other words hold it to just the amount of extra poundage that the baby, the amniotic fluid, the placenta, and the additional blood volume entailed in pregnancy could be predicted to tally by the end of the nine-month period. Thin mothers had smaller babies than fat ones did, and small babies were easier to deliver than large ones. The argument seemed unanswerable.

Recent research on two separate fronts, however, has cast serious doubts on the wisdom of this regime. In the first place, there is evidence that babies born to mothers who have been artificially (or otherwise) underfed during pregnancy may not have achieved optimal brain development at birth. In comparison to other parts of the body the brain has already achieved fully a quarter of its adult size at the moment of birth, and if there has been any lag in development before birth the deficiency may never be made up. If so, effects on I.Q. and other mental functions may prove to be irreversible.

Protein deficiencies in the diets of pregnant rats are known to reduce newborns' brain size by some 23 per cent; and while no such drastic reduction is found in human newborns, there is evidence that the size of the spleen, liver, and adrenal glands is significantly affected by the mother's protein intake during gestation. Thus while it may not be true, as the old wives maintained, that a pregnant woman is eating for two, it is also not true that she is only eating for one; the truth of the matter from a metabolic viewpoint clearly lies somewhere in between.

Under the circumstances, maternal nutrition is emerging as one of the most important of the many checks and balances that play their part in the genetic unfolding of the unborn child. The baby in the mother's womb is in her but not of her; complicated homeostatic relays between the mother's tissues, her immunological system, and her endocrine glands have been called into play at the moment of conception to back up the fragile hospitality that exists between them. Changes in one partner to the resulting symbiosis bring about automatic changes in the other; and the once widespread assumption that the growing fetus is a sort of genetic automaton, responding to inarguable commands from its own genes and chromosomes and none other, has had to be considerably revised.

The relationship between the mother's food intake during pregnancy and the developmental and nutritional status of the newborn baby at birth thus have increasingly come to be seen as two sides of the same coin; the developing fetus lives almost entirely on glucose, and the mother's ability to regulate the level of glucose in her blood during pregnancy is critical not only for her own well-being but for her baby's as well. Insulin is the hormone secreted by the pancreas in order to keep blood sugar at a constant level in the circulating blood, and during pregnancy the fetus is totally dependent on the mother's insulin supply, since the baby will not be able to manufacture any insulin of its own until at or slightly before birth.

But on closer analysis the simple linear relationship between these two neatly articulated systems is not as straightforward as it seems. For with the fetus growing at the predictable headlong velocity that it must in order to achieve a healthy size at term, insulin output in the mother will have to go up a little bit each day, just to keep in step with the ever-increasing demand for blood sugar from the developing fetus; and in the process of adjusting to this built-in escalation of nine months' duration, the mother's own blood-sugar-regulating machinery may well get out of hand. For this reason pregnancy itself has been called a "diabetogenic" state, meaning that the very fact of being pregnant increases a woman's chances of developing diabetes over and above that of the population at large.

The effect is one that is probably heightened by each succeeding pregnancy like the cumulative error built into a chronically over-heated economy by its own inflation rate. And if the response does not disappear soon after the baby is born, it is clearly one that is going to cause trouble for years to come; for from now on, every time the new mother eats a meal containing carbohydrates and sugar, and thus floods her circulating blood with glucose, the beta cells of her pancreas will respond on cue by secreting their by now predictable surplus of insulin. If the feedback circle involved in this operation is behaving "normally," her glucose level will obediently fall in response to the oversupply of insulin, and she will feel hungry well before her actual nutritional status gives her any really good reason to.

And if at this point, like Mrs. X in the diet-candy commercial, her will power is no stronger than that of the common run of humanity, she will respond to her hunger by eating, and to eating by getting fat—or perhaps even fatter than the rest of us would do under the same set of circumstances, since insulin itself seems to increase the permeability of cell membrane to glucose and other nutritive molecules. As of this moment, then, the young mother we have conjured up will, with Mrs. X, be well on her way to joining the ranks of the fat getting fatter—unless she is very careful about her diet for many years to come.

Weight gain in pregnancy is not a foregone conclusion and varies widely in different parts of the world and in different cultures. F. Hytten and E. Leitch reviewed studies of the phenomenon on a world-wide basis and found that what was considered normal weight gain in various countries (that is, changes from prepregnant weight which eventually resulted in full-term normal infants born alive) ranged all the way from zero, or even a slight net weight loss, to a total gain of about 50 pounds. After sifting their data for adequacy of method and measurement, the authors concluded that on an over-all, world-wide basis, the average weight gain from the beginning of the first trimester until the end of pregnancy was on the order of 27.5 pounds.

A caution is in order here: Most of the data finally included in Hytten and Leitch's tabulations were from countries which keep the most trustworthy health statistics in the first place; but this fact probably introduces a bias of its own. For it is in the nature of trustworthy statistics to emanate from the more industrialized and technologically advanced countries of the world, and at this moment in history most of these countries are clustered in the Northern Hemisphere, where babies and their parents are considerably larger than a random world-wide human sample would be. Weight gain in pregnancy is therefore probably higher in such countries too, a factor that should of course be taken into account in considering these norms and drawing conclusions from them.

The whole issue of weight gain in pregnancy obviously has cultural as well as biological implications. Clearly, women whose normal life-styles entail a bare minimum of physical effort and a comfortable surfeit of good food will tend to gain more weight than women who go on working strenuously and eating stintingly up until shortly before the moment of giving birth. But no matter what ethnic or geographical group a woman hails from, or what subsistence activity she practices (whether it is standard day-in, day-out housework, U.S. suburban style; slash-and-burn Melanesian yam horticulture; or birch-twig-broom street cleaning à la Russe), women all over the world seem to be specifically designed to gain at least a modicum of extra weight during pregnancy, no matter how fat or thin they may have been to begin with.

The reason for this panhuman, cross-cultural phenomenon is probably to make allowances for a certain indispensable caloric reserve or even surplus against the hour of childbirth, when the mother is no longer going to be capable of carrying on business as usual, and will have to hand over her normal food collecting and food processing duties to someone else in the community until she gets back on her feet. Evolution has apparently not left the provisioning of the mother and the newborn baby during this period wholly at the mercy of the economic and emotional contract between the new mother and the father of her child (who may be absent, on the outs with her, or even conceivably dead at the time the baby is born). Fortunately for the new mother and for the future of the species as a whole, a certain margin of safety has been built into the system here in the form of the mother's own adipose tissue reserves. Nature has arranged matters so that, even without another human being to provision her, the mother and her newborn child can survive the lying-in period, at least for a while, on the mother's own subcutaneous food reserves alone.

This biological fail-safe factor is apparently world-wide. Indian women working side by side with men on tea plantations (women who are, incidentally, much smaller and more delicately built than their European counterparts, and whose babies are therefore not surprisingly among those with the lowest birth weights in the world) gain a modicum of weight during pregnancy over and above the amount that can be accounted for just by the products of conception alone; and they manage to do so without any change from their prepregnancy diet or any measurable reduction in their daily physical workloads, which may be arduous. The same thing is true for women in Gambian villages, where the backbreaking work involved in planting, cultivating, harvesting, and transporting the rice and millet that form the mainstay of the diet of both sexes is consensually defined as women's work. In Gambia pregnancy does not exempt a woman from the day's work, and babies are often born in the rice fields, at several hours' hot and humid march from home. In both these cases weight gains are considerably less than the 27.5 pounds' average postulated by Hytten and Leitch, but they are still on the order of 12 to 15 pounds and, in terms of the size of the women (and their babies) in both the Indian and the Gambian groups, they represent an impressive increase of total body weight, seemingly conjured up out of the nutritional thin air of the nonaffluent postcolonial tropics.

The lesson is obvious: Contrary to prevalent medical formularies, it pays a woman to have some flesh on her bones if she wants to get pregnant in the first place and bear a baby to term in the second. Recent research suggests that there may even have to be a certain critical minimum of fat tissue on deposit to the cells before adolescent girls can start to menstruate and, by extension of course, to conceive and bear children too. All over the world, girls of every ethnic group and culture show a sudden weight spurt at puberty: Fully half of this gain consists of subcutaneous fat. Rose Frisch and R. Revelle theorize that the weight gain in girls at or just before puberty may represent the need to bring this adipose tissue reserve up to some crucial level in order to turn on the various interlocking hormonal systems that must all be in good working order before menstruation can begin. (While it is true that boys have the same adolescent growth spurt as girls, in boys most of the newly added tissue deposited during this period is made up of muscle and bone; in girls much more of the added tissue is deposited in the form of fat. Before puberty girls have 10 to 15 per cent more fat than boys do; but by the end of adolescence this differential has increased to the point at which they have twice as much fat as boys.

The opposite side of this coin is the case of *anorexia nervosa*, a psychosomatic disorder seen mostly in adolescent females who, although vastly underweight, see themselves as fat; the disease is heralded by—and sometimes masquerades as—excessive "dieting." Here the close relationship between fat reserves and reproductive readiness shows up in an inversion of the process, like a photographic negative, confirming the well-documented observation that when adolescent girls (or sexually mature women for that matter too) lose substantial amounts of weight, menstruation may be one of the first casualties of the change in weight, returning only years later when weight is back up to a certain minimum. Psychiatric theory holds that *anorexia nervosa* constitutes a sort of somatic refusal of sexual maturation and motherhood; but in cases of simple environmentally caused starvation and malnutrition the hormonal effect is exactly the same. Commentators like Frisch, Revelle, and J. MacArthur conclude that a minimum reserve of fat tissue is one of the first anatomical prerequisites for proper functioning of women's reproductive systems. Without it ovulation cannot go forward and conception cannot take place.

While individual weight gains at puberty can vary tremendously, most girls tend to gain an average of 16 kilos (35.2 pounds) of stored fat between the ages of nine and fifteen; Frisch and Mac-Arthur estimate that the 144,000 calories tied up in a weight gain of this magnitude are roughly what would be needed to sustain a successful pregnancy and three months of postpartum breast feeding without serious energy drain on the mother, her unborn fetus, and—of necessity—the newborn baby at the breast. If this arithmetic is correct, the additional fat stored in the normal girl's body over and against that of boys at puberty might represent a sort of built-in "granary" programmed into the mother's physique by nature so as to ensure the species' continuity even in the face of severe short-term famine, social isolation, or abandonment. The flip side of this equation is that, when the food supply is too stringent to fatten up that year's tally of future mothers, the girls stay thin and their wombs stay empty. Something approximating direct evidence for the rightness of this theory exists in provable form in recent statistics from Europe: In the Dutch famine of 1944 the birthrate fell to roughly half its previous level, and many women stopped menstruating altogether until the end of the war.

The arrangement is one that makes excellent ecological sense: People who live in nutritionally marginal areas would probably be even harder pressed than they already are if it were not for some such built-in and more or less self-regulating restraint on reproduction when times are bad. Twentieth-century technology and relief measures in the form of food drops and emergency missions may alter this ecological control process a little, but probably not for long; and men's predilection for fat women in certain cultures may date from the observation that a woman with a little padding around her hips has a better chance of conceiving and bringing live children into the world than one without. But even without the benefits of modern science and computer modeling, it must have seemed clear in such cultures once upon a time that, at a certain point in body-fat economy, an underfed woman will simply stop reproducing. At this point the tribal or social group whose generative future is vested in her body will have to choose between extinction, major technological innovation, or, as a last resort, simply pulling up stakes and moving to—literally—greener pastures, in hopes of fattening up the tribe—and especially its women.

Starvation is the mother of invention, and contingencies of this sort may have been among the critical cues for the great human migrations of prehistory, on the one hand, and for major technological breakthroughs on the other. Just such a scenario has been posited, for example, for the enormous technological upheavals and population displacements of the so-called Neolithic Revolution, when man switched from a predominantly hunting economy to a predominantly farming one in Southeast Asia, the Middle East, and southern Europe. At the beginning of this far-reaching ecological crisis in human history, the melting glaciers and warming climates of Europe, Russia, and Asia led to extinctions of enormous herds of cold-adapted game animals on which the human hunters who were among our immediate ancestors in the Northern Hemisphere had been almost totally dependent for food, clothing, and the raw materials for certain indispensable tools.

To develop new food resources Mesolithic hunter-gatherers of the Northern Hemisphere had to turn to agriculture, and in the process a revolutionary new way of life for the entire species was not long in following. With this new subsistence invention, food could now be saved and stored up against lean times. Granaries were invented; food surpluses accumulated. Women began to get pregnant more dependably and to reproduce at shorter and shorter intervals, and one of the first population explosions in human history was on. The total human population at the height of the Ice Age stood at about 3,000,000 souls, scattered across three and possibly four continents; by the end of the Neolithic Age and the agricultural revolution it had burgeoned by a factor of ten.

Presumably, ecological feedback mechanisms like the one outlined here between fertility and the prevailing food supply do not happen by some sort of metabiological magic, but are set in motion by simple hormonal or humoral triggers in the fertile woman's blood. Nobody knows what they are, but an educated guess would be that there is some kind of early-warning system during which the woman's nervous system registers inadequate levels of essential nutrients in her circulating blood, and responds by turning production of certain vital hormones down below the bare minimum needed to start, orchestrate, and carry out the various endocrine relays involved in ovulation and menstruation. Whatever the process is, it appears (fortunately) to be a reversible one. In other words, when the woman's diet improves and the crucial level of nutrients rises in her blood again, the same monitoring system that went into action in the first instance to turn ovulation off will now register this new information and respond to it by turning hormone production back up again in all the appropriate organs. The stage is now set for conception to take place and for the human demographic curve to continue its normal—and by now somewhat frightening—upward curve.

By the end of puberty, women's considerable handicap in the anti-adipose tissue marathon has been set for life; and while the role of the female sex hormones in weight gain has never been clearly understood, there is good reason to suspect that they must play a major part in the process. How they do so is not certain. Estrogen by itself seems on balance to have a somewhat muddled effect on weight gain and loss; in some cases estrogen therapy has been used to cure obesity, while in others it has been suspected of causing it. A synthetic estrogen compound, diethylstilbestrol, was until quite recently routinely added to beef cattle feed in order to fatten the animals up, speed tissue growth, and get them to market well ahead of their own normal developmental schedule. Estrogen seems to have an affinity for the fat cells in certain tissues and certain parts of the body. Fat breasts represent localized sites of high estrogen receptivity (quite apart from the receptivity to estrogen of the mammary gland itself); so do the buttocks and hips. Estrogen acting in tandem with insulin, on the other hand, is known to have an even more potent effect on fat deposition than estrogen alone. It is probably this powerful combination that is at the root of the pregnant woman's difficulties with unwanted weight gain. As pregnancy progresses so does estrogen production; and this, added to the normal day-by-day escalation of insulin supply as it rises to keep abreast of fetal blood-sugar demand, may be all that is needed to tip the balance in favor of outright obesity.

But if not, there is always progesterone to tilt the scales. Progesterone, which is, like estrogen, secreted generously throughout pregnancy but especially so toward term, has been experimentally implicated in weight gain (at least in rats), and it is progesterone that is credited with the monthly weight gain that some women are troubled by toward the end of their menstrual cycles too. Progesterone levels in the nonpregnant woman are low until about the midpoint of the cycle, at which time ovulation takes place, an egg is released by the ovaries, and progesterone—whose function it is to prepare the uterus for implantation by the fertilized egg—rises dramatically. From a biochemical viewpoint, progesterone seems to have a very similar molecular structure to the androgens, and like these male hormones may stimulate the building of muscle, bone, and organ tissue too. The voracious appetites that some women develop during pregnancy or in the last week before menstruation may reflect this androgenlike effect of progesterone. (Experiments with rats show that the response in adipose tissue is not a specific one but works on and through many different body systems at once. Animals given supplementary progesterone tend to drink and eat more, excrete less water from their tissues, move less often than usual, and navigate more ponderously when they do so.)

Taken together, the three major hormonal triggers to overweight (insulin, estrogen, and progesterone) are probably a normal hazard of any pregnancy; but their cumulative effect over the course of several pregnancies may be ruinous for women with a special susceptibility to them. After two, three, or four babies, such a woman's metabolic and endocrine machinery will have mastered the unhappy capitalism of obesity, learning to make much out of little in the process. Too much: For it is an article of faith of our time and culture that a woman cannot be either too rich or too thin; and unless women with this kind of adipose tissue economy—the Mrs. X's of the Western world—learn to live on judiciously restricted diets for the rest of their childbearing years, they may unhappily keep on gaining unearned caloric income from very little basic adipose tissue capital for the better part of their adult lives.

Other women, with other endocrine economies, will fare better. But until we have better ways of measuring the interplay between all the factors involved in the process, guesses about individual vulnerability and risk factors will have to remain post hoc, and by then it may be too late to interrupt the vicious cycle and straighten it all back out. In the meantime, a fair guess might be that basal metabolism must play some significant part in the proceedings, and a seemingly favorable factor for women about to have babies is that basal metabolism normally increases during pregnancy by a factor of about 5 per cent—which should be all to the good. On closer inspection, though, this advantage turns out to be somewhat equivocal. In the first place, basal metabolism in pregnancy increases least in women whose metabolic rates were lowest to begin with. And in the second place, the relationship between fat tissue, which is the chief repository of energy reserves in the body, and muscle, which is one of the chief consumers of these stores, is one that varies characteristically as between men and women—with the variation being of course largely in favor of men.

Men have proportionately more muscle and other lean tissue than women do, and their higher basal metabolic rates are directly related to the need to keep this large muscle component well supplied with the oxygen it needs to carry on its work. Fat tissue, on the other hand, needs much less oxygen to fuel it, and is altogether metabolically less active than lean tissue is in the first place—a fact that is rather pointedly illustrated by the finding that adipose tissue has a lower specific temperature set point than muscle, bone, and organ tissues do.

(An interesting footnote to this difference is the fact that men and women seem to react differentially to heat and cold. Although body temperatures for both sexes are normally about the same, the common observation that men seem to be less heat tolerant than women, and women less cold tolerant than men, may have its origins in this significant difference between fat and muscle in the two sexes. The higher basal metabolic rate of men generates more internal body heat than the low metabolic rates of women do, and makes them feel hot at ambient temperatures at which women feel comfortable or even a little cold. Once the battle of the thermostat has been joined it becomes difficult to settle the issue without resort to argument; but the fact of the matter is that the two sexes simply do not bring the same sensory equipment into a cold room. Women's thicker layers of subcutaneous fat insulate their internal organs handily, but have the paradoxical effect of also insulating their skin surfaces from the original, internal source of body heat; and while heat perception is probably monitored directly in the brain, cold is sensed first in the skin. Women therefore feel cold first, worse, and longer than men do, even though both sexes may register an identical 98.6° on identical thermometers in the same room at the same hour or even moment of the day.)

Men's high ratios of muscle to fat are probably always in their favor to some extent in the matter of weight control, while women's high fat-to-muscle ratio exerts a built-in throttle on the rate at which a woman can mobilize her own fat reserves even during pregnancy, when metabolic rates normally increase. Fat tissue demands and gets less oxygen than lean tissue does and this has a dampening effect on all basic body chemistry as well.

The difference in lean and adipose tissue that characterizes male-female differences in body build was probably evolutionarily a long time in the making; even so there is some reason to believe that it may not be totally impervious to change. If so, the deus ex machina may turn out to be cultural. Longitudinal studies of average weights for men and women have begun to reflect an interesting reversal of a historically venerable pattern; American women's average weights were three to four pounds lower in 1964, for example, than they had been thirty years earlier; while men's average weights increased by roughly the same amounts. Since both sexes are getting taller, height can be ruled out as a determining factor in the change. What seems to be happening is that a gradual change in the activity patterns of the two sexes has been taking place, at least in the predominantly urban population from which these statistics were culled. In other words, women have been getting more active (and perhaps more diet conscious) in the last three decades, and men less so.

The number of labor-saving devices that have proliferated since the end of the Second World War has probably cut less deeply into the energy output of middle-class women, paradoxically, than into that of middle-class men; it still takes a person (usually a woman) to push a vacuum cleaner, "man" a floor polisher, and carry laundry loads back and forth from the hamper in the bathroom upstairs to the washing machine in the cellar two flights down. And if this work takes the place of services that in many middle-class houses were once routinely performed by maids or laundresses, the woman who has fallen heir to the machines is going to be subject to a net caloric and energy deficit in the long run. In research on women's work roles, sociologist Ann Oakley found that the number of hours women spent on housework in the urban United States went from 51 per week in 1929 to 77 per week in 1971, in spite of (or perhaps even because of) the proliferation of "work-saving" devices that became available in the interim.

On the other hand, in households where much of the heaviest

women's work may well once have been done by servants, men's abdication to the machine has been much more radical than women's has. Men no longer shovel coal every winter morning to keep a furnace going, and the advent of power mowers, snow blowers, power saws and drills has meant a total energy increment to middle-class men who once had to perform these calorically very costly jobs by hand. In the context of middle-class urban and suburban culture, at least, the technological revolution has therefore tended to raise the physical activity levels of women, while lowering the physical activity levels of men; and the statistics cited here may reflect this basic biosocial shift toward a creeping sedentariness among males.

With this shift in the time-honored pattern of sex role activities, North Americans and Europeans have made a major departure from their Ice Age beginnings as hunters with a life-style that favored fatness (and sedentariness) in women, and leanness (and hyperactivity) in men. The roles are now equalized, if not reversed; it is men who sit indoors all day in the environmentally homogenized and physically undemanding climates of temperature-controlled offices and factories, while women perform the more physically strenuous work of keeping house and raising children.

Or do so, that is, until they get pregnant and their relatives and obstetricians tell them to "slow down." Visibly pregnant women are probably the last people in America for whom a man (or even another woman, for that matter) will still give up a seat on a bus or a forward place in line. For it is one of the protocols of the Western subculture surrounding pregnancy that women in advanced stages of gestation should stay off their feet; and what insulin, estrogen, and progesterone acting singly or together could not accomplish by themselves, folk wisdom may handily end up enforcing anyway. Admonished to take a load off her feet and spine, the pregnant woman may therefore, especially during the last three months before she gives birth, end up leading as sedentary a life as the average male white-collar worker has come to do—with predictable results for her figure and for the profit pictures of some of the best-selling nostrums of the American diet industry.

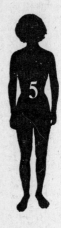

5 Somatotype: Butchers, Bakers, and Harvard Men

William Herbert Sheldon's well-known typology of body build was published in 1940 and minted three useful new words for the language of body size and shape: Sheldon believed that people's physiques could be classified as either predominantly endomorphic (fleshy, light-boned, and well-padded), mesomorphic (muscular, broad-shouldered, and skeletally sturdy), or ectomorphic (long-legged, skeletally fragile, and linear), according to how large a dose of each of these three basic somatic factors were present in the individual's general physical make-up.

Working from nude photographs of a total sample of 4,000 male college undergraduates, Sheldon and his associates assigned a value of 1 to 7 for each of these three components to every subject in their sample. Theoretically it should not have been beyond the realm of possibility for a person to have a high reading in all three factors: An individual could conceivably be, that is, very fleshy, very stocky and muscular, and very long-necked and leggy all at once. The beauty of Sheldon's work, however, was its demonstration that this situation in fact hardly ever arose. The people in Sheldon's sample tended on the whole to be higher in one of the three components, or at the most two; rarely if ever did they achieve equally high ratings for all three. The message of such research is, meanwhile, that human beings come in all shapes and sizes, and that if we were not being so constantly constrained to bring ourselves into line with "the norm" by diet, exercise, and the optical illusions created by well-cut clothes, it would not be as burning an issue as it is to know exactly what that norm may happen to be at any given moment in time and space and cultural concordat.

Even the ancestral prototype is, at the moment, in question. It is an axiom of Darwinian theory that evolution is irreversible; a lucky adaptation, once it is knit into the warp of a new species' master plan, can never be unraveled from its taxonomic woof. But although species and individual organisms can never return to the ancestral status quo, neither can they escape from it; and the systematics of human descent continue to define us as a species in terms of our nonhuman and our not-quite-human ancestors. We are bigger than Australopithecus, leggier than Neanderthal, brainier than *Homo erectus*. There may even be missing links still undiscovered, buried deep in the detritus of landslides and flood plains and glacial moraines, or out of sight underwater along the continental shelves of Europe, Asia, and Africa, waiting to be dug up. It is in the meantime a sobering realization that we know more about the evolution of the horse, taxon for taxon, than we do about the evolution of our own forebears.

Under the circumstances it takes a brave spirit to reconstruct a family tree and a morphology for *Homo sapiens:* The data are not all in, and it goes without saying that it is always unwise to construct a whole taxonomy on the basis of a single and possibly unique specimen. Who knows, for example, whether the sole skeletal survivors of Swanscombe or Steinheim were fair type specimens for their groups as a whole? Anthropologists still live under the shadow of Piltdown Man—a sophisticated forgery whose anthropoid jaw and human cranium once came close to leading a whole generation of paleo-osteologists and other specialists down the garden path of erroneous scientific ascription. Consider for a moment the man on the street, that classificatory and ethical abstraction: Would we care to pick one of him at random and base our description of the whole species on that one particular face and body alone?

And yet, you have to begin somewhere; a sample of one is better than no sample at all, and for some of our protohuman ancestors we can do considerably better than that. Australopithecus bred true for several millions of years; so did *Homo erectus*. Neanderthal man did not fare quite so well in terms of generations but left recognizable bones behind him over a wide-enough range in space and a narrow-enough span in time to make himself useful to paleontologists in a general way. Meanwhile the urge to classify goes on. *Homo sapiens* himself is an inveterate collector, a cataloguer of things, creatures, and events—including himself and such of his ancestors whose bones have endured long enough to be tabled and counted.

As far as anyone knows to date, the species arose in Africa, an offshoot of the primate family tree. Since the bloodlines of man's immediate hominid ancestors are still up for scholarly certification, it seems pointless to offer any interim taxonomical report at this time. One of the first recognizably manlike creatures, meanwhile, for whom a respectable fossil record has actually been established is the small upright ape Australopithecus, or "southern ape," whose brain capacity was only about one third to one half as big as modern man's, but who had already clearly gotten up onto his hind feet to walk, thus freeing his hands for carrying, throwing, tool making, and other more or less typically human pursuits. If this creature was in fact an ape, he was like no ape this generation of zoologists has ever seen or heard of.

From the viewpoint of body shape and size, the adult Australopith (as he is sometimes called), who weighed some 60 pounds and stood about four feet high, represents a comparatively delicately built body type: The Pygmies of the African rain forests, for example, stand only slightly taller than these averages (four feet eight) but weigh considerably more (96 pounds). In terms of general body dimensions, if current reconstructions are not too far from the mark, Australopithecus was probably about the same size and shape as a normal nine- or ten-year-old child of our own species, and may have had roughly the same body proportions too.

At the risk of making an anatomical mountain out of a taxonomic molehill, it can probably be said that modern man's first progenitor on the hominid family tree was a smaller and more delicately built version of the subequatorial Pygmies of our own era. And although

Australopithecus himself may be about to cede pride of place in the human pedigree to a more advanced type of fossil man (the much discussed hominid recently discovered by Leakey, about whom a great deal of learned sound and fury has been raised in academic circles within the last few years) this generalization still holds; for although his head was slightly larger than the classical Australopithecus, Leakey's candidate had roughly the same body proportions as his better-known and more widely studied contemporary. Whichever of these two creatures is finally assigned primogeniture and is definitely established as the last of the missing links between man and ape, it is therefore probably safe to say that he was less massive and weighty than any ethnic or geographic version of *Homo sapiens* around today. In keeping with our tropical beginnings (mean annual temperatures 5,000,000 years ago probably stood some 20° F. higher in Africa and elsewhere than they do today) the ancestral species was a comparative lightweight and, except for low leg-to-torso ratios, a moderate "ectomorph" in Sheldon's terms.

Around 1,500,000 years ago or thereabouts, when Australopithecus and his compatriot, *Homo habilis,* had been established in Africa for some time, sudden climatic changes began to occur the length and breadth of the planet, with dramatic consequences for many species—including presumably our own. Temperatures began to oscillate widely between the equable tropical norms to which our apelike ancestors were primarily adapted and temperate or even downright frigid annual means, to which they certainly were not. At one extreme swing of this climatic pendulum the snow line on Mt. Kenya stood some 5,000 feet lower than it does today. Closer to sea level, intermittent cool, wet weather later breathed life into the desert. The Sahara bloomed, and what had once been an impassable no man's land to the north of Australopith's home range became a momentarily fruitful and navigable terrain.

The ancestral genus may have chosen this moment in prehistory to migrate north, mile by thoughtless mile. It was in all probability a perfectly unconscious decision. Roaming bands of hunter-gatherers nowadays exploit territories of about a 6- to 8-mile radius, and randomize the direction of the day's hunt by simple cultural rituals, like throwing dice or reading an animal's entrails for omens; and our prehuman ancestors may have done the same. With much of the water in the oceans being gradually siphoned off into the ice sheets which were beginning to spawn the great glaciers of the last Ice Age, previously submerged continental shelves were suddenly above water, and land bridges to Europe emerged out of the waters of the Bosporus, opening up a whole new continent to the creature working his piecemeal way north through history. By 400,000 years ago some form of man (probably *Homo erectus*) had certainly made his way into what is now Hungary; and by 150,000 years later his offspring were firmly ensconced in Europe at least as far north as the Thames River valley in England. At the time that Swanscombe man made camp on the shores of the Thames not far from present-day London, elephants and rhinoceroses shared his woodland habitat.

This European version of our own ancestors had a brain case and cranial capacity almost on a par with that of modern man, but his face may have been a bit more primitive. Both males and females were around five feet tall, with long, straight legs, though perhaps somewhat less useful hands than we have now. Massive neck muscles supported a very thick-boned skull; in all probability *Homo erectus* was not only bigger than Australopithecus but chunkier and more muscular than his hominid precursor had been.

But the climate under which *Homo erectus* established himself in Europe proved to be short-lived; the great Scandinavian glacier was on the advance, and the resulting glaciation marked the birth of a new and enigmatic subspecies of man in Europe: the famous and still mysterious Neanderthal man, a cousin or poor relation of to-day's European populations, and very possibly one whose genes are still viable and active by replicating themselves in our own gene pools today.

Neanderthal is the cartoon cave man of secular iconography: a brutish specimen and figure of prehistoric fun. Although his brain capacity was as big as or bigger than that of modern man, the shape of his skull and his chinless and low-browed face gave him the look of a throwback to his early Australopithecine forebears. He was, climate and opportunity permitting, a meat eater. Evidence of ritual burials he practiced, and of well-organized ambushes of large herd animals he masterminded, leave no doubt that Neanderthal was at least as intelligent as his immediate precursors in the human line. He had to be. Isolated between the Scandinavian glacier to the north and the Swiss glacier to the south, classical Neanderthal's life in Europe had become an increasingly difficult one. Morphologically, Neanderthal man in Europe was a mesomorph. He stood slightly over five feet tall with a long, deep-chested torso and relatively short arms and legs. The curvature of his long bones suggests a species-wide susceptibility to rickets, hinting that Neanderthal may have evolved in a climate for which, having brunet hair, he was pelagially ill prepared to get enough Vitamin D from the sparse sunlight available to him in cloudy, glacial Europe. His hands and feet were short, but his torso and the forebones of his arms and legs were heavily muscled: In spite of his stature Neanderthal must have been a redoubtable hunter, hauler, hurler, and woodsman. By analogy with circumpolar peoples living today, it seems safe to suppose that he lived in small family groups or compounds, holed up for the long winter in caves or dugouts with little privacy and not much in the way of formal civic constraints. So, although Neanderthal's burliness of build suggests the character and reflexes of a fighter and a brawler, ecological signs and portents favor an alternative reading: This strong and possibly silent hunter (Neanderthal's language capabilities have been the subject of much scholarly debate) buried his dead with affection and care, and learned the humanizing lessons of communal living at close hand.

Neanderthal "disappears" from the European fossil record around 35,000 years ago, and his geographical range is pre-empted at this time by a race of human beings virtually indistinguishable from modern man. This sudden (and, as such things go, unprecedented) transition from one physical type to a very different one is the major overriding mystery of man's prehistory on the European subcontinent. No drastic or obvious shift in ecological circumstances can be called to account for it; for while it is true that there was a temporary improvement of climate around 38,000 years ago, Neanderthal had survived and prospered in other interglacial periods before this one, and even turned the adaptive pressures during them to good account. There was meanwhile no sudden or even very noticeable shift in the prevailing fauna: The reindeer and wild horses Neanderthal had always hunted were still widespread, and there is no evidence of any sudden virulent pandemic disease at large in Europe. In fact, life in the small and isolated nomadic bands of Ice Age Europe make it highly unlikely that any epidemic of major proportions could ever have gotten a serious toehold on more than one or two local groups at a time: Epidemics need crowds and migrants to batten on, and Paleolithic Europe was simply too sparsely populated to sustain a serious plague.

Nevertheless, and for whatever reason, a new hominid variant and a new physical type was now abroad in Europe and the Middle East. This creature was very close to the preferred northern European ideal of the present day, being tall, long-legged, and rather rugged in the face: Cro-Magnon man is so skeletally similar to Scots and Scandinavians of the present time that it has been suggested that these modern peoples may well be the ethnic inheritors of a Cro-Magnon stock who once lived much farther south in Europe and who may have moved north during the Mesolithic era (*ca.* 9000 to 3000 B.C.), following the great herds of reindeer which had already inspired so many of the famous cave paintings and bone carvings of Spain, France, and Russia. Though probably somewhat taller and larger than the peoples who inherited his somatotype, Cro-Magnon man was virtually indistinguishable from resident Europeans living around the edges of the North Sea today. He was, in Sheldon's scheme, a mesomorphic ectomorph; and, if we can accept the artistic record in evidence, his gene pool included a fair number of genes for endomorphy too, at least in women: The Venus figurines bear witness to this variation in body build.

"Evolution," writes Jacques Monod, "seems always to be fulfilling a design, to be carrying out a 'project': that of perpetrating and amplifying some ancestral dream."

In the case of our own species, if there is such a dream it is a picaresque one: For every adventurer who climbed the mountain because it was there, there must be at least another hundred or so who climbed it to see what was on the other side.

The creature who struck out northward across the Sahara a million years or so ago was in many ways not the same as the one who finally arrived and set up camp on the banks of the Thames some 750,000 years later. During this time man's habitat was getting progressively colder, and like other animals that crossed the Anatolian highlands into Europe with him at the beginning of the Günz glaciation, man was getting larger in response to changing climate, food supply, and other ecological imponderables. But the increase in relative brain size outpaced the growth of other body organs. Climate, novelty, and perhaps simple curiosity had conspired to keep this evolving species on its toes. If the ancestral African model had resembled a sort of adult nine-year-old, 500,000 years later the nine-year-old had come of morphological age. Australopithecus had grown up. The species no longer lived, looked, or behaved as it had earlier.

Speciation tends to proceed centripetally—creatures are most like themselves at the center of their original habitat and least so at the perimeters of the home range. Out at the edges of a territory the weather is not what it was in the homeland, flora and fauna are unfamiliar, and individuals who cannot adapt to new ways are weeded out of the local gene pool in childhood or adolescence. If Australopithecus was a small-scale ectomorph, Neanderthal was clearly a classical mesomorph; and Cro-Magnon's gene pool included its fair share of genes for endomorphy, if we can believe the evidence of the Venus figurines—although the standard model was probably a rather mesomorphic ectomorph, tall, broad-shouldered, and long in the leg. The plasticity of human size and shape has thus clearly been one of the most useful adaptive devices in the anatomical history of the hominids from their very earliest beginnings.

But speciation takes place in time as well as space, and by the time the ancestors of modern man were firmly established in Europe, Southeast Asia, and China, Australopithecus himself was already extinct as a species; the men of the last glaciation belonged to a new species, *Homo erectus,* and those who drove the Neanderthalers out of Europe (or perhaps simply married them to death) were another species altogether: *Homo sapiens.* The new version is indistinguishable on morphological and artifactual grounds from man as we know him today. Africa, repopulated from the north by *Homo sapiens,* buried its prehuman past under the detritus of new civilizations spreading southward from the Mediterranean littoral; Africans of today and of the last million or so years bear no resemblance to the earlier hominid generations from which we are all ultimately no doubt descended. There is thus only one species of man alive today, but the versatility and plasticity of this single taxon is almost as impressive as the versatility of numbers themselves. Men come in all colors, shapes, and sizes, and Sheldon's taxonomy of body types is only the latest in a long series of classificatory efforts that has tried to pin down the details and sort people into types by body morphology, physique, and temperament.

Somatic typecasting of this sort—somatotyping, in Sheldon's terminology—is at least as old as Hippocrates, whose "phthisic" and "apoplectic" prototypes described two basic variants of human physique in ancient Greece—the first linear and vertical, the second broad and horizontal. Ernst Kretschmer, a nineteenth-century psychiatrist, drew the same general distinction, dividing the population up into "pyknics" on the one hand and "asthenics" on the other, with a third category, "athletics" falling somewhere in between.

As a general rule, the question of body type has almost always gone hand in hand with notions of personality theory of one sort or another; until Freud, the idea that our characters are inseparable from our physiques, and that our psychological temperaments must have something fundamental to do with our physical habitus, was more or less taken for granted by all concerned. The jolly fat man, the pugnacious muscleman, and the skinny aesthete have been stock characters of Western literature for centuries. Sancho Panza's belly reveals his character, and Don Quixote's cadaverousness has cultural resonances of a totally different sort. Falstaff is only half true to his own stereotype as a greedy sensualist; Shakespeare was immune to stereotypes and understood, well in advance of his times and the medical science of his age, that the "grave gapes thrice wider" for fat people than for thin ones, or that sighing and grief can blow people up like bladders. Falstaff comes onstage as the usual happy sensualist, the jolly fat man; but the author and Prince Hal knew better; they have seen the depression under the glad-handing and the apartness under the bonhomie.

But Shakespeare's was a voice in the wilderness; the notion that physique mandated personality went on and on. P. Naccarati early in this century found a low but persistently significant correlation between intelligence and linearity of body build; and ectomorphs, said Sheldon, are "cerebrotonic"—that is, nervous and brainy. Pound for pound, more of the ectomorph is composed of nervous-system tissue; ectomorphs are therefore dominated by their nerves and heads. The situation contains the germs of its own fragility: Kretschmer had already established that the majority of his schizophrenic patients were asthenic (lean and long-legged), while a majority of his manic-depressive patients were pyknic (short and round).

Interestingly enough, this distinction has stood the test of time, replication, and sophisticated statistical analysis. Whatever biochemical magic is at work behind the somatic scenes to make the Don Quixotes of this world long and skinny, the Sancho Panzas short and fat, seems at the same time to predispose them toward one or another of the basic ways that man has of going mad—if and when that misfortune arises; and it was Sheldon himself who pointed out that paranoids tend to be mesomorphs more often than ectomorphs or endomorphs.

Freudian and other "environmentalists" can be counted on to recoil from the implications of this kind of analysis, but on closer inspection it may seem that they have no very good reason to. A strictly environmentalist argument can be made for the case that fat cuddly children grow up in different emotional environments than nervous bony ones do; that mothers and nurses react differently to babies who love their food than to those who pick at it; and that brawny baby mesomorphs can be a trial to sedentary mothers or a delight to sporty ones. It needs no great stretch of the imagination to conjure up the psychological consequences of such interpersonal transactions on young children whose personalities are still in the process of being forged. Every man should be allowed to go to heaven in his own way, says the proverb; by the same token we may all be preassigned our unique ways of going mad, or of being sad and glad and bad. If that way turns out to owe much to our basic temperaments, only the most orthodox of environmentalists will be surprised.

Life crises strike differently at the fat and short than they do at the long and thin. It is one thing to be fair, fat, and forty, another thing to be svelte and "of a certain age." Mesomorphs (and endomorphs) grow up early and fast; their long bones may have stopped growing by the age of fourteen or sixteen (earlier for girls, later for boys), and their secondary sex characteristics may begin to show up while they are still in grammar school. Depending on the value the culture they are growing up in decides to place on a hairy chest or a well-filled bustline, this precocity will be rewarded or punished on the social scene. Generally speaking (and this probably applies even to cultures as youth-oriented as our own) anything that smacks of early maturity in the peer group tends to be overvalued in the young. We spend the first years of our life wishing we were older than we are, and the last years wishing we were younger, and it is probably in the nature of most thirteen-year-olds to envy an age-mate's mustache, first menstrual period, or pubic hair. These precocities confer status in a youth subculture which, having no direct access as yet to money, power, or educational one-up-manship, still vests status in the physical basics themselves: height, physical strength, and any provable kind or degree of sexual precocity.

While the short-legged mesomorph and endomorph are flaunting their physical precocity among their peers, the ectomorph is taking his own good time about growing up. Although getting longer and longer in the leg, the ectomorphic boy's chin may still be innocent of fuzz, the ectomorphic girl has probably not had her first period yet and may be the only one in her class who still doesn't have to wear a bra. These disparities in rates of maturation are either devastating or bracing, as the case may be; and they make themselves known just at that time of life when young people are most apt to feel themselves on display and naked unto their enemies anyway. Again, no psychoanalytic or environmentalist explanation need be invoked to account for the differences in adult temperament between people who come of age early in adolescence versus those who only reach their full growth in their late teens or early twenties. Their psychological and cultural experiences will not be the same—and neither, it stands to reason, will their personalities.

The interplay between physique and character is thus not as simple or as simpleminded as the early constitutionalists painted it or as the Freudians still consider it to be. We are the sum and substance of all our experiences—and these include our hormonal and humoral experiences as well as our social ones. The sex steroids that speed the adolescence of mesomorphs to an early anatomical conclusion are biochemical compounds like any others, and they act on the central nervous system as other chemical compounds, including drugs, do: Pimples and nocturnal emissions are not the only disadvantages of too much androgen in the circulating blood. Drunk on their own hormones as on some newly discovered amphetamine, adolescents may be prey to bizarre moods and cravings. Teachers and parents rationalize the resulting disturbances in characterological terms; the adolescent, they say, is "not himself." Ectomorphs may fare even worse than mesomorphs and endomorphs in this respect. They grow more slowly than other children and may thus have to put up with chronic overdoses of their own hormones over much longer periods of time than endomorphs and mesomorphs do; the mood swings engendered along the way may then become so standard that they end up being incorporated into the adult personality in a way that the more short-lived ups and downs of the other two somatotypes never do.

Recent research in human genetics suggests that the major genetic differences between two taxonomic families—chimpanzee and man, for example—may be due not so much to differences in specific genes of the two species in question (man and chimp appear to have an astonishing 95 per cent of their total complement of DNA in common) but to the timing with which one set of genes gets activated and turned off as opposed to another. This possibility will seem less startling if we remember that the foreshortening of the skull in certain dogs such as boxers, pugs, and terriers, and the dwarfing of the legs in dachshunds, depend on minute shifts in the timing of embryonic bone development between these breeds; an excess of one particular hormone over another during the fourth week of fetal life will affect the bony development of the skull, while the same excess at a different developmental moment will exercise the same foreshortening effect on the legs, depending on which part of the skeleton is under most intense growth and elaboration at that particular point in intrauterine time. The "neotenous" baby face of the adult rain-forest Pygmy, and the snub-nosed, childlike, and wide-eyed face of the Lapps and certain European mountain dwellers, have by the same token been attributed to this kind of selective infantilization of the bones of the head and limbs, caused by as yet unanalyzed factors in the intrauterine timing of certain hormones that direct the rate at which one organ system develops as opposed to another. The genes that the Pygmy and the long-legged Masai cattle herders to the north of them share in common may amount to fully 99.9 per cent of their total chromosomal resources; but the timing which dictates the sequence in which one gene is made operative as opposed to another can make all the difference between the six-foot Nilotic peoples of East Africa and the four-foot-eleven Bushmen of the Kalahari.

By the same token the relatively underdeveloped state of the human infant at birth, as opposed to that of apes or many other mammals, and the resulting prolonged childhood to which his helplessness at birth condemns him, have made all the difference in the species' need and ability to learn, to teach, and to pass culture down from one generation to the next. Similarly, differences in hormonal timing between endomorphs, mesomorphs, and ectomorphs within the same culture cannot be without social and intellectual consequences of their own. The cuddliness of endomorphs has physical as well as social origins, as do the braininess and introversion of ectomorphs, and the high activity and drive levels of mesomorphs. But these physical antecedents have various social consequences; mind and matter, physique and temperament do not operate independently of each other in other orders and phyla, and it would be more surprising than not to discover that they did so in man, alone of all the animals.

Sheldon himself was fascinated by the psychological correlates of body build, and although he was unable to put many of his speculative ideas to the test of cold statistical analysis, it was probably rather for want of time and support than for want of hypotheses to test. Sheldon's own approach to the subject matter was eclectic: he had got his Ph.D. in psychology in the 1920's and added an M.D. from the University of Chicago in 1934. After a brief teaching stint Sheldon established himself, first at Harvard and later at Columbia under the auspices of their respective medical schools. His *Varieties of Human Physique* was published in 1940; *Varieties of Temperament* appeared in 1942, and *Atlas of Men* in 1954. Although Sheldon's name has been and continues to be one of the most frequently cited in the social-science and medical literature, Sheldon himself has been slow to receive the official imprimatur of either the medical or academic establishments, and his most lasting contributions will probably prove to have been neither in medicine nor in psychology, but in the field of human biology, where a modified version of his technique is still being applied today—especially in Europe.

As Sir Peter Medawar recently pointed out, the popular stereotype of the white-coated scientist, cool if not cold of mien and unflinchingly objective of mind, could not be farther from the facts of the matter; there are as many kinds of scientists as there are bakers and candlestick makers, ranging from collectors and classifiers to detectives and explorers. And in this roster Sheldon should probably be classified with the collectors. His habit of giving totem signs and designations to the various somatotypes—as e.g. "Pacific walrus" for the human male 6–4–2 somatotype ("Bigger than his Atlantic brother, a little longer, and has a discernible neck; gentle by nature, walruses can fight back powerfully when attacked . . .") and "Wasps" for the male 1–2–6 ("Slight, delicate fellows, crushed by your lightest step. Yet they can sting")—did not go down well in the broader scientific community; and Sheldon's concepts and methods came in for more than their fair share of criticism. In the process, some very rigorous methodology was applied to his data; and, to the general head scratching of the social science community, many of Sheldon's most arrogant assertions proved to test out rather well after all.

The hub of the problem was Sheldon's contention that an individual's behavior ought to correlate closely with his somatotype. Sheldon's "evidence" for this belief was his own intensive psychological appraisal of subjects he and his team had already somatotyped. The possibility of bias in a situation of this kind is undeniable: It is human nature to find what you set out to look for and to overlook or discount whichever of your discoveries seem to conflict with your own pet theory most.

Other investigators, fired by his ideas, set out to measure the gap between Sheldon's assertions and real-life events. Irvin Child of Yale undertook the job of testing Sheldon's behavior-somatotype relationship under stringent laboratory conditions—a stricture Sheldon himself had never seen fit to apply. Child gave 532 Yale students who had already been somatotyped by Sheldon's team a questionnaire about various behavior items and personality characteristics of theirs. Students were asked to rate themselves on items which ranged from "Gets to sleep easily" and "Tends to be complacent about himself in his relations with the world" to "Likes cold showers" and "Prefers a few very intimate friends to having many friends." The results vindicated Sheldon's assertions in almost every instance—though by no means as strongly as their originator might have liked. Nevertheless the correlations were significant enough—and occurred in a large-enough number of test items—to warrant the conclusion that physique does have some unique influence on behavior and personality.

The agonizing question in modern social science is always "How significant is it?" Statistical methodology assigns an arbitrary level of co-occurrence for two related items before they can be considered reliably or even reportably significant; in principle, two things have to occur together only slightly more than 50 per cent of the time for their co-occurrences to be considered as causally bound up in each other; but in practice the two events should co-occur much more frequently than this to be considered "highly significant" and strongly causally self-entailed. Most of the correlations found by Child were at too low a level of significance to meet such standards. For example, out of 96 predictions based on Sheldon's formulations, 77 proved to go in the expected direction; but of these, only 20 were highly statistically significant. Still, for a piece of research based on such admittedly speculative and intuitive concepts as Sheldon's, correlations like these are not to be sneered at: Though Sheldon may have overstated his case somewhat to begin with, the case itself is a good one as it stands.

An interesting quirk of Child's data is that ectomorphs and mesomorphs (especially the latter) bear out the predictions Sheldon made for them much better than endomorphs do—suggesting either that endomorphy is less binding on character than the other somatotype components are, or that Sheldon's perceptions about the character of endomorphs was less brilliant than his perceptions about the other two types. Sheldon himself is reputed to have been a classic ectomorph (or 2–4–5 in somatotype shorthand) and, as an exceptionally good-looking man in his own right, may have cast all ectomorphs in his own image and sized them up accordingly.

Child's research was the first in a series of like-minded investigations; over the years, fired by Sheldon's concepts on the one hand and Child's data on the other, various investigators have had a hand at filling in the gaps, and differences of somatotype have been statistically correlated with a wide range of other variables—including physical disease, psychological aberrations, and occupational preferences—with uniformly interesting results.

In a study published in 1962, Albert Damon, investigating the epidemiological aspects of somatotype, found for example that women with diabetes tended to be fatter and less mesomorphic than healthy, nondiabetic controls. The same sort of body configuration was found to characterize women with uterine cancer; while, on a more general level, cancers of the female reproductive system (i.e., breast and cervical as well as uterine cancers) were found to be somewhat more prevalent in women with more distinctively feminine body builds than they are in women with more masculine figures. These correlations, like all those reported here, were "significant" but not overwhelmingly so, and the author made no attempt to, and lays no claim to trying to, work out the physiological whys and wherefores of the reported correlations. Estrogen has long been suspected of playing some auxiliary role in the development of female-reproductive-system cancers, but it has never been demonstrated that women with more feminine body shapes have higher levels of estrogen than those without, and until further research is done along these lines, the relationship between hyperfeminine figures and cancers of the female reproductive system remains up in the air.

In men, on the other hand, while there seems to be no evidence of correlation between reproductive-system cancers and body build, somatotype did prove to be a reliable predictor of heart disease; heart attacks at an early age befall fat mesomorphs significantly more often than they do men with other body builds—including endomorphs, whose fat is apparently not as great a risk factor, in and of itself, as the combination of fat and muscle in fat mesomorphs. This is perhaps the most important and most significant point to have been overlooked by the actuaries and to have been (unintentionally) bowdlerized by too broad a reading of their data: Heart-attack victims are not so much fat as they are fat, muscular, and lateral in body build.

Damon's findings in this area have been seconded by other investigators, notably B. Lindegård in Sweden, whose own research along these lines brought him to the corollary conclusion that a long-legged and lanky build is as good a coronary disease insurance as anyone can get. Linear ectomorphs are the least likely candidates for heart disease of all the somatotypes at all ages and in both sexes. Another researcher doing work in this field, Per Bjürulf of Norway, found that coronary atherosclerosis in males was significantly correlated with both muscularity and with size of fat cells in an individual's adipose tissue reserves, but not with the number of fat cells present. Since the number of fat cells, as opposed to their size, is probably a function of the individual's genes, while their size is a function of his feeding habits, we can probably conclude that it is not the born endomorphs who are most at risk in this situation, but the mesomorphs who have fallen on evil dietary ways later in life and have let themselves run to fat in a way to an extent that their bodies were not originally programmed to negotiate.

Like Lindegard, furthermore, Bjürulf found that leg length and height correlated negatively with heart disease; in other words, the longer and leaner an individual is the less likely he is to have heart disease of any kind. These separate lines of research are in remarkable agreement with each other, and should prompt a new look at the famous *Build and Blood Pressure Study* of 1959, in which all kinds of overweight are lumped together in a rather simplistic and uncritical reading of the statistical facts. Endomorphs who have been losing sleep over the mortality tables may therefore breathe a (cautious) sigh of relief; mesomorphs whose muscle has recently tended to turn to fat may, however, have to remind themselves that there is still cause for alarm. (Ectomorphs were already, presumably, pretty relaxed about the whole question anyway, and may go on being so if findings like these continue to come along.)

(Recently, data from the famous Framingham study on heart disease have shown that blood factors, which are presumably under some sort of genetic control, may be crucial to individual susceptibility to heart and artery disease. Certain blood lipids, like cholesterol and the low-density lipoproteins, seem to contribute to the widespread plaque formation in the arteries which causes both heart injury and stroke; others, the high-density lipoproteins, appear to have an exactly opposite effect and may even play a sort of scavenging role inside the arteries, by clearing away pre-existing plaque after it has formed. These blood factors are probably related to the sex hormones, since women have higher titres of the high-density, scavenging lipoproteins in their blood, and lower titres of the low-density ones, than men—at least until the age of menopause. And it may well be that there are similar relationships waiting to be teased out between the hormonal factors in heart disease and the hormonal variables in body build as well—relationships which may in turn account for the risk factors of different somato-types when it comes to atherosclerosis, heart infarction, and stroke.)

Among other disease or disease syndromes that seem to fall unequally to the lot of mesomorphs and ectomorphs is their differing prognoses in tertiary syphilis: Mesomorphs are more apt to suffer from general paresis in the late stages of syphilis, while ectomorphs are especially susceptible to *tabes dorsalis,* or spinal cord degeneration, in the late stages of the disease. In diabetes, late-onset patients are generally much more endomorphic than childhood-onset cases. Diseases which proved, on the other hand, to have no relationship to body build at all were acne, asthma, and ulcers—a finding that should help lay to rest the popular stereotype of the lean and hungry ulcer patient once and for all.

Cigarette smoking, on the other hand, is related to somatotype only in a roundabout way, if at all: Damon found cigarette smoking to be positively correlated with leanness in a group of male smokers carefully matched for occupation and general ancestry (in this case, all subjects' grandparents were Neapolitan Italians). This correlation may stem, however, from the fact that smoking speeds up metabolism by a factor of about 10 per cent on the average, so that in any given group of people the smokers "naturally" tend to be thinner than the nonsmokers. Since we know from other sources that more smokers die of lung cancer than nonsmokers do, meanwhile, any correlation between lung cancer and leanness may on closer inspection turn out to be bent through this incidental metabolic prism. In this connection, though, it is interesting to note that epidemiologists have long suspected a correlation between the elongated and narrow-chested physiques of ectomorphs and the scourge of tuberculosis. Scientists have speculated that the small chests and low lung capacity of classical ectomorphs may make them more vulnerable than other body types to lung infections in general and to TB in particular; it now appears that the literary stereotype of the emaciated nineteenth-century consumptive reflected a perfectly realistic clinical norm. Short, fat, and muscular people tend to be more resistant to TB than long skinny ones are, a fact that may have something to do with adaptation to cold and overall resistance to respiratory disease in the various body types.

Somatotype has proved a rockier terrain to mine psychologically than physically: Mental correlations to body build are harder to pin down than epidemiological ones. Sheldon himself was convinced that such correlations existed, and his own research linking temperament to physique yielded a correlation that was fairly significant—significant enough, that is, to bolster the morale of fellow thinkers and to arouse the skepticism of nonbelievers. Meanwhile such research as has been done in other laboratories tends to confirm Sheldon's conviction that mesomorphs are extroverts, noisy and physical glad-handers; and that ectomorphs are indeed cerebrotonic or brainy. Studies on endomorphs, however, continue for some reason to be few and far between.

P. K. Bridges studied the reactions of students to test situations and found that ectomorphs facing exams have significantly higher corticosteroid metabolites in their circulating blood than mesomorphs do—the implication being that their general anxiety level is so high that their adrenal glands work overtime in the face of an impending psychological crisis. In the same research situation, ectomorphs also evidenced higher self-reported anxiety, and psychological tests confirmed the self-reported data. While no one likes to take a test, ectomorphs seem to like test taking even less than the rest of us do, and to suffer more physical and psychological distress as a result of the test situation.

Bridges's study, incidentally, conducted as it was among medical students at the University of London, brought to light the interesting and unexpected finding that endomorphs were in short supply in this population altogether, compared, that is, to Sheldon's group of New England college students and to the American population at large—a curious finding, and one that is echoed by Richard William Parnell, who did similar research among Oxford undergraduates. For whatever reasons, English university students seem not to be as variable in physique as American undergraduates are, or as people in general are, at least in the United States; they tend to cluster much more evenly in the mesomorphic and ectomorphic range of the scale than Americans do—either because Britons are a less polymorphous (and/or less endomorphic) lot than Americans to begin with, or because the British university student population is somehow preselected for leanness by virtue of other extraneous factors (like social class, unconscious bias against fat people on the part of admissions officers and other educators, or whatever).

Fascinating research has been done on the occupational and professional choices of the different somatotypes. Parnell found that British degree candidates in scientific subjects tend to be tall and slender mesomorphs; while in America, Stanley M. Garn and Menard M. Gertler reported that research workers in a factory tended to be much more ectomorphic than men in other job categories in exactly the same industrial setting. Other researchers have reported very similar findings. Carl Seltzer's research in Boston established the finding that among superior students at Harvard, those with the less masculine and less mesomorphic builds tended to concentrate in humanities as opposed to the natural or social sciences. Testing the same phenomenon in other groups, Seltzer found further that 26 per cent of army chaplains, 20 per cent of communications officers, but only 15 per cent of army draftees, 10 per cent of Harvard grant study awardees, and 8.5 per cent of chain-store managers had low somatic masculinity ratings. There would thus seem to be at least some slight basis in fact for the popular stereotypes of physical frailty and sissification among men whose occupations take them out of the hurly-burly of commerce and set them to deal with the things of the mind on a daily occupational basis; though what one is to make of the Harvard award students in this scheme of things is puzzling. Of course no one of these figures is impressive enough in and of itself to warrant any dogmatic and across-the-board conclusions about what makes one man a preacher and another an athlete; the findings are there but they are tenuous. Believers will go on believing, and skeptics will go on doubting; meanwhile it is to be hoped that the data will keep coming in and at some future date will be strong enough to speak for themselves.

"Our minds are constantly wrought on by the temperaments of our bodies," wrote John Dryden; and in trying to define the interface between them and refine the statistical raw material that studies like Parnell's, Seltzer's, and Bridges's have mined, psychologists have gone off in several promising directions. Pursuing the fine line between psychological performance and physique, T. R. Schori and C. B. Thomas of Johns Hopkins School of Medicine administered Rorschach tests to a total of 228 medical students who had been previously somatotyped by J. L. Angel of the Smithsonian Institution. The famous Rorschach inkblot test consists of a number of varicolored inkblots symmetrically blotted down the middle in which people can, and on request do, make out more or less meaningful shapes of things or creatures according to the dictates of their own personalities and perceptions. Because there are no "right answers" to the Rorschach test the individual taking the test is theoretically projecting images from the *terra incognita* of his own mind's eye onto the nonpictorial inkblots he is being presented with, and one of the premises of the testers is that far from being totally random and idiosyncratic, responses to individual cards will tend to sort themselves out in a pretty predictable way, depending on the personality traits of the individual who is doing the responding. So reliable has this sorting process proved to be over the years that the Rorschach test is often routinely used for diagnostic purposes at psychological clinics and in psychiatric evaluation in general; but until Schori and Thomas's work it had not been used to assess personality differences between somatotypes.

The authors' results were provocative and promising. The only significant correlation they were able to establish between the Rorschach response and the basic somatotype was that in general endomorphs had significantly more so-called "form-related" responses than the other somatotypes did; there was no difference between somatotypes, however, on such factors as intellectual productivity, human movement responses, or a tendency to see whole configurations as opposed to details.

The rationale behind any projective test is that people will tend to bring their own basic personality traits to bear on their perceptions of unidentified images; the high "form-related" responses of endomorphs thus suggest, in the language of the test protocols, an underlying tendency to produce order out of chaos, to reduce ambiguity to some rationally bearable level, and to organize the disjointed, heterogeneous imagery of the inkblot into something more legible and sensible than it appears to be at first blush. Sheldon was not actively involved in research at the time this study was carried out, but it is a safe guess that it would have pleased him. He himself had already classified endomorphs ("viscerotonics," in temperamental terms) as reality-oriented, comfort-loving people; of all three temperaments they are the most domesticated and conventional, the least tolerant of uncertainty and unnecessary confusion in the world around them.

Like the tendency of obese subjects to perseverate in psychological experiments (and, by extension, in day-to-day living situations out in the real world as well), the tendency of endomorphs to produce form-related responses to a series of vague and programmatically meaningless inkblots on Rorschach cards is one that gives many psychoanalytically oriented psychologists pause. Why should fat people be any more inclined than thin people to impose structure and regularity on the formless outlines made by splotches of ink haphazardly blotted between two folds of the same sheet of paper? If anything, the popular stereotype of the obese as slugabeds and slatterns would seem to suggest an opposite kind of response (although, in all fairness to the psychoanalytic theorists, their handy assumption that at the symbolic level most things do double duty as their own opposites makes this sort of inversion not only thinkable but even highly probable).

Cognitive peculiarities like these, however, pose serious questions for non-Freudian thinkers, and a new breed of psychological analysts seems to be coming forward to deal with such findings on a more common-sense level than the Freudians. Workers like Stella Chess have turned to studying the role of temperament in basic behavior patterns and in the game plans of babies and young children. Human beings in this view are like house pets and other animals in that they have temperaments, and temperament in the true sense of the word can never be fully accounted for or explained away on the basis of childhood traumas or unique biographical experiences. Regardless of what tragedies or strokes of fortune do or do not befall any one of us at an early age, and regardless of what success, luck, and talent we can lay claim to later on as individuals, most of us have characteristic moods, levels of awareness and arousal, and feelings of well-being inside our own skins. In the aggregate, these form the signature we sign to the raw data of our daily experiences. People recognize us by our moods and modes of feeling as they do by our faces; our prevailing mood or affect is the seal we set on the events of our daily lives. Sheldon's conviction that temperament is largely grounded in physique is the other side of the coin of the Freudian assumption that the leitmotiv of biography is the individual's neurosis, psychosis, or character disorder. The truth probably lies somewhere in between these two extremes. At the very least, systems theory has taught us to be suspicious of the old chicken-and-egg model of cause and effect; trying to assign a beginning or an end point in complex matters like these can be a thankless task.

For those who believe in such things, meanwhile, differences between somatotypes have been traced all the way back to underlying differences in body biochemistry. Although we all manufacture more or less the same chemicals in the blood-and-tissue factory of the human body, we manufacture differing amounts of them and, in some cases, differing versions of the same chemical molecules. What these differences add up to in terms of behavior, life-style, and occupation is a question that absorbed Sheldon and formed the cornerstone of his life's work. Certainly the logic of size and shape is ungainsayable in many human endeavors. Teamsters and loggers need muscle and stamina to do their jobs; the basic physical equipment of the mesomorphs is often their occupational stock in trade. Secretaries and accountants need patience, orderliness, and—in strictly physical terms—the ability to sit in one spot for about seven hours a day without going stir crazy. While not all ectomorphs are poets, research workers, or Harvard fellowship grantees, any more than all mesomorphs are teamsters or football players, the statistical odds in favor of an individual of any one somatotype making a living in one field over and against another are probably far from random or gratuitous. The sedentary worker's fleshiness is probably at least as much a cause of his occupational choice as it is an effect of that choice: For while it is true that staying in the same place all day tends to make you gain weight (unless you reduce your caloric intake accordingly), it is equally true that only certain kinds of people can be counted on to put up with the enforced inactivity of the typical clerk's, tailor's, or secretary's job to begin with. Mesomorphs tend to feel caged and restless when confined to a circumscribed place for any length of time, and the six, seven, or eight hours a day that the shoemaker puts in at his last or the typist at her desk would tend to drive the plowman to distraction and the long-distance runner to tics and skin rashes.

Sheldon's own research established that there is a full 20 per cent difference between the average basal metabolic readings of mesomorphic ectomorphs and those of mesomorphic endomorphs. The active thyroid glands of mesomorphs may go far toward explaining their need for action and physical discharge of nervous energy. The sluggish thyroids of endomorphs, on the other hand, may explain their muscular laxness, their resistance to physical effort, and their general physical and psychological imperturbability. There are other, measurable physical factors involved in this kind of personality difference. Sheldon cites autopsy reports showing that the mean intestinal weight of endomorphs is significantly higher—1,473 g.—than that of mesomorphs—1,085 g.—or ectomorphs—786 g. The corresponding difference in lengths of the gut of the three different somatotypes is comparable. Endomorphs have not only relatively but absolutely much more visceral tissue devoted to the ingestion, processing, and digestion of their food than either of the other two somatotypes does. In physiological terms this means that the endomorph spends more of his time, blood, and energy processing his food, on a lifetime basis, than either of the two other somatotypes does. The general enervation and sluggishness that are said to go hand in hand with a good digestion may thus be contributing factors to the prevailing mood and affect of the typical endomorph and may in turn have something to do with the endomorph's deserved reputation for serenity, unflappability, and indolence. With or without an assist from other endocrine systems (insulin, for one example; the sex steroids, for another), endomorphs, everything else being equal, should therefore make good mothers, fathers, doctors, nurses, and cooks.

The ectomorph's large expanse of skin and nervous-system tissue, on the other hand, compared to that of the other two somatotypes, disposes him to irritability and the sensitivity of a quivering tuning fork which, in the presence of a good and well-trained mind, should give him the basic somatic wherewithal for life as an intellectual or a dreamer. Introversion is the price Sheldon believed ectomorphs might be expected to pay for the few hundred thousand or so extra nerve cells designed into their extra surface complement of bare skin: Too much unedited information irritates and distracts the ectomorph, whose typical postural rigidity and twitchiness are the somatic defenses he must mount against too steady an inflow of unsorted and unprocessed stimuli. Experience has theoretically taught him that he can reduce all that environmental noise to a bearable level only by getting off alone somewhere with a good book, a pet project, or a poem to compose. Seltzer's and Parnell's work on the somatypes of research workers and doctors of philosophy, cited earlier, confirmed Sheldon's hunch that we should look for the ectomorphs of this world in the more secluded corners of it.

Statistical survey research confirms the tendency of each somatotype to cluster in different sorts of jobs, at least in part as a result of temperament and body build. J. M. Tanner's work in England showed that a class of officer cadets at Sandhurst was significantly more mesomorphic than a group of Oxford students of the same age and sex, but significantly less so than a similar group of student physical-education teacher trainees. And even within a given profession, somatotypes tend to specialize in the same direction as in the population at large: Earnest Hooton, for example, found that in the regular army, the least muscular and fattest soldiers wound up in supply and administration more often than they did in more active specialties. It should come as no surprise meanwhile that truck drivers as a group are more mesomorphic than otherwise; driving a heavy truck on cross-country routes is not a job for the physically frail, the mentally sluggish, or the absent-minded and jittery. At the same time, however, champion truck drivers turn out to be even more mesomorphic than their normally mesomorphic colleagues are, so at least one of the ingredients in the special success of superior driving performance is the basic physical equipment that the driver brings to the job in the first place. Will power, ambition, and personality in themselves may not be enough to turn the trick—a somewhat unsettling notion in a culture that posits motivation and other psychological imponderables as the sine qua non of professional excellence in any field.

Of course muscle alone is not the only determining factor in physical strength, but it is certainly a major one: When height and weight are factored out, for example, weight proves to account for 25 per cent of total dynamometric strength, while size of muscle mass and the total amount of muscle account for the remaining 75 per cent. Sheer grit and determination probably account for less in this equation than the Protestant ethic has encouraged generations of American bodybuilders to believe. Muscle size is a highly heritable commodity, and in the absence of mesomorphic ancestors it is doubtful that even Charles Atlas could have developed the biceps and pectorals for which he was justly famous. But with the preponderance of muscle tissue that the mesomorph brings to his task go certain other physiological pluses that may be useful too, including smart reflexes and overall resistance to fatigue.

Such qualities are at a premium in precisely those occupations that have traditionally been dominated by males throughout most of human history, and in which men will probably continue to outnumber women in the immediate future as well. Woodcutters, weight lifters, and long-distance truckers all prove to be not only more mesomorphic than men in other professions but also lower on the whole on "gynomorphy" (femininity of physique) according to A. Damon and R. A. MacFarland, among others. Elsewhere, M. J. Karvonen's study of outstanding occupational performance in woodcutters established the same sort of finding that Damon had noted among truck drivers. The champion woodcutters in Karvonen's study were taller and more mesomorphic than their peers, with their extra length concentrated chiefly in their torsos and not in their legs. The ideal woodsman's strength is concentrated in his arms and in his trunk, and the axe of the twentieth-century forester is wielded with much the same set of muscles, and much the same kind of dynamometric heft, as that once brought to bear by Neanderthal man as he went about his daily work in the Paleolithic forests of central Europe.

Body shapes and sizes have a history as well as an anatomy of their own. Neanderthal's bowed but probably brawny forearms and richly muscled hands must have served a woodsman's and a spearsman's purpose; in the forested highlands of interglacial France and central Europe the antediluvian "mesomorph's" talents would have been in obvious demand. Later, other ways of making a living brought other somatotypes into fashion; herdsmen need physiques different from those of tillers of soil or hunters of game. Just as temperament models occupation, ecology models physique, and the fossil evidence points to the conclusion that throughout hominid prehistory speciation has almost always followed shifts in climates and life-styles. The history of physique therefore reflects the history of the species itself in capsule form; and perhaps some day if we are lucky we can reconstruct a record of hominid and human temperament from the evidence of the fossil record itself.

Sheldon would not have shrunk from the task; it was his own conviction (and less facetiously upheld than it may sound) that Christianity had ushered in a new fashion in bodies as it had in consciences: Based on a sample of some 124 paintings of Christ displayed in Boston museums in the 1940's, and including works from a cross section of schools, centuries, and aesthetic traditions, Sheldon noted that as depicted in Western art, Jesus emerges as a man with a mean morphological first component (endomorphy) of 2.2, a second component (mesomorphy) of 2.6, and a third component (ectomorphy) of 5.4. Christ is, in short, a classical ectomorph, with a third-component score that puts him in a class by himself when compared to the rank and file of ectomorphic Harvard undergraduates of Sheldon's day—let endomorphs, mesomorphs, and less outspoken ectomorphs make of this finding what they will.

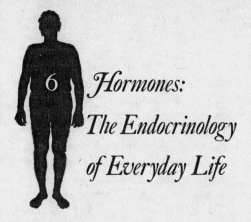

6 Hormones: The Endocrinology of Everyday Life

To people raised on the idea of progress, evolution figures as a straight line at best, or at worst as a sort of rising curve, with lower life forms down at one end of the trajectory and higher forms up at the other. Progress implies a climb, with or without any imaginable end in sight. The truth of the matter is probably a lot less orderly, less linear, and less progressive than we suppose. In nature, and especially in biosystems, things seem to evolve crabwise toward no visible or prefigured goal, and sometimes only hindsight reveals the upward nature—if any—of the advance. By contrast, in individuals, homeostasis, even stasis, is the rule: Once growth is completed, any further progress would represent a sort of disaster. Gigantism is a case in point. Obesity is another.

Nowhere is this lesson more painstakingly spelled out than in the one-step forward, two-steps back system of hormonal checks and balances that govern so many of our body processes. The adult organism is a biological conservative, if not a downright reactionary; and the body in its natural wisdom craves homeostasis the way plants crave light. At the level of the individual, evolution is always a risky venture. The body mistrusts "progress," and rightly so; in the context of an individual life there is really only one apotheosis after birth—and anyone in his right mind tries to stave that one off as long as possible. On the contrary, everything in the ordinary course of daily living is normally always seeking to return to Go; and it is only at the species level that evolution can really take place without catastrophe. Hormones are part and parcel of the body's self-policing and self-pacing; they are the biochemical messages we send ourselves to keep our life processes in line. There are hormones, antihormones, and anti-antihormones; the details of these interlocking systems are only half known and understood to date, and the complexities are still coming to light almost around the clock.

Hormones are large protein- and fat-based molecules which are found in only slightly different variants throughout the animal kingdom; they are put together from bits and pieces of amino acids in our daily food on hereditary instructions from our genes, or (during fasting) from the proteins in our own lean tissues and blood. Like blood cells, antibodies, and drugs, hormones circulate freely in the blood until they hit a target organ, provoke the predesigned response, and generate feedback. Feedback is often in the nature of output of another hormone. Too much insulin in the circulating blood, for example, provokes a call for glucagon to counteract it; too much growth hormone may signal the brain for more somatostatin, etc.

The fine evolutionary line between one-celled animals and complex, many-celled ones probably marks the point at which hormones first came into biological existence in the great planetary zoo. One-celled animals need very little data to proceed on; light, dampness, pressure from the outside world comprise all the signals the amoeba needs to make its way from birth to death: Food itself becomes the signal to feed; critical mass becomes the signal to divide and reproduce.

Things get more complicated once that single cell begins to branch out and specialize. Impressed with the extreme ancientness of a substance called cyclic AMP in zoological history, biologist John Bonner came to the conclusion that this was the Ur-hormone, the basic and primordial substance that came into existence as a means of bridging the gap between one cell membrane and the next and so transmitting information from cell to cell. What in our own bodies serves as the basic chemical grammar of oxidation and energy exchange within the cell was once long ago in the evolutionary scheme of things the principal messenger between the cell membranes of one single-celled animal and the next.

Bonner's work on the cellular slime molds—the so-called social amoebas—seems to show the point in evolutionary history at which this basic metabolic operation became a hormonal one. Slime-mold amoebas are one-celled animals, but for purposes of breeding they periodically stream together into collections of upward of hundreds of thousands of individual amoebas which proceed to gather themselves into the shape of a slug and then crawl off in search of food and breeding grounds. Once the slug has found a likely spot, it upends itself and assumes the shape and stalkiness of a rooted plant, with a mass of generative spores at its uppermost tip, all contained in a globular bulb not unlike the flowering end of a weed. When the spores from this bulb are blown about by the wind or otherwise dispersed, each one can start a whole new generation of social amoebas, and the whole mysterious ritual of transmogrification from one-celled, solitary homesteader to multi-celled community on the grand scale begins all over again.

The drama is a fascinating one not only because it shows how changes may be rung on individuality and collectivity in the biological world, but because the force that seems to organize and orchestrate this dazzling metamorphosis is not "instinct" or "environment," but something manufactured *in situ* by the amoebas themselves, a chemical factor on the surface of the amoeba's outer membrane which seems to act like a chemical attractant or glue and which, after years and years of painstaking research, Bonner was finally able to identify as cyclic AMP.

We are—as vertebrates, as mammals, and especially as human beings—many eons removed from the slime molds and many gene sequences beyond them in the scope and complexity of evolutionary happenstance. But biochemically we are still all brothers and sisters under the skin; and the force that impels the social amoebas to foregather and organize into a social slug in order to feed and breed his left eidetic tracings in the rhythms of our own bodies. Like the slime mold we depend on hormonal action and interaction to synchronize the rhythms of our lives from birth through growth and maturity to old age. It is hormones that carry the genetic instructions of all our inner biological clocks, telling us when (and how much) to grow, when to prepare ourselves for procreation, hibernation, defense—and feeding. As individuals, no two of us are ever quite alike in the amount, timing, or intensity of the hormonal surges that orchestrate these basic behavioral responses and synchronize them to the ongoing events of life in the real world. No two human beings will ever produce exactly the same amounts of a given hormone in response to exactly the same inner or outer cues, and keep on producing that precise quantum for exactly the same length of time. And yet substantial behavioral effects can hang on the difference. One extra microgram of epinephrine (adrenaline) in the blood can make the difference between which of two otherwise fairly matched gladiators will best the other in a fight; variations in the amount of progesterone secreted by a pregnant woman can make the difference in carrying a child to term or aborting in the first few months of pregnancy. A split-second lag in the release of glycogen from storage in the liver can be a matter of life and death to an animal contemplating flight from a natural predator. Less dramatically but no less significantly, the hormones which govern other basic responses to real life (including the events inside our own bodies) can have noticeable effects on our own behavior, our bodies, and our temperaments; and all this can proceed with or without significant repercussions in our social lives and lifestyles to match.

To say therefore, as many authorities do, that hormones do not affect obesity is to deny the primordial role played by hormones in organizing and editing all our basic responses to life and the world around us. Bound up as they are in the most basic daily rhythms of breathing, rest, tissue oxygenation, growth, and reactivity to things in the world outside, hormones in fact form the basic regulators of all our cellular rhythms—including those that dictate how and when we feed, convert our food to fuel, and call up fuel reserves from storage as the need arises.

If the slime molds were the first animals to invent the idea of chemical regulation of basic life rhythms, no other species since then has been able to make do without this invention, and the basic chemical designs of individual species' hormones allow us to reconstruct some basic evolutionary trajectories across phyla and species. Growth hormone, for example, is essential to all vertebrates except birds; thyroxin may have an even more august evolutionary history, since it is essential to life in all vertebrates and some invertebrates as well—and can be used interchangeably in all vertebrates without arousing the host animal's immunological defenses. Insulin, on the other hand, although it is found in all vertebrates, occurs in slightly different forms from genus to genus and from species to species, suggesting that it is somewhat younger or newer in the evolutionary scheme of things than the more widely interreactive thyroxin and growth hormone are.

On the whole, though, so chemically similar are the hormones of other mammals to those manufactured by the human body that we can (and do) use thyroxin from cows and prolactin from sheep to fill the prescriptions that treat human hormone deficiencies. But while certain nonhuman hormones can have clearcut target-organ effects in man, others do not; it is an interesting footnote to the special complexity of human growth hormone, for example, that while it can produce measurable effects in animals other than man (including fish and frogs, as well as other mammals) only growth hormone from his own or possibly a few other primate species can have any measurable effect on target cells in man.

The similarity of our own hormones, meanwhile, to those of many other animal species illustrates the probability that these biological molecules are as old as the hills and in some cases perhaps a good bit older. Hormones can thus be said to have evolved with the very earliest free-moving organisms, long before the species as we know them now came into existence in the forms in which we now know them, and to have kept pace—or even to have paced—the magnificent zigzag by which the various life forms made their way inchmeal up the Linnaean tree from slime mold to *Homo sapiens*.

To say that hormones have nothing to do with obesity is to deny the central role played by at least three—and probably several more—of these very ancient chemical hieroglyphs on the evolutionary record. It is to deny the central role played by insulin, for example, in blood-sugar regulation and cell glucose absorption; of growth hormone in regulating the rate of fatty-acid release from adipose tissue cells; or of thyroxin in setting the rate at which we burn oxygen in the cells. Other hormones involved in fat breakdown are ACTH and epinephrine (although to date these have been studied mostly from the point of view of their effects on the brain and the sympathetic nervous system). Glucagon, a substance that acts as an insulin antagonist and counters insulin's fattening effects at the cellular level, is also a potent fat mobilizer. Testosterone is a tissue-building hormone, and as such has an indirect but important effect on fat accretion too; the female hormone estrogen seems to play a more inscrutable role in fat formation, even in the parts of a woman's body that are particularly sensitive to it, such as the breasts and hips.

Even minor variations in the amounts of these hormones circulating in the blood will obviously have to have some sort of effect on the rate at which one individual builds fatty tissue up and another individual tears it down; and sooner or later these effects are apt to be translated into something that can be logged and measured on the average set of bathroom scales. Discounting the role of hormones in weight gain or loss is therefore a disingenuous practice on the part of the diet doctors, and one that probably ought not go unchallenged, no matter how well intended it may be.

From the dieter's point of view there are two major groups of hormones to contend with: those that help to build up fat on the one hand (the lipogenic hormones), and those that help to break it down on the other (the lipolytic hormones). Insulin takes pride of place in the first group. Insulin is one of the crucial hormones—if not the crucial one—involved in the process of cell nutrition. The primary purpose of insulin is to transfer glucose across the cell membrane into the cytoplasm of the cell itself; where insulin is inadequate, low, or nil, diabetes eventually results. Untreated juvenile diabetics, to prove the point, may become seriously emaciated; the inability of their fat cells to take up fat and store it reduces the untreated juvenile diabetic, literally, to skin and bones—even though he or she may be getting enough, or even more than enough, to eat and drink. In obesity just the opposite takes place: Food intake is high, blood sugar is high, and the pancreas keeps pouring out insulin to control the high blood sugar—with the end result of increasing fat uptake in adipose tissue cells, and increasing poundage on the scales.

Glucose is the basic substance needed by the body to transfer energy and set up the various chemical reactions involved in cell maintenance, reproduction, and repair; but getting it out of the bloodstream and into the cells can be a problem (it is *the* problem in diabetes) since the process doesn't take place by simple osmosis, or absorption through the cell walls, as many other vital supply transfers do. Insulin seems to have evolved as the answer to this workaday problem in the biochemistry of living organisms; in some way not well understood at the present time, insulin acts on the cell membrane to make it much more permeable to glucose than it would otherwise be, and therefore speeds up the transfer of glucose from the circulating blood into the cell itself.

The absence of insulin is lethal, and results in diabetic coma. But too much insulin can be unhealthy too, because it eventually results in a lowered blood-sugar supply, overstorage of nutrients in the tissues and, sooner or later, a self-perpetuating form of hunger and overeating in response to the chronic blood-sugar insufficiency. Which came first—the overeating or the overproduction of insulin—is the chicken-and-egg dilemma which obesity research has sought to, and with luck eventually will, learn how to unravel.

The fashionable hypothesis is that people overeat for psychological reasons, thereby incur an overabundance of insulin, and then learn to live, however gracelessly or gracefully, with the consequences. There is some evidence, though, that matters are not quite so simple. Certain obese individuals seem to have a marked cellular insensitivity to insulin; it takes more and more insulin on their parts to get less and less glucose out of their blood and into their cells than it does in other people. Glucose hunger in the cells of some individuals can trigger changes in the brain which tell them it is time to eat; and they will go on doing just that, regardless of how much glucose may already be at large in the blood. Albert J. Stunkard found that hunger contractions in the stomach do not turn off even when the blood is loaded with sugar; they only do so when the sugar effectively reaches the insides of the cells, as it does when glucagon is added to the glucose-insulin mix being infused into the subject's blood.

All cells are sensitive to insulin, but adipose tissue cells seem even more responsive to insulin than most, and there is some question whether fat synthesis anywhere in the body could take place in the first place without insulin to help it along. Even dietary fat circulating in the form of unassimilated fat globules, or chylomicrons, in the blood probably gets an assist past the cell wall and into the cell interior from insulin: J. H. Bragdon and R. S. Gordon have shown that ingested fat is taken up much more readily into the tissues of recently fed animals than it is into those of animals who have not had a meal for some time. The difference between the fed animal and the unfed one is the amount of insulin already circulating in the blood. The same thing is true for carbohydrates. Test-tube studies show that when insulin is added to rats' fat cells in a petri dish, carbohydrate uptake is much more active and much speedier in its effects than it is in cultures without the added insulin.

One of the major fat-promoting effects of insulin, though, is one that is rarely mentioned in the medical literature and may deserve more attention than it usually gets. This is the sedative effect that insulin produces as it goes about moving sugar into the cells and simultaneously removing glucose from the blood. Throttling down on glucose supplies to the brain, which happens when blood sugar is low, may have the effect of inducing faintness and confusion if the deficit is severe; when the deficit is not quite as serious as all that the individual may just feel drowsy and relaxed. To the subjective sensation of sleepiness may then be added the objective physiological fact of a damped-down circulation and resulting loss of available oxygen in the tissues—a soporific home brew with a built-in vicious circle of its own: To get more energy, the individual may decide he needs more food; or his brain may decide it for him. These metabolic ripple effects make sugar (and insulin) an excellent sedative. For an animal with good ecological reason to store excess fat and curtail excess activity (hibernators, for example), this kind of double-barreled energy conservation program makes excellent sense. But in an animal like modern urban man, who is obviously already living well within his own lipid means to begin with, and with no foreseeable major ecological catastrophe or shortages in sight, the syndrome is clearly maladaptive. The sedative effects of sugar and insulin for the overweight are therefore probably among their most insidious side effects.

While insulin is probably the single most important fat-building hormone in man, it is far from being the only one. It is, however, the best-known and the most easily documented one. It is also the most straightforward in its fattening action. Cortisol and other glucocorticoids (cortisol being the most important one in man) have opposite effects on feeding depending on whether they are in good supply or poor supply: High doses curtail appetite, while low doses increase appetite. Both these effects may be regulated by insulin; cortisol seems to enhance the insulin insensitivity of cells, and it has been hypothesized that this may trigger the release of more and more insulin to compensate. Cortisol has another role to play in body tissue metabolism: It controls water balance and blood pressure. The so-called buffalo-hump obesities that are characterized by a moon face, by fat build-up on the nape of the neck, and by relatively larger fat accumulations on the upper part of the torso than the lower are usually related to cortisol overproduction.

The other endocrinological fatteners—with two notable exceptions—are those that act in opposition to and serve to put the brakes on hormones whose basic work it is to mobilize fat; they are therefore not so much fattening agents as antislenderizing ones. Somatostatin, for example, is a recently discovered hormone that seems to have been designed specifically to turn off the production of growth hormone, the great fat mobilizer; and certain brain hormones or "neurotransmitters" which oppose the effects of the adrenal hormones probably achieve much the same purpose, whether that is what they were originally designed to do or not. Glucagon, the insulin antagonist, belongs to this category too; recently it has been proposed that it is really glucagon excess, and not insulin deficiency, that is responsible for the major symptoms of diabetes.

Various other fat-promoting hormones with a less roundabout modus operandi than these seem to be sex-related, and while insulin may be the culprit for the species as a whole, women have a special handicap in this respect: Progesterone, prolactin, and estrogen are all produced in much greater quantities, and with far more visible side effects, in women than in men. The consequences for weight gain are obvious, if not downright banal. Women are fatter than men both relatively and absolutely, a biocultural accident that both sexes have had to learn to live with more or less gracefully over the centuries.

But here the certainties end and the uncertainties multiply. Since the estrogens are women's hormonal signatures in all mammal species, we would expect to find some clear-cut causal relay between body fat on the one hand and estrogen output on the other. The relay is undoubtedly there, but it has proven to be harder to pinpoint than it ought to be. Far from the neat causal (or vicious) circle that most researchers once expected to find, all the evidence seems to go the other way. High estrogen levels tend to depress appetite, not boost it. Midway through the menstrual cycle, when ovulation occurs (and estrogen is highest), food intake is low and glucose is easily metabolized. At the onset of menstruation, on the other hand (when estrogen is lowest), food intake is high, glucose turnover is sluggish, and appetites are apt to skyrocket. Another anomaly: Researchers have demonstrated that (at least in rats) the male hormone testosterone tends to promote fat formation, while the female hormone estrogen inhibits it. Contrariwise, instead of promoting fat formation, estrogen tends to promote connective-tissue build-up, especially in the organs that are sensitive to it, the so-called target organs, including the breasts and the uterus.

These data come from studies on laboratory rats; but there are human parallels. In the estrogen-high stage of women's menstrual cycles, for example, enzyme activity in all target organs increases across the board, and all cell proteins—including messenger DNA, transfer DNA, and ribosomal cell molecules—increase significantly in human breast, uterine, and liver tissues. This lean-tissue build-up is probably achieved at the expense of fat build-up. Directly or indirectly, estrogen exerts a curb on insulin, and when estrogen levels fall off at menopause, insulin inherits a clear field in the hormonal battlescape. Middle-aged spread is an estrogen deficiency disease of women with faulty insulin balance, and can be and sometimes has been treated accordingly.

The powerful effect of estrogen's role in body-fat metabolism clearly works to women's advantage in one way, whether or not it ultimately proves to work for or against them on the bathroom scales: In contrast to the male hormone testosterone, estrogen promotes the formation of unsaturated fats like the B-lipoproteins at the expense of saturated ones like cholesterol and the triglycerides—and this difference in the actual chemical composition of men's and women's body fat (as opposed to the way in which such fat is characteristically distributed around their bodies) seems to give women significant protection from arterial disease. The result is that as long as estrogen levels are high (that is, until menopause) women's arteries remain healthier than men's, and their death rates from strokes and heart disease remain lower.

The clue to estrogen's major effect on fat, however, will probably turn out to lie in its long-term effects on insulin production and regulation. Paradoxically, these may prove to be exactly the opposite of estrogen's short-term effects—at least in women of childbearing years. Animal and human tests show that one result of long-term overexposure to high estrogen levels (as during pregnancy or hormone therapy, for example) may eventually be a seriously reduced glucose tolerance. By a kind of rebound action, insulin may go into overproduction as the body strives to get sugar out of the blood and into the cells—including, of course, the adipose tissue cells. In other words, although in the short run estrogen may act as an insulin antagonist, too much estrogen in the blood for too long a period of time may have just the opposite effect. And, to make matters worse, there is also some evidence that basic precursors of the all-important energizing hormone thyroxin may be turned off, or at least throttled down, by excess estrogen in the circulating blood—thus interfering with the normal rate of fat and oxygen turnover in the body in still another way.

Another female hormone that seems to have a more or less direct influence on actual fat formation is prolactin, which acts in tandem with insulin itself to persuade the cells to take up fat and glucose. Prolactin is secreted late in pregnancy and throughout the nursing period in women, and as its name implies, one of its functions seems to be to insure an adequate breast milk supply for the duration of nursing. In its effect on fat synthesis and release, prolactin takes over at that point in the reproductive cycle where progesterone leaves off. If it is progesterone that is at the basis of the weight gain that is found in pregnant women all over the world, regardless of the mother's diet and the caloric cost of the work she does while she waits out the nine months till confinement, it is probably prolactin that regulates weight gain and loss in nursing mothers and in women who have never borne children at all. Like progesterone, prolactin works hand in hand with insulin; injecting either prolactin or progesterone into rats raises their appetites and increases their food intake. But this effect may depend on the presence of estrogen (it is seen only in females, not in males), and even —at least in birds—on the time of day.

From the zoological—not to mention the sexual—point of view, the word prolactin (i.e., milk-promoting) is a serious misnomer; although first discovered and chemically isolated in human beings, the same hormone is now known to appear throughout the vertebrate phylum including those vertebrates—fish, amphibians, reptiles, and birds—where it could not possibly turn on lactation in the mammary glands for the simple reason that these animals do not nurse their young and therefore of course have no mammary glands to nurse with in the first place. Prolactin's overriding function seems to be not (as was first supposed) to entrain milk production in the pregnant and lactating breast, but to regulate fat build-up and depletion in time with other basic reproductive rhythms. This holds true for males as well as females, in a sense; for it turns out that even in mammals, prolactin is produced in significant quantities in males as well as females.

Like growth hormone, prolactin in both sexes shows daily rises and falls related to mealtimes and periods of fasting. Unlike growth hormone, though, prolactin seems calibrated not only to feeding cycles involved in fat storage and release, but also to reproductive cycles. This is true in both higher and lower vertebrates, and experiments have proved that the time of day is critical for prolactin's action: Depending on whether animals were given prolactin injections at one time of day or another, its effects on fat stores in the body might be diametrically opposite. This finding holds true for mammals as well as birds, amphibians, and reptiles, and suggests very strongly that prolactin must serve in some way to regulate—or perhaps even to trigger—seasonal (and daily) migratory patterns of the animals in question. The system is a complicated one and is closely calibrated to the production of corticosteroids. For example, zoologist Albert Meier and his colleagues at Louisiana State University found that when white-throated sparrows were given daily injections of corticosteroids alternating with prolactin at various time intervals, manipulating the timing of these two hormones produced significant behavioral changes in the sparrows as well as even more notable changes in body-fat stores. With a time lapse of twelve hours between the two injections, for example, the birds showed "growth of the reproductive system, heavy fat stores, and nocturnal restlessness oriented to the north under the open sky." At eight-hour intervals, on the other hand, the birds showed inhibited reproductive-system growth, depleted fat stores, and no nocturnal restlessness at all; and when the two injections were given at four-hour intervals "prolactin stimulated increases in fat stores and induced nocturnal restlessness that was oriented to the south under the open night sky.'' Since the experimental birds had all been kept in continuous simulated daylight to remove any effect that alternating dark and light cues might have had on their behavior, the results could only have been due to the administration of the hormones themselves, and not to any naturally occurring stimulus in their environments.

Men are not sparrows and do not migrate and reproduce according to the season or the time of day. But they do gain and lose weight in characteristic circadian cycles, and their weight gains and losses are to some extent at least contingent on levels of hormones like prolactin and growth hormone in their blood and target organs. Meier himself is alert to the effects that the rise and fall of natural hormonal tides may have on fat storage in the obese, and speculates how prolactin and other hormones might be manipulated some day to help people lose weight. Students of the problem might keep it in mind that drinking water inhibits prolactin release, while naps and stimulation of the breasts (at least in women) encourage it. (Studies like Meier's meanwhile raise the hope that the day may not be too far off when we will know enough about the circadian rhythms of corticosteroids and prolactin in our own species to be able to tell people who want to lose weight that a little judicious lovemaking, followed or preceded by a nap as the case may be, may prove to be a good antidote to obesity, depending on the time of day.)

Fortunately for the future of the eighteen-inch waistline and the whittled hip, there are hormones which mobilize fat from its bulging storage depots regardless of the time of day as well as hormones that deposit it there; and on balance there are more of the former than there are of the latter, although this may come as a surprise to people who have been stubbornly overweight for the better part of their lives. Thyroxin, epinephrine, pituitary growth hormone, and glucagon are all fat mobilizers with proven roles in the liberation of fat from adipose tissue pads; many of them act as direct antagonists to insulin (though it is possible that when we know more about them we may find out that the shoe is, evolutionarily and historically, at least, on the other foot, and that insulin developed later as a means of keeping fat mobilizers in their place). Thyroxin should probably head the list of the fat-mobilizing hor-

mones. The thyroid gland sits at the base of the throat and manu-
factures two hormones (thyroxin and tri-iodothyronine) which dictate the speed at which oxygen is burned and energy exchanged and
degraded in all the cells of the body. Sluggish thyroid glands produce sleepy people, pasty skins, brittle hair and nails, cool cells.
Probably one of the reasons for the increase of fat in people as they
get older is that thyroid activity slows down and basal metabolic
rates tend to drop off progressively with increasing age; after the
age of 25 you would have to lower your caloric intake by about .5
per cent per year, year after year, just to avoid getting .5 per cent
fatter per annum as you get on in years. This slowdown sets off a
vicious circle; fat tissue has a somewhat lower basal metabolic rate
than bone, muscle, and organ tissues do, so the fatter you get the
more of this metabolically lazy tissue you have to contend with and
the less metabolically active tissue there is left to contend with it. It
is of course in the nature of a vicious circle to go on and on, and
this one can only be interrupted by either subtracting calories from
the system or adding activities to it. Adding thyroxin itself is not,
apparently, the answer, unless there is a gross and obvious thyroid
deficiency to begin with; otherwise, the added thyroxin from outside sources simply cues the body to turn its own output down accordingly in response.

Actually, obese people often have elevated, rather than lowered,
basal metabolic rates, as a direct result of the added protein that is
part of the enlarged fat cells their bodies contain (as well as whatever added muscle and connective tissue they may have had to
produce over the course of time to keep all the added fat tissue in
working order). In other cases, especially those where the genes are
simply not programmed to provide bigger and better muscles in the
first place, or where life is too sedentary to produce them in the
second place, the ratio of fat to lean tissue may exert a significant
brake on metabolism itself and the result is a low basal metabolic
rate that may be mistakenly ascribed to thyroid deficiency.

Once doctors came to understand that it is probably the fat in the
obese person's body composition that lowers over-all basal metabolism, and not the other way around, they generally gave up the
somewhat self-defeating practice of prescribing thyroid extract to
overweight patients in hopes of speeding up metabolism and increasing fat mobilization from the adipose tissue stores. Most peo-

ple left to their own devices have more or less steady thyroid hormone outputs no matter how fat or lean they are; this varies as a function of age, health, and other imponderables, but substituting an artificial supply of thyroid hormones for a natural one might well have exactly the opposite effect from the one intended and end up by progressively shutting down production in the gland itself in increasingly easy stages.

In addition to its general role in heating up energy reactions inside the cell, thyroid hormone seems to play a more localized role in the gut, by increasing glucose absorption through the intestinal wall, so that more sugar becomes immediately available to the liver and the circulating blood. This is probably a side effect of thyroxin's major function as an oxygen booster, but the result is no less dramatic for all that; and because this effect is involved in the basic biochemistry of the cells it comes as something of a surprise to learn that there are certain organs left totally unaffected by the thyroid hormones: in the brain, the retina, and the testes, oxygen uptake seems to be immune to the gross effects of too much or too little thyroid hormone, posing an interesting physiological (and evolutionary) riddle still to be plumbed.

Another important function of the thyroid hormones is to promote tissue growth and physical maturation. One of the first indications doctors have of thyroid deficiency in a young child is failure to grow properly. Bones and central-nervous-system tissue are in the high-risk category here. Depending on what age the child or baby may have been when the deficiency developed, the bones may have stopped growing, hair may be scanty, and mental functioning may be below par. If caught early enough all these effects can be reversed by giving the child thyroid hormones. In adults the same general sort of thing can occur, but since growth is not still going on the damage is less global, less noticeable, and less direct.

Possibly one way of understanding the dramatic effect thyroxin and tri-iodothyronine have on growth is that they seem to work in tandem with another hormone which directly governs the rate at which phosphorus and calcium become available to the bones for uptake into the soft cartilaginous parts of the bone that are still actively lengthening. This hormone is specific for tissue growth—not fat—and has been called growth hormone in recognition of that fact. Also, although it affects all tissues, growth hormone seems to play an especially important role in protein transfer from blood to muscle cells: Animals injected with growth hormone transfer nutrients from their blood into their muscles much faster than uninjected animals do, and presumably than they normally would. Too much growth hormone therefore, as might be expected, produces outright gigantism. This feature of growth hormone, taken together with its bone-building qualities, would seem to make it the elective hormone of muscle men and circus giants; and conceivably the gene or genes that code for relative amounts of growth hormone could account for family and even group (or race) differences in body size. But however this hormone actually does its work, it seems to need thyroid hormones to be fully effective: When the pituitary gland (where growth hormone is secreted) is surgically removed, the animal can function normally with daily doses of growth hormone—but only if the thyroid gland itself is still intact and functioning.

For purposes of obesity, though, the salient aspect of growth hormone is its role in fat mobilization—a role so striking that confusion still reigns as to whether growth hormone itself, or some submolecule of it, may not constitute a specific, ad hoc fat-fighting hormone whose absence spells obesity and whose presence confers svelteness. The pharmacological dream of a fat-control pill as reliable and easy to take as the birth control pill is one that has kept many endocrinologists working late nights in the labs for decades; the last enthusiasts to be heard from are the human chorionic gonadotrophin promoters, whose research, first publicized in Italy, burst on the public in the pages of fashionable women's magazines in the sixties and still seems to be finding favor in various get-thin-quick programs today. If there is something to be said for human chorionic gonadotrophin as a fat mobilizer, though, that something may be nothing more or less miraculous than its molecular resemblance to growth hormone, of which it constitutes what biochemists call an active analogue. (A word of caution is in order here: Aside from the undisputed fat-mobilizing action of growth hormone and its chemical analogue, chorionic gonadotrophin, it also has the property of promoting excessive connective tissue growth, and could thus have an unfortunate effect on cartilage in the face, the earlobes, and the hands; while in adolescents and young adults who may still be growing the effect on bone growth itself might conceivably amount to a lot more than the would-be weight loser had ever bargained for.)

Growth hormone is, as the name implies, the hormone that governs actual growth; without it we would all be dwarves; too much of it and we would be giants. The genes that code for height and bone size probably act through growth hormone; but growth hormone does not magically disappear from the bloodstream as soon as we reach maturity—the pituitary glands of middle-aged and old people secrete growth hormone too. Something in the target cells seems to turn the tissue-building action off after a certain age; but the hormone itself continues to circulate, and incidentally to mobilize fat from storage, as long as the organism goes on living, and as long as there is still fat to be mobilized. Growth-hormone deficiency in children results in dwarfism and delayed sexual maturation; in adults it is more likely to result in an excess accumulation of fat. Insufficient protein in the diet can result in a growth-hormone deficiency, as it can in the deficiency of any of the protein-based hormones (including glucagon, insulin, and a host of hormones manufactured in the pituitary which determine when and how much of the sex steroids and adrenal hormones are to be manufactured), a point that should be noted by dieters, especially the more enthusiastic ones.

An interesting peculiarity of growth hormone is that it is usually excreted during sleep, and sleeplessness of any great length of time may therefore curb its release. (Jet fatigue may therefore have pernicious effects on the waistline, and so may long-term insomnia.) And, as with insulin, there is evidence that obese people respond differently to growth hormone than normal people do; J. Roth and his colleagues have shown that under conditions that would normally trigger growth hormone release (i.e., rapid fall in blood glucose, prolonged fasting, and hard physical activity) some obese adults fail to respond with the normally expected growth hormone rise. The well-known inability of many obese subjects to mobilize free fatty acids under strenuous fasting conditions may have something to do with this abnormal growth hormone response. Interestingly, according to adolescent obesity specialist Felix Heald, this lack is not observed in obese adolescents, but only in obese adults—suggesting that adolescent obesity may indeed be more amenable to correction than adult obesity is, a viewpoint that was once enshrined in folk wisdom as the belief that obesity in adolescents was just "baby fat" and nothing much to worry about—and one which may therefore merit some judicious latter-day rehabilitation as fact.

It has become useful in recent years to look at the body as a great information-processing system: Compared to the giant multiterminal computers of major universities and industries, the human body itself represents a miniaturized computer miracle, running on closely printed instructions from the genes, preprogrammed from conception, and self-edited throughout a person's life-span. The sun comes up; we yawn, stretch, and get out of bed. Skin temperature drops, cueing the hypothalamus to send out a call for more heat from the thyroid gland; thyroxin floods the system, oxygen burns in the cells, and slowly but surely the body thermostat climbs back up to 98.6°. This is only the first hormonal chamber music of the day. Other environmental cues provoke other, equally complicated and minutely self-calibrating hormonal responses.

One of the most dramatic examples of this kind of information relay—from the real world to the skin, from the skin to the brain, from the brain to the hormones, and from hormones to the blood plasma and out into the vast living, breathing computer network of the living body—is the so-called flight-or-fight response: the famous behavioral syncope in which we either freeze or take to our heels in response to sudden danger perceived in the outside world. Epinephrine and norepinephrine are the hormones secreted by the inner part of the adrenal glands to organize action in the face of clear and present danger—well before the brain has really had time to come up with a thoughtful, well-reasoned response of its own. The effect of that sudden surge of epinephrine in the blood is to damp down the action in the bones, gut, and skin, and shift blood to the muscles, nerves, heart, and brain itself. In the liver gene action is speeded up. RNA, the substance which codes for cell activity, doubles in liver cells in response to adrenal hormones; glucose storage and extraction goes into high gear as the organism prepares for emergency supplies to the nervous system for flight or fight. All this activity requires fuel; and with digestion and feeding closed down for the emergency, the body must call on its own fuel stores for processing into back-up energy supplies. Epinephrine is the hormone that does the job, by its specific and almost instantaneous action on the fat stored up in adipose tissue cells.

Cold, pain, anxiety, stress, glucose hunger, and hemorrhage all have the same effect. All activate epinephrine (and/or norepinephrine); and research suggests that it is the intensity of the effect, rather than its actual psychological import, that calls the adrenal hormones into high gear. Epinephrine appears in all vertebrates and in some invertebrates as well, and it is chemically interchangeable across species, suggesting its relative antiquity in biological life. Although it is apparently not absolutely essential for day-to-day life, the organism has no way of responding to emergencies, or to extremes of heat and cold, emotional crises, or sudden spurts of hard work without it; and it would therefore seem to be essential for all but the most blissful and uneventful of lives. Histamine, acetylcholine (a brain neurohormone), morphine, and trauma all stimulate epinephrine release; all therefore may indirectly trigger fat release from storage, too. Nicotine has exactly the same effect on epinephrine release, and people who stop smoking therefore may have a hormonal as well as behavioral reason for gaining weight.

There may be easier ways to trigger fat release, however. R. Cleghorn and his colleagues have shown that free fatty acids in the circulating blood can rise by a full 286 per cent in response to stress—and the stress need not be life-threatening, either: a stressful interview, a tough oral exam, having a vein punctured for blood tests, or even just thinking about work to be done can do the trick. Mediating the resulting release of free fatty acids from adipose tissue depots is epinephrine; fat people may draw their own conclusions about how much anxiety they care to put up with in the course of a day's occupation.

Anger, incidentally, may or may not have quite the same effect on adipose tissue as fear. In a series of fascinating studies on psychiatric patients, using medical students as a presumably nonpsychotic control group, D. H. Funkenstein discovered that paranoid schizophrenics, whose emotional tone is one of rage and suspicion about their fellow men, tend to have significantly greater norepinephrine than epinephrine levels in their blood. On the other hand, psychotic patients—in whom anxiety, rather than anger, is presumably the major emotion—produced significantly more epinephrine than norepinephrine in response to stress. To find out whether this hormonal difference was specific for the person or just for his mood of the moment, Albert Ax conducted experiments in which perfectly normal persons were selectively either angered or scared. The results showed that norepinephrine in a given subject tended to be related to anger; the same subject responded to the feeling of fright, on the other hand, with raised levels of epinephrine in the blood. Although other investigators have challenged some of the specifics of these studies, it would seem for the time being that a fair case could be made for the hypothesis that epinephrine is the hormone of fear, while norepinephrine is the hormone of anger. A particularly charming bit of research in this field involved the relative preponderance of the two hormones in ice-hockey players, and produced the finding that goalies tended to have higher epinephrine counts while their more ostentatiously bellicose teammates had higher norepinephrine titres.

Norepinephrine, incidentally, is chemically and molecularly a precursor of epinephrine, and whether there are any conclusions to be drawn from this molecular happenstance for the (psychological) primordiality of rage over the (biological) primordiality of fear—or vice versa—remains to be seen. The puzzle this poses has interesting tie-ins with the question of hunger and feeding; norepinephrine receptors in the hypothalamus can stimulate an animal to feed or stop feeding, depending on the amount of hormone they happen to be binding at any one time. Nature, in fine, seems to have worked out the circuitry for anger and/or fear so as to cut in on the circuits for hunger and satiety—or at least to operate at the same voltage and amperage as the latter—an interesting bit of brain-body wiring that will be dealt with in more detail in a later chapter.

The same thing could be said equally accurately about the circuitry that involves release of fat from adipose tissue deposits in response to emotional cues. In experiments with medical students and psychotics (a classical couple of paired opposites for this sort of research, incidentally) Cleghorn had found that although fear is an excellent fat releaser, anger itself plays no such useful role in the mechanics of releasing free fatty acids from adipose tissue cells: Dieters may draw their own inferences from this conclusion, and count to ten or not as they see fit.

Epinephrine and norepinephrine are produced in the medulla, or inner part, of the adrenal gland; the cortex, or outer part, may have its own role to play in body-weight regulation too, but if so it is a somewhat subtler one. Aldosterone, a hormone produced by the adrenal cortex, is intimately involved in sodium and potassium balance in and between the cells, and affects weight mainly through its effect on the amount of water held in the body so as to keep these elements in proper equilibrium with each other. Too much salt can affect fat deposition as well as body weight: High sodium counts at the cell walls seem to markedly improve the cell's ability to take up glucose, so that the more salt available to the tissues, the more likely they are to incorporate whatever sugar may be on hand too—a good thing for people with a weakness for foods like peanut brittle or cheesecake (which are almost as long on salt as they are on sugar) to keep in mind.

ACTH (adrenocorticotrophic hormone) is manufactured in the pituitary and governs the production of the adrenal cortical hormone cortisol. It exists in all vertebrates, with slight chemical differences from species to species, and its molecular structure suggests that it is subject to considerable individual variation between one person and another, since only twenty-three of its grand total of thirty-nine amino acids are directly responsible for its physiological action. ACTH is an insulin antagonist; deficiency of ACTH can therefore cause increased sensitivity to insulin, resulting in more glucose being transported across the cell walls, and hence greater overall storage of sugars, proteins, and fats. ACTH deficiency symptoms include sluggish pituitary function (with resulting skin pallor, infertility, growth failure), frigidity and impotence, and low blood sugar. The strong pull exerted by ACTH on available supplies of Vitamin C may explain why Vitamin C itself seems to act in some ways as an insulin antagonist and (indirectly) as a fat mobilizer: The greater the available supply of Vitamin C, the more copious the ACTH output is apt to be, and the resulting restraint on insulin production—which works to the dieter's obvious advantage—may therefore depend on the amount of Vitamin C the organism can lay claim to—albeit in a very roundabout fashion.

Last but not least in this complex array of hormones and hormonelike substances that affect the body's ability to gain and lose weight, and the ease with which it manages to do either, is a substance that has had a sort of now-you-see-it, now-you-don't history in the annals of hormone research: to wit, the so-called fat-mobilizing hormone (FMH in endocrinological shorthand). Beginning in the 1930's a flurry of important inquiries seems to have set biochemists off on the trail of an elusive fat-mobilizing substance in the pituitary glands (and urine) of various mammal species, including rats, pigs, and man. This substance, which first came to endocrinologists' attention in the anterior pituitary glands of cattle and later was also gleaned from the pituitaries of hogs, rats, and human beings, showed up reliably as well in the urine of animals who had been starved or severely fasted for a period of at least 24 hours. Various names were suggested for this new discovery. Adipokinin, lipotropin, and fat-mobilizing hormone are among the many suggestions, and the failure to establish a nomenclatural consensus about it reflects as clearly as anything else can do the even more basic failure to establish the substance's unique molecular and biological identity at all.

Among endocrinologists, though, there seems to be fairly widespread agreement that some lipotropic (i.e., fat-burning) hormone manufactured in the anterior pituitary gland of most mammals does exist, and that it gets produced in large quantities during the early days of a fast; that once it gets mobilized it acts to release fat from adipose tissue depots under the skin; and that it has the paradoxical effect of putting a strong brake on appetite, thereby acting very much as a sort of innate, homegrown amphetamine of the body's own devising. This effect may have something to do with the hunger-free state some people report during the first few days of a strenuous diet, just when, to all intents and purposes, they should be feeling their worst hunger pangs; and there is evidence that in the obese this mysterious factor works poorly—if at all. This may be one of the reasons the fat get fatter, and stay fatter longer, than other people do: their adipose tissues may simply be less responsive to this house brand of anorectic than other people's fat depots are.

There is evidence both pro and con regarding this hypothesis. For example, J. A. Stevenson and his co-workers found that in obese rats who became ravenous when appetite centers in the brain were surgically damaged, an injection of FMH got a much better response than it did in normal rats, as measured by the increase in blood levels of free fatty acids. In man, on the other hand, T. M. Chalmers, A. Kekwick, and G. L. Pawan found that in six obese patients with general anterior pituitary deficiency, a three days' regimen of 1,000 calories per day (90 per cent of it in the form of fat) failed to produce any appreciable amounts of FMH in the urine at all.

The first published reference to the mysterious fat-mobilizing hormone seems to have seen the light of day in 1930, in a report on the effects of a beef pituitary extract on laboratory rats; when injected with extracts of this substance from the pituitary glands of cattle, laboratory rats responded with release of fat from storage and, accordingly, with high levels of free fatty acids in the blood. Two years later a similar study showed much the same effect in rabbits, and meanwhile, in 1931, the German endocrinologist H. Schäfer had made the appropriate connection between the increase in blood and liver fat and the decrease in adipose tissue fat that was being seen in the various species of animals tested. An interesting aside from these early experiments was that the animals who received injections of the pituitary substance in question seemed to be eating less than the animals who received no such injections; whatever the substance was, it appeared to have a marked effect on appetite. Further experiments confirmed the original finding that there was indeed something in the pituitary extract being investigated that acted on adipose tissue to release fat, and on the brain to inhibit feeding in the process.

Other interesting findings began to pile up on the heels of the earlier ones. Chalmers, Kekwick, and Pawan found that reducing carbohydrates in the diet was at least as important as reducing calories in inducing FMH activity: With diets of 1,000 calories a day or their equivalents, FMH began to come into play only when carbohydrate intake was less than 100 grams, and went up progressively as carbohydrate intake went down.

Another fascinating but somewhat puzzling fact that happened to surface in the course of the ongoing experimentation was that injection with the pituitary extract seemed to reduce blood calcium levels in injected animals to very low, and possibly even dangerous, values. (Since calcium and magnesium are among the minerals which govern muscle contraction—including the rhythmic contractions of the heart muscle—dieters would therefore perhaps be well advised to up their calcium intake if they are going to reduce their carbohydrate calories drastically and thereby activate FMH.)

For the next few decades biochemists and endocrinologists addressed themselves to the painstaking task of isolating the active factor in the pituitary-gland extract that was having such a remarkable effect on their lab animals' fat reserves. Although FMH seems to exist quite widely throughout the species that have been tested for it so far, there appear to be important molecular differences between species with respect to this hormone: FMH from pigs works well, for example, on rabbits and guinea pigs, but not on rats or mice. The pituitary gland in all animals sits at the base of the brain and secretes at least six recognized hormones whose individual action is so powerful that in some cases their specific effects can be registered when even as little as one part of the hormone is present in 20 million parts of whatever solution it is dissolved in. By extensive biochemical assay of this kind, D. Rudman and F. Seidman determined in 1958 that the hypothesized fat-mobilizing substance was molecularly and physiologically distinct from any of the other six familiar active hormones already known to be secreted by the pituitary gland (i.e., growth hormone, thyroid-stimulating hormone, adrenocortical hormone—ACTH—and the three gonad-stimulating hormones, prolactin, luteinizing hormone, and follicle-stimulating hormone). But whether the new substance constituted a genuinely new molecular entity or, alternatively, did not simply mark the action of two or more previously known hormones triggered into acting together in a new way by the onset of starvation (or by exercise itself, as J. Roth and his co-workers at the Bronx Veterans' Administration Hospital determined in 1963) remained pretty much up in the air.

Some investigators believed staunchly that what was involved was a newly discovered and hitherto wholly unknown substance; other researchers had their doubts, and began to adduce evidence that the new substance was in fact some biochemical variant of growth hormone itself. Both Zvi Laron in Israel and O. Trygstad in Sweden, though using different chemical assay methods, found that by breaking down the growth hormone molecule with various mechanical devices and chemical agents, they could produce a substance which was a much more powerful fat releaser than ordinary growth hormone alone; whether this was the elusive "new" hormone itself could not for the moment be proclaimed with any real certainty. But with this new finding the burden of proof has shifted to the positivists in the other camp and, as matters stand now, the general consensus among clinical (as opposed to molecular) endocrinologists seems to be that the mysterious fat-mobilizing substance is to be considered a kind of maverick growth-hormone variant, unless and until somebody can come along to prove the contrary. If and when they do, the medical and pharmaceutical sweepstakes promise to be high.

Incidentally, the recent diet fashion of using human chorionic hormone extract to bring about weight reduction, while much decried by responsible physicians, banks on the fact that a fetal form of growth hormone found in the placenta of newborn babies acts as a powerful fat mobilizer when injected into the blood of grown-ups. The so-called chorionic factor has a nomenclatural and molecular history almost as fuzzy as that of the hypothetical FMH itself, and may, on closer analysis, prove to be (as may FMH) some special variant of growth hormone too and not a hormone in its own right. (One argument against this theory, and in favor of the quiddity of the new substance, is that both it and human chorionic gonadotrophin have the curious property—unlike growth hormone—of cutting appetite dramatically, even when calories are drastically curtailed, although some skeptics have suggested that this appetite-suppressing effect may be due to nothing more or less exotic than ketosis. In ketosis, incompletely burned fat molecules in the bloodstream have been known to induce nausea, perhaps in much the same way and of much the same sort as that queasiness we may feel after eating a high-fat meal, since in both cases—albeit for exactly opposite reasons—the blood is temporarily full of incompletely metabolized fats.)

The difficulty in both cases may, however, turn out to be semantic as well as biochemical. Growth is something that apparently takes place and can only take place in the presence of a certain back-up amount of fat; hence the poor growth records of children in the poverty areas of the world. The fat-mobilizing aspect of FMH may thus be entirely secondary, at least from Nature's point of view, to the tissue growth and repair that is the original purpose for which the fat is being mobilized. As diet faddists and would-be ectomorphs, we may all have blinded ourselves to the real purpose of those unwanted bulges under our skin: They are there to make sure that we have something to live on and make repairs with when there is nothing else in the form of food coming in for that purpose from the environment.

Growth and fat may be all one thing to Nature (there is some evidence that even in acute starvation the body will still hang on to some last modicum of fat and sacrifice muscle tissue in the process to preserve it), but they are of course two totally different things to the harassed dieter (and his or her physician)—as different, in fact, as night and day; as different for that matter as guilt and self-esteem. Perhaps if we could reach the synthesis in our semantics that our bodies seem to have mastered in their physiology, we could accommodate our minds to the idea of a substance that manages the neat trick of burning fat in order to build other tissues up. If and when we do, the tantalizing hairline between "growth" hormone, on the one hand, and "fat-mobilizing hormone," on the other, may go the way of all other unnecessary mental baggage as well. In the meantime, though, we have no choice but to live with the paradox as it stands—or to live with it, at least, until the biochemists tell us differently, once and for all, by announcing the distinctive molecular structure of the hypothetical new hormone and synthesizing it successfully in their laboratory retorts.

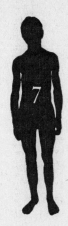

7 *Physiology:*
"Ventrem Omnipotentem"

—Rabelais

The idea of using fat for fuel did not begin with man and mammals. Almost from the beginning of life on earth, fat has had a handy biological role to play as a means of storing reserve fuel supplies for organisms programmed to make their livings on the move. This statement is no less true for plants than it is for animals. Stationary plants store their nutritional reserves in the form of carbohydrates; but plants that depend on scattering and reseeding to reproduce themselves use lipids to nourish the next generation's germ cells just as animals do: seeds, pollens, and nuts all store their reserves in the form of fat.

By the same token, larval forms of certain insects may carry a grand total of 90 per cent of their weight around in lipid form; locusts and monarch butterflies, for example, prepare for the long-distance migrations on which their species' destinies depend by orgies of preflight feeding—and fat deposition—that can last for several days. Among birds, the long-distance migrators may fatten themselves up by a factor of 25 to 30 per cent in the space of a week before striking out across lakes, inland seas, and great intercontinental bodies of water toward their winter quarters. And salmon returning from the ocean to their ancestral spawning grounds upriver may swim at a rate of 52 miles a day, against countercurrents, rapids, and cataracts; they do not stop to feed during their journey but draw entirely on their stored lipid reserves to sustain them in their literally uphill flight against gravity, rocks, and river currents. Sharks, another order of long-distance swimmers, store fat in their livers for the long haul. The weight of a shark's liver as it sets out on a journey can account for fully one quarter of the animal's total body mass, and the shark may weigh in with a lipid content of as much as 90 per cent at the time it embarks.

Except for camels (who, to quote one observer, must be among the bearers of one of the largest and most impressive fat organs in the natural world), higher forms of vertebrates tend to store their fat less locally than fishes do, so that, in many familiar species at least, fat ends up being distributed all over the body more or less evenly (except in the limbs and extremities, where it might interfere with locomotion). But in the process of spreading out under the skin, fat seems to take on new uses and begins to serve functions which it may not originally have been intended for in the evolutionary scheme of things. With a solid girdle of fat under the skin and around parts of the viscera, insulation and even active heat production may now handily be added to fat's primary use as a storage depot. George Cahill suggests that in view of the metabolic give and take that is always going on inside active fat tissue, the layer of fat that exists between our innards and our skin should be characterized not so much as a thermal interlining, but as a kind of electric blanket with a cellular power supply and voltage of its own.

In animals that spend long hours in punishingly cold environments (whales, Alaskan fur seals, and Japanese pearl divers to name a few), the storage function of fat may be equaled or even surpassed by its tremendous thermal advantages. The bull of the Alaskan fur seal, for example, who leaves the frigid circumpolar water for two months of every year to breed, may lose up to 200 pounds of fat in the space of one short Alaskan summer on dry land; and when it comes to human beings, the notorious fleshiness of Easter Islanders and the original Hawaiians has been ascribed by anthropologist Carleton Coon to the fact that their life-styles involve spending considerable amounts of time in the chilly medium of sea water. The excellent showing of female Channel swimmers over and above male competitors may be due to a similar mechanism: Women's natural superiority in the matter of subcutaneous fat gives them a clear odds-on advantage in the cruelly cold waters between the Atlantic Ocean and the North Sea.

Whatever its thermal qualities may be, fat is ideally suited for the economics of fuel storage reserves by virtue of its unique nutritional cost-effectiveness. Gram for gram, there is almost twice as much nourishment in a unit of fat as there is in one of carbohydrate or protein. By the law of parsimony, fat is therefore clearly the biochemical medium of choice for storing the most energy in the least amount of space for animals and organisms that make their livings on the move.

Seen under the microscope, adipose tissue bears a touching resemblance to bubble bath. And, at slightly higher magnifications, like nothing so much as tapioca packed globule to globule in a stringy intercellular glue streaked with narrow filaments of connective tissue, blood vessels, and nerves. Waxing or waning as the case may be, human fat cells individually, and fat tissues in general, are admirably designed to provide a versatile living inner tube, inflatable or deflatable as required, with the minimum stress and strain both to the skin on the outside that encloses it and the viscera on the inside that it encloses.

Animals vary somewhat in the anatomical arrangements they may make between fat and other tissues, and the relationship between the skin, the fat, and the underlying muscles and fascia are rather distinctive in human beings. In most species (including most primate species other than man) fat and lean tissue are less adherent than they are in man, and Frederick Wood Jones has speculated that the difference may be due to man's hairlessness, and to the fact that fat is therefore virtually the only form of reliable built-in insulation man can depend on anatomically when the temperature drops. Other species have fur, feathers, and certain ingenious vascular blood-shunting devices in their bag of cold-weather tricks, but man (and some of his livestock—notably pigs) has virtually nothing between him and the elements but his fat and his skin, and this may be one of the reasons that fat adheres so stubbornly to underlying fascia in human beings.

(It is this adhesiveness, probably, that accounts for the kind of dimpling effect that has been dubbed "cellulite" in the annals of the reducing industry. The term has been applied to the puckering or dimpling of fat that occurs in the buttocks and thighs of overweight and usually middle-aged women, and has become such common coin that it would be pointless at this late date to try to expunge it from the dieter's vocabulary. Although there is no such word medically, the condition it has reference to is one that unfortunately can and does exist. What apparently happens in "cellulite," so-called, is that the ribbons of connective tissue which serve as pouches for large groups of fat cells in a sort of honeycomb arrangement underneath the skin lost their elasticity and shrink with age; the overlying skin which is attached to these fibers then contracts to measure, and, if the size of the fat cells encased in them does not shrink to match, a kind of overall dimpling occurs like the dimpling on the surface of a golf ball. The cure for this is simply to reduce the size of the empouched fat by dieting, and thereby shrink the fat cells inside their pockets of connective tissue back down to the limits of the shrunken connective fibers themselves—an undertaking that does not actually call for extraordinary measures like massage, excessive water intake, or peculiar diets; any good old-fashioned reducing regimen will do the trick.)

Within the human body, fat follows a growth curve, and has an interesting cellular history of its own. The precursors to the cells that will begin to fill up with fat toward the end of the nine-month gestation period, as the fetus comes closer and closer to the moment of getting born, are embryonic blood vessels; in fact, when totally emptied of their lipid reserves—as they may be in acute starvation, for example—fat cells may, according to F. Wassermann, go back to producing blood cells again, thereby reverting to basic embryological type. Fat itself, however, is one of the last kinds of tissues to be manufactured in intrauterine life. About halfway through development, in the normal course of events, when the fetus is around 150 days old, small flat lentil-shaped cells will begin to take form under the skin around the baby's shoulders and neck, and above the kidneys; but not until about the third week before birth will these cells actually round themselves out and begin to fill up with fat. If the baby is born prematurely these cells will not have had a chance to fill up, and the paradoxically ancient and wrinkled look that results will not go away until the baby's fat cells have caught up with the rest of his tissues in the developmental timetable.

Local fat pads around the baby's shoulder girdle, the breastbone, and the kidneys are the first to be laid down and probably the first to be used up in the normal course of postnatal life. They are somewhat darker than the fat in other parts of the baby's body, and have a richer blood supply than other fat does; this tissue, the so-called "brown fat" of all newborn mammals, seems to have a highly specific function to serve during the immediate postnatal period, and that function is largely a thermal one. At birth the baby has to leave a surrounding temperature of 98.6° F. and adapt to the prevailing room temperature of the nursery, the bedroom, or the birth hut as the case may be. Birth is a chilling experience, at least for the newborn; and Western culture doesn't help much by taking the baby away from its mother and putting it into a crib, far from the source of metabolic heat that it has been accustomed to for the better part of nine months. Brown fat apparently serves to bridge the gap between the temperature of the cozy intrauterine incubator and the cooler world beyond the womb; it is a form of fat that we have in common with most, if not all, of our mammalian kin on the Linnaean family tree, and animals (and presumably babies too) who are raised in less than thermally adequate postnatal environments tend to use up their brown fat stores much faster and more dramatically than those who are kept comfortably warm throughout the neonatal period.

Fat—either brown or white—is among the last tissues to be laid down in the developing fetus, and there is some question as to whether we come into the world with our full complement of fat cells all finished and assembled at birth, or whether overfeeding in infancy may not actually stimulate the infant's body to produce not only more fat, but also more fat cells to store the additional fat in as well. Research carried out by physicians Jules Hirsch and Jerome L. Knittle at Mount Sinai Hospital and Rockefeller Institute in New York seems to suggest that there is no fixed limit on the number of fat cells a baby can produce at birth, and that feeding the newborn infant above and beyond the minimum call of parental duty may cause his or her fat cells to divide exponentially, thus starting the baby off down the rocky road to adult obesity at an avoidably early age.

Hirsch and Knittle studied the fat pads of male laboratory rats whose brains had been surgically incised in an area called the hypothalamus, which is known to control feeding and satiety; rats lesioned in this part of the brain develop ravenous appetites and soon eat themselves into an obese state. The authors killed these animals at various stages in their postoperative careers and found that, as expected, all the lesioned animals had gained respectable amounts of weight and fat. But the gains were of two distinct kinds. In some of the animals there were abnormally high numbers of fat cells for this particular genetic strain; in others they found only the normal number of cells but each cell was enormously oversized. How much of the over-all surplus was due to increased numbers of fat cells, and how much was due to a simple increase in the size of the pre-existing cells, depended on the age at which the animal had first started to gorge. If the animal had been less than 15 weeks old when it was operated on, the number of its fat cells was grossly excessive; if the animal was operated on after 15 weeks, however, the resulting obesity was due to an increase in the size of each individual fat cell, with no over-all increase in the number of fat cells themselves.

Next, turning their attention to adult human beings, the authors found what they considered to be a very suggestive similarity between the "cellularity" of people who had been obese since childhood versus those who had gotten fat somewhat later in life. Fat people whose obesity dated back to the age of ten or earlier had significantly more fat cells than fat people whose obesity had a shorter history. The authors speculated that this difference could have stemmed from different early-life feeding experiences between the two groups just as it had in rats: The overfed child may be adding fat cells to his basic adipose tissue stock that no amount of self-restraint and will power later in life will ever be able to melt away. The underfed child, conversely, may get just as fat as the overfed one if he overeats when he grows up, but dieting will bring him back within reasonable adipose bounds in short order.

Hirsch and Knittle's research on the "cellularity" of obesity first saw the light of day in medical journals in the sixties, and was almost immediately taken up by the popular press as a rallying cry for the dietmongers, for its implications meshed nicely with the therapeutic and social-science orthodoxies of the moment. During the fifties and sixties it had become increasingly fashionable to blame children's chubbiness on their parents, just as it had been the fashion in an earlier day to blame the hapless parents for their children's skinniness. This position was not without difficulties of its own; anyone who has ever watched an overeager mother force-feeding a balky infant (or trying to) cannot help having some doubts about the magnitude of the parent's role in this procedure, as opposed to the child's. More to the point, though, than the strong personal styles that undoubtedly exist in infants' eating habits is the fact that Hirsch and Knittle's theory rests to some extent on the anatomical and cellular maturation patterns of rats. But the cellular development of rats follows a timetable quite different from that of humans and other primates. Unlike human beings, according to D. B. Cheek, the deposition of fat in rats is normally delayed until just before puberty in both sexes; while in human beings fat, as we have seen, begins to be deposited one month to three weeks before birth, increases to its maximum velocity at twelve months, and is normally quite completed at three years. After that, any increase in the fat complement of the body is due to an increase in fat-cell size—with perhaps some additional cells being formed at or just before puberty.

The rat model may therefore not be appropriate when it comes to adipose-tissue growth in man. This is not to say that overfeeding in infancy may not have other untoward effects on human shape and size, including speeding up the maturation rate and stimulating certain hormonal subsystems that may lead to trouble with fat metabolism later in life. But much of human growth research seems to point to the conclusion that overnutrition early in life has at least as great an effect on organ size—and hence on stature and general robustness—as it does on adiposity itself.

Meanwhile, the carefully controlled studies of identical twins raised on different dietary regimes that would be the only way of proving or disproving Hirsch and Knittle's conclusions are not being, and probably never will be, undertaken. This is because, given today's antifat *Zeitgeist,* no respectable pediatrician steeped in the orthodoxies of our day and age is apt to recommend overfeeding a baby in the interests of basic research, any more than pediatricians of an earlier era might have prescribed underfeeding for the same purpose. In the meantime, generalizing from rats to humans in this as in many other areas of scientific research remains an iffy undertaking; similar as the two species may be in their eating habits, social life, and demographic histories their actual physical growth patterns and tissue morphologies may be too dissimilar to provide useful analogues for each other in these particular instances.

As we saw earlier, there are age, sex, and ethnic differences governing the amount of subcutaneous fat an individual is born with and may have to reckon with on an anatomical basis throughout the rest of his life. Adipose tissue has a life cycle of its own. Starting with a very slight lead in infancy, girls outmeasure boys in amount of trunk and limb fat at birth and continue to do so as they get older, until, at adolescence, their adipose tissue depots—at least in the arms and legs and across the back—are roughly double that of boys. (This is especially true in Caucasoids.) Women, in this country at least, go on depositing fat until well into their fifties; men reach their maximum weights (and their maximum proportional amounts of fat) between the ages of 35 and 54. Since muscle tissue in both sexes probably stops proliferating sometime around the end of adolescence or the early twenties, the presumption is that any weight gain in adult life is apt to represent a net increase in the fat content of the individual, rather than any increment in lean tissue mass.

The increase of fat with age seems to be a world-wide phenomenon, and since it is one that shows up in relatively economically depressed, "thin" cultures as well as nutritionally lavish, "fat" ones, it may have more to do with species-wide physiological aging processes than with either cultural or economic ones. Fat can be a useful appendage in older people who have to hunt or swim for a living, and may also provide them with some margin of nutritional safety when they are no longer as agile and competent at these skills as they were in their younger days. (One curious reversal of this pattern of increasing fat with age is apparent in the Witoto of the Amazon River basin, but this may be the exception that proves the rule: according to Nicole Maxwell, Witoto children run to fat in childhood and are given the leaves of a mysterious medicinal plant to chew on at the first sign of chubbiness; as a result they rarely grow up to be fat as adults.)

Metabolism falls off slowly from age 20 onward at a rate of about .5 per cent a year, and active bone, muscle, and organ tissue decreases accordingly. Unfortunately, therefore, just maintaining the same weight throughout adult life and middle age, even for those who are lucky enough to manage it, is tantamount to increasing the relative amount of fat versus lean tissue in a given person's body. Unless you are prepared to weigh some 10 percent less in your middle years than you did at the end of puberty, the chances are that you are going to be considerably fatter at age 45 than you were at age 20, even if you weigh exactly the same as you did then. Unfortunately this arithmetic applies to men as well as women; the male hormone androgen stimulates muscle growth and is probably one of the major causes for the preponderance of sheer brawn in men vis-à-vis women in the younger age groups. But both men and women manufacture androgen in varying amounts throughout life, and by about the sixth decade of life the two sexes are much more evenly matched hormonally than they will have been at any time since preadolescence. Their skin-fold caliper readings go up accordingly, signifying an increase in trunk and limb fat for both sexes; their creatinine excretion rates go down at the same time, signifying a concomitant loss of lean tissue. The implications of this increasing parity are that men at middle age begin for the first time in their lives to be almost as fat prone as women.

"The organism," writes Jacques Monod, "is a self-constructing machine." We go on putting ourselves together and taking ourselves apart on a lifetime basis; physiologically, we are in constant chemical ferment all our lives. This means that tissues are never static, even after they have stopped growing and the organism has reached its adult, "finished" form. Even the unyielding and undeformable bone tissue that seems to hold it all together is constantly breaking down and being re-formed around its own axis; and one half of the protein in the liver is turned over regularly and completely every seven days.

Paradoxically fat, which grows and diminishes visibly within measurable units of time and space, is one of the least metabolically active of all the tissues in our bodies. Compared to most other tissues it has fewer nerve endings in its cells and uses less oxygen to maintain itself than other tissues do; when we reckon its energy turnover relative to other kinds of body tissues, fat turns out to have a specific basal metabolic rate of some 5 per cent less than lean tissue does. This relative inertia is now usually called upon to explain the sometimes low basal metabolism of the obese. Theoretically the basal metabolism of obese people should be much higher than normal (and often it is) since they have *in toto* so much more tissue to carry around with them and maintain than people of normal size do. Depending on the ratio of lean tissue to fat in an obese person's body, though, basal metabolism can be either abnormally low or abnormally high. At one time it was generally assumed that low basal metabolic rate was the precipitating factor in obesity itself; but now it seems much more likely that the low metabolic readings of the obese—if and when they do occur—may be an artifact of the low energy output of their fat tissue itself; if fat people did not have so much adipose tissue to lower their over-all scores, their basal metabolic readings would quickly revert to normal, or so the theory goes.

But although fat cells exchange energy more slowly and stingily with the rest of the organism than other kinds of cells do, it would be unwarranted to conclude that the exchange is minimal or nil; the system is in a constant state of metabolic give and take with the organism as a whole. Fat is always being stored with the right hand and withdrawn from storage with the left; the two processes involved in this exchange take different pathways, and obesity and thinness would seem to add up less to a straight-line equation between input and output than to a constant trade-off between deposits and withdrawals. Some of us are more efficient fat storers than others; some of us are more efficient fat burners; and the difference depends on a complicated mix of variables, including genes, activity levels, age, hormones, nerves—and, of course, food intake itself.

It is the rallying cry of overweight patients in the diet doctors' waiting rooms that everything they eat goes to their hips; today's spaghetti dinner is tomorrow's middle-age spread, a conversion so predictable that if we didn't know any better by now we might naïvely assume it was a simple expression of the law of gravity, as at least one wit has suggested. But the facts are not so simple, and much of current nutrition research has focused on the details of that inevitable trajectory. If it remains unarguable that the food we eat does indeed take the straightest line it can from the mouth to the hips or the belly, it is still a matter of some clinical interest to determine just how it gets there, how long it takes to do so, and why.

Energy—physical energy—is produced by fission. On a grand scale this process is the one that is visible in the ill-famed mushroom cloud of an atomic explosion; on a microscopic scale the same sort of thing is always going on inside us, where enzymes tirelessly trigger the oxidation and breakdown of the various hydrocarbon chains our foodstuffs are made of. Inside our bodies the fissioning process is small-scale, invisible, and noiseless; but in both cases the physical end product of this fission is energy—either in the form of heat, pure and simple, or in the form of chemical energy that powers muscles and nerves.

The ability to raise body temperature through feeding is one that is shared by all warm-blooded animals. Cattle, swine, rats, goats, and U.S. Army men all eat more when the temperature is low than when it is high, and the reverse is equally true: at environmental temperatures of 90° F. feeding begins to slow down in all these animals, and by the time rectal temperatures reach 104° (which is not an unheard-of reading, incidentally, for a man doing strenuous exercise for more than a few minutes at a time) virtually all species stop feeding entirely. This state of affairs is true not only for man and other homeotherms but for such disparate creatures as toads, single-celled paramecia, and honeybees (although the critical temperature maximum for a honeybee may not be quite the same as it is for a toad—or, of course, a man).

Even in perfectly neutral thermal environments, though (i.e., environments in which the organism is neither gaining nor losing heat into the surrounding air), food has a marked effect on body temperature; the temperature difference between a fed animal and an unfed one in the same cage, in the same room, at the same time can vary by as much as one full degree F. This difference is due to what is called the specific dynamic action of food, and it varies a little—though not very much—according to what kind of food one eats. Eating proteins, which are somewhat more complicated to break down inside the body than carbohydrates or fats are, tends to raise body temperature very slightly more than these other two basic food components do. But this difference has probably received more attention than it deserves in the popular literature about nutrition; the point to remember is that all foods raise body temperature, and that, as Thoreau once put it, "the expression 'animal life' is nearly synonymous with 'animal heat.' "

Heat loss is, for this reason, one of the major occupational hazards of starvation. Ancel Keys put conscientious objectors on semi-starvation diets under carefully controlled conditions at the University of Minnesota in the 1940's, and found that even at the height of warm summer weather his subjects complained of the cold and slept with as many as two or three blankets on their beds at night. Other warm-blooded animals may have the same problem in cold weather; the Connecticut Audubon Society reports that on an empty stomach a bird like the chickadee will not be able to survive more than twelve hours at zero temperatures; while on a full stomach the same bird can make it through the night at temperatures of 40° below zero.

The thermal effect of the specific dynamic action of food tends to be somewhat less for large animals than it is for small ones; large animals have a greater body mass and a larger total tissue amount than small ones, and they therefore use up more oxygen per unit of surface area than small ones do. In the process, whatever minute rise in temperature may occur from ingesting and processing food itself may tend to get lost in the overall metabolic shuffle. Since the heat-monitoring part of the brain in the hypothalamus is finely attuned to variations in body temperature regardless of whether these variations are brought on by eating, by oxygen consumption through exercise, or by a local heat wave, a large animal's hypothalamus may not be able to draw quite as fine a line as a smaller one's will between the relatively minor signals coming to it from the digestive tract—with the result that the large animal may take much longer to feel satiated (or warmed up) than the smaller one does, and may therefore go on feeding longer than a smaller animal would be apt to do under the same set of thermal circumstances. Everything else being equal, this would be all to the good: Big animals need more food than small ones do and it is therefore advantageous for them to go on eating longer, and eat more at each sitting, than their smaller conspecifics would. Like all good systems, though, this one has its drawbacks, and one of them may be obesity.

One of the many ways in which fat people differ from the nonfat, as F. Rolly and others have shown, is that they seem to be much less responsive to the thermal effects of the specific dynamic actions of foods they are digesting than normal people are. In fact, a whole range of abnormal reactions to cold and heat have been brought to light in the obese: Fat people do not raise their basal metabolic rate in response to a drop in the environmental temperature as fast or as efficiently as nonfat people do, for example; this means that both food-induced temperature rises and cold-induced temperature drops are slow or feeble in the obese. The defect is probably an effect of the insulating capacity of fat tissue itself, which has such low thermal conductivity that it may take fat people up to ten times as long to lose body heat in response to a drop in the temperature as it does normal ones. M. B. Kreider, describing some of the vicissitudes of cryotherapy (a process in which patients' body temperatures are lowered to make them more receptive to cancer chemotherapy), reports the case of one extremely obese man who needed a total of twenty hours of precooling to get his body temperature down to the required 90° F., as opposed to the two- or three-hour period that the same procedure takes in normal people. By the same token, and perhaps for the same reasons, fat people do not release free fatty acids from adipose tissue depots in response to cold stress at the same rate and to the same extent as normal people do. But whatever the reason for the abnormal response, the result is that the obese person's hypothalamus is apt to have become insensitive to what may well be one of the major triggers to satiety in the mammal brain; and he may therefore go on eating long past the time when he has really had his fill.

Fat or thin, the body uses the heat generated by feeding to keep its thermostat satisfied at some species-specific optimum operating temperature; and it uses the energy produced in the process to get on with the day's work. That work may be as minimal as the effort invested in keeping the lungs inflating and deflating on schedule in a patient in a deep coma, or as stupendous as the effort required to move megaliths by hand across miles of difficult terrain for henge or pyramid building in Neolithic England or dynastic Egypt. But in either case the process is exactly the same, biochemically speaking. Food—whether recently ingested and therefore already in the alimentary pipeline, or stored away long ago for emergency use in the fat cells, or even (in a pinch) locked up in essential protein tissue in an otherwise calorie-depleted and effectively starving animal—will be continuously and ploddingly broken down into its chemical subcomponents, with the energy release in the process being converted to use for the body's next task, however big or small.

Here again, there are notable differences between the obese and the nonobese. Glucose injected into the forearm muscles of obese subjects has been shown to move into the muscle cells at a much slower rate than it does in nonobese subjects. On the other hand, oil injected into obese subjects disappears from the blood much faster than it does in nonobese people. M. Hetenyi interpreted his findings on the speedy disappearance of fats from his obese subjects' blood to mean that the fat he was injecting into them was going directly from the blood into the adipose tissue cells and thus bypassing the usual metabolic pathways. Taken together, findings like these suggest that the obese may be especially good at processing fat and especially bad at utilizing sugar in their muscles and other lean tissue cells—thereby putting them in obvious double jeopardy from the point of view of laying down new fat.

The intricately integrated chemical factory that our bodies consist of is on a 24-hour-a-day production schedule and requires a constant flow of energy to keep production going; but although mammals cannot spend their whole lives feeding, the daily biochemical show must go on, and the animal has got to have a constant supply of energy on tap regardless of whether or not it happens to have a full mouth or a full belly at just the particular moment when a specific molecule is needed to produce a new cell, lengthen an old one, or patch up an injured one. All animals therefore have to have some arrangement for reserve energy storage, whether it is external like the honey in the bee's hive, or internal, like the subcutaneous fat depots of mammals. For any given feed, therefore, a certain number of calories will be put to work right away for the organism's immediate metabolic needs. The brain and muscles run on glucose, and if it has been a long time between feeds, glucose extracted from the most recently eaten meal will bypass the usual storage conduits and go into immediate action in the bloodstream for delivery to the cells.

But almost any fair-sized meal will be apt to contain more calories than the organism actually needs at any given moment just to keep it going; and these extra calories will in the normal course of events follow the complicated food processing and sorting cycle all the way from the esophagus to the fat cells—which thus, gradually, day by day, will come to contain the infinitesimal (or, alas, not so infinitesimal) surpluses of the hundred or so square meals the animal may have eaten in the last days, weeks, or months. This process is daily, repetitive, and continuous, and it takes place in thin and normal-sized creatures just as it does in those who are visibly over-weight.

In the normal course of events, all food that enters the system is subject to some degree of processing in the digestive tract, and no matter what form the food first appears in, the liver, faced with short-term surpluses of any kind, will convert the supernumerary calories to fat and send them back into the blood for uptake by the adipose tissue. Some foods do go through the pipeline faster than others, though. The stomach, like a sort of static centrifuge, sepa-rates the three basic kinds of nutrients into concentric layers with fats outside, proteins next, and carbohydrates in the middle. Carbo-hydrates metabolize fastest and are the first to leave the stomach and enter the small intestine for uptake into the blood. A sweet or starchy meal therefore pacifies hunger faster (but less lastingly) than a meal that includes protein and fat. Proteins metabolize at a somewhat slower rate than carbohydrates do; while fats stay in the stomach long after the other two kinds of foodstuffs have found their way out of the stomach and into the duodenum. One of the most persuasive things that can be said for a balanced meal is, therefore, that everything else being equal, it tends to both kill hun-ger faster and keep it at bay longer than a meal that consists of only one kind of foodstuff to the exclusion of one or both of the others.

Minerals have a digestive timetable of their own. While we do not extract calories and energy from them, minerals are the not-so-incidental fellow travelers of almost all the foodstuffs we eat and, like the vitamins that have got to be on hand before most enzymes can go into action in the actual food-processing system, minerals are integral to cellular homeostasis and to the proper functioning of all organs in the body. Minerals are not involved in the food-processing cycle itself, though, except at the cellular level; most of them are therefore taken up by the tissues in almost exactly the same chemical form they were originally ingested in, and may show up in the tissues within minutes of being eaten. Potassium and iron, for example, can appear in the cells almost instantaneously. In one experiment, iron in cattle fodder was tagged with radioactive particles to make it traceable by scanner, and was shown to have taken only five minutes from the time it was ingested before it reappeared in measurable quantities in the cow's milk. By the same token, isotopes of sodium can show up in the sweat of the human hand in a little under seven minutes after eating.

Protein, on the other hand, must be carefully smelted down by the small intestine into its amino-acid subcomponents before the body can turn the meat, eggs, milk, fish, and other protein foods we eat to its own metabolic account. This process is begun in the stomach (where food is churned to a neutral, almost liquid mash) and completed in the small intestine; and while we don't know exactly how long the process actually takes, particles labeled to make them detectable by isotopic scanning devices can be picked up in the urine about 24 hours after the meat they were attached to was originally eaten. Nitrogen is a by-product of all animal proteins, and this time lapse probably represents a delay of some hours over actual uptake of other parts of the same protein meal by the tissues themselves. The protein from food cannot be stored in a metabolically useful form for more than about 24 hours at a time, and therefore a minimum daily intake is required to replenish the supply of essential amino acids that we need to have on hand on a daily basis.

Fats, which—like proteins—can in most cases only be taken up by the body after some tailoring to human metabolic needs, are the last to leave the stomach and tend to slow down digestion all along the line. A high-fat meal will load the blood with fat particles for some three to five hours after it was ingested, but the rate at which adipose tissue proceeds to extract fat from the blood and lymphatics, and incorporate it into the fat cells themselves, seems to vary a lot from individual to individual. How long it takes for a single fat globule to get all the way from the stomach, through the intestinal wall, and into the adipose cells is a matter of conjecture, but probably depends to some extent on hormone levels, muscular activity, and the general biorhythm of the individual involved.

The readiness of adipose tissue to clear fat particles from the blood and incorporate them into the adipose tissue cells is a highly personal matter too. At one extreme are those individuals who take up fat so fast and efficiently that the difference between a diet snack and a gourmet dinner shows up the next morning on the scales in the form of a real weight increment; at the other end of the continuum are those people who cannot store fat in their cells at all. As a result their blood is chronically full of dangerously high levels of lipids and cholesterol with no place to go except—probably—to the insides of the arteries, and to other organs where it is just as useless, if not downright dangerous. Obesity itself, far from being the cause of high blood-fat levels as it has sometimes been suggested, may in fact be a sort of desperate solution to the body's dire problem of extracting excess fat from the blood before it can damage the circulatory system, and stash it where it can do no harm—though the effort may be a self-defeating one in the long run. For the short run, however, the faster your body can remove fat from the circulation and set it aside in adipose-tissue cells, the less risk you may run of having that same fat end up on the inside of your arteries, interfering with normal blood flow and engendering high blood pressure and coronary infarcts in the process. (On a long-term basis, of course, the picture is somewhat cloudier; if overeating is chronic, the net result will be to keep blood lipids high on an intake basis anyway, and the consequences, in terms of arterial occlusions, will be just the same as if the adipose tissue were not doing its job of clearing fat from the blood.)

It should be emphasized that the fat we actually eat is not the only foodstuff that ends up being incorporated into the adipose tissue cells as lipids. Given the independence of the two simultaneous and ongoing processes of metabolism—breakdown of foodstuffs into their basic nutritional components on the one hand, and build-up of lipids for storage on the other—any food that is eaten that is in excess of the body's immediate caloric needs is going to end up as fat in the adipose tissue depots. This includes protein foods as well as carbohydrates and fats themselves; and it is just as true for thin people, moreover, as it is for fat people. In fact it makes very little difference to the body what chemical form the surplus comes *in* under; in the matter of energy storage it is quantity, not quality, that counts, and too much is too much, whatever chemical composition it may happen to have. "Too much" may need some redefinition too. Unless you happen to eat your luncheon sandwich while pole-vaulting or logrolling, the 500 or so odd calories that it contains are always "too much" for your body's particular needs at that particular moment, and some percentage of those calories is going to go the fat-building route through the liver and into the blood and adipose tissue. The body keeps its books on a two- or three-day basis, but probably does not keep running accounts of breakfast, lunch, and dinner deposits and withdrawals. There are therefore always likely to be temporary surpluses—and, if all goes normally, deficits and surpluses will balance out at the end of two or three days.

Depending on how much you eat, how many cells there are in your body, how fast those cells are dividing, wearing out, and building themselves back up, and how much or how little energy your particular body requires for running through the whole metabolic process from beginning to end, there will eventually be more or less fat left over for storage in the adipose tissue cells themselves. Fat build-up and fat breakdown take different energy pathways and use different chemical reagents to get their work accomplished. The two processes are nevertheless so similar that they were once thought to be simply inversions or mirror images of each other; it is now known, though, that they require quite different chemical reagents, as well as different reaction sequences, to play their respective roles. Physiologist David Green has made the interesting discovery that fat build-up requires manganese to complete its cycle; fat breakdown on the other hand uses magnesium at the same point in the inverse metabolic reaction.

This being so, it may help to understand why some of us are likely to be better fat builder-uppers, or synthesizers, while some of us are better fat dismantlers, or catabolizers, than others. Blood supply, nerve endings, and amounts and kinds of hormones are all implicated in the basic biochemistry by which the body converts food to fuel and stores the surplus as fat; and no two of us, unless we are identical twins, are apt to have the same quantities and qualities of these things on hand metabolically—nor the same foodstuffs in our diets for them to work on even if we did. Differences in ways of laying down fat are obvious even at the simple observational level of evidence. We all have our own unique fat patterns, idiosyncratic lumps and lean spots to which our bodies revert—sometimes maddeningly—according to their own genetic blueprints. These idiosyncrasies undoubtedly follow genetic programs which may or may not ever get carried out to the letter in real life, depending on how much we actually eat. Fat cannot form in areas of the body where there is no underlying adipose tissue to begin with; and where there is a lot of this underlying tissue it will tend to reach its own level like water in a container, if and when we overeat.

The actual mechanics of fat synthesis and breakdown are still being documented. When we gain weight we tend to gain weight all over our bodies, not just here and there; and although some parts of our bodies may have a disheartening tendency to fatten up before others (or even at the expense of others—a common-enough complaint of flat-chested women among others), still the process is always rigorously symmetrical: the extra inch that lands on one side of a woman's hips or thighs is in the normal course of events going to be inexorably mirrored and reproduced on the other. This mirroring or symmetry of both the waxing and waning process suggests that the whole thing is under some form of neurological control: Otherwise gravity and other local, one-sided variations in pressure, use, or exercise would tend to lump fat on one side of the body or even at one particular spot at the expense of the other. Interestingly enough, the same neurological control that applies to fat seems to apply to bone and muscle tissue synthesis as well; according to Albert Damon, long-distance truck drivers, whose right legs and feet normally receive much more exercise and traction in the course of their daily work than their left legs do, show no appreciable size differences in the bone and muscle of the right leg over and against that of the left, suggesting that normal muscle development is symmetrical even when the mechanical stimulus for that growth comes almost entirely from one side of the body, and even though actual strength, as measured by a dynamometer, may be less in the underused leg than in the exercised one. (Fat, incidentally, is less easily mobilized from some spots of the body than it is from others, with calf and forearm fat being much less subject to size changes during dieting, so that these spots are usually the last to lose their fat in the course of any reducing diet.)

How the neurological control of fat actually works is still a matter of conjecture. Actual nerve endings in fat cells are few and far between, but they do exist, and cutting them can have disastrous effects on the ability of the individual fat cell to give up its lipid content in response to starvation, exercise, or hormonal command (although not, unfortunately, on its ability to store new fat, which does not seem to depend on nervous impulse, or at least not to the same extent). The clue to the neurological stimulus for both fat storage and fat breakdown is the way in which "denervation" (cutting the nerve that leads into the fat cell) can interfere with the symmetry of the body's over-all fat stores. When the nerve endings to only one side of the fat pad are cut, the disconnected tissue suddenly enlarges on that side of the body alone, while the corresponding fat pad on the opposite side of the body stays the same size or, if food is withheld, may even get smaller. In rabbits this effect can be measured within the first 24 hours after the nerve-cutting operation, and the process goes on for about two weeks before the tissue seems to reach some natural saturation point and level off of its own accord.

Other unmistakable clues to the role played by nerve fibers in fat storage and release are emerging from the evidence of certain disease states and from the anatomical sequels to central-nervous-system injuries. Paraplegic patients, for example, may be virtually emaciated in the upper parts of their bodies above the point where the spinal cord was originally injured, but may still have abnormal amounts of fat in adipose tissue pads below the point where the injury took place. In the same way, fatty tumors (lipomas) sometimes appear in areas where the patient may have suffered neuritis in the past; and the appearance of such lipomas on symmetrically opposite parts of the body following injury to a given segment of the spinal cord is another case in point. Even in neurologically intact tissue, for that matter, F. Hausberger has shown that cauterizing a small area of one fat pad on one side of an animal's body produces mobilization of fat not only in the cauterized tissue itself but in its mirror-image counterpart on the other side of the body as well.

Neural connections may explain the where, when, and how much of an individual's fat patterning; but another thing that may help to explain individual differences in fat synthesis and breakdown is the role of those specific enzymes that help to break down fat in any given person's body. In certain rare and exotic hereditary diseases, researchers have been able to show that a minor defect or deviation in a single gene can cause tragic results in the form of the so-called lipid storage diseases. These disorders (Gaucher's syndrome, Niemann-Pick disease, and Tay-Sachs disease to name a few) take the form of unnatural lipid build-ups in the bone marrow, liver, and spleen, and sometimes in the brain as well. Bones disintegrate and break under this stress, blood refuses to clot properly, joints swell, and mental retardation is not uncommon. Death ensues at an early age, usually in childhood. Roscoe Brady's painstaking research into these disorders shows that they are caused by the absence of an enzyme that in genetically normal subjects breaks down a kind of fat called glucocerebroside into its respective glucose and lipid molecules.

As so often happens in the history of medicine, new knowledge about fatal diseases can throw a sort of reflected light on nonfatal disorders, and even on normal functioning as well, although this is usually a more long-drawn-out and low-priority order of business than disease research itself. Enzymes have long been known to play a role in fat breakdown in normal, healthy individuals; M. A. Riczak described one such enzyme; others soon came to light, and a group of investigators led by University of Pennsylvania physician Albert I. Winegrad confirmed the hunch that the enzyme lipase, when added to tissue slides of fed and starved rat adipose tissue cells in petri dishes, had a definite fat-degrading effect. This effect was strongest in the tissues of diabetic rats, which may throw some light on the notorious inability of diabetics to hold on to their fat reserves, especially triglycerides. Other enzymes like lipase have been shown to have specific abilities to break down other kinds of fat molecules (including monoglycerides, stearates, etc.). Some of these enzymes are manufactured in the gut, and others in the pancreas, including the one that breaks down cholesterol. It is easy to see how a deficit of one or more of these enzymes could complicate the business of losing weight or, alternatively, how overproduction of others could be expected to speed it up; and human beings are almost certainly going to prove to be as variable in this aspect of their metabolic functioning as they are in so many others.

So far the work that has been done on lipases has been exploratory and hasn't established much in the way of hard-and-fast knowledge about such enzymes except to delineate their chemical structure and to establish the fact that they exist. Brady's work on the exotic enzyme that breaks down the special fats involved in Gaucher's syndrome and Tay-Sachs disease suggests the possibility that low levels of other enzymes designed by nature and evolution to break down other fat compounds (up to and including those that go into storage in the adipose tissue cells that cushion our bellies, buttocks, and thighs) might be conspicuous by their absence in the relatively benign fat-storage disease that obesity itself amounts to.

Run-of-the-mill obese people are not victims of out-and-out genetic misfortunes like Tay-Sachs or Gaucher's syndrome; but whatever the cause of their own fat-storage problems may be, they have been experimentally shown to have enzyme peculiarities not present in thin and nonobese people. D. Galton, for example, observed that the fat cells of obese patients do not oxidize a certain enzyme called alpha-glycerophosphate dehydrogenase at the normal rate; the left-over enzyme molecules are therefore chronically available in surplus quantities for fat synthesis and fat storage. Brady showed that the fat-synthesizing activity of the same enzyme fell to much lower levels when these patients went on diets and there were therefore, presumably, fewer calories left lying around for it to work on. But in other obese patients, whose obesity was directly attributable to pituitary and hypothalamic disorders, dieting had no effect on enzyme activity at all, which suggests that it may work only in people whose weight problem is basically a physiological and metabolic one, as opposed to people with a central-nervous-system, or "regulatory," disorder.

Paradoxically, it takes just as much energy to build fat up as it does to tear fat down, but with one essential and biochemically crucial difference: Fat build-up does not demand oxygen, and therefore, if your oxygen supply is low for any reason, the course of least resistance for the body may be to form new fat rather than break down old fat for energy and heat. The person whose body has been programmed by its genes, hormones, or life-style to play this rather thrifty metabolic trick may as a result feel a constant low-grade fatigue that is due not so much to a heavy output of work and effort as to a short supply of oxygen in the lungs and in the circulating blood. The chronic tiredness of the obese, often put down to the effort of dragging too much extra weight around, may in fact be due to the happenstance that he or she is storing more and more fat at the expense of less and less tissue oxidation and energy release. If so, the only way to relieve the tiredness may be to get up and take a brisk walk, wash a floor, or cut a cord of firewood. Metabolically, this kind of oxygen fatigue can only be aggravated by resting and can only be cured by working; the way to beat the system in this case is therefore to goad the oxygen-using pathways in the body into action, either by vigorous physical effort or by embarking on a course of carefully considered fasting. And/or, in extreme cases, starvation.

The suggestion is not quite as frivolous as it sounds—either medically or metabolically. Short-term starvation (say of one or two days' duration) is the quickest way there is of shutting an anaerobic (nonoxygen-using) operation down, and triggering an aerobic (oxygen-using) one into high gear. In the process, unfortunately, a certain amount of good lean protein tissue (from the skeletal muscles, chiefly) will certainly have to be sacrificed; but some healthy adults can manage the loss without dire consequences, provided they are getting a good daily input of minerals—including salt, calcium, and potassium—which might otherwise be in danger of getting lost along with the protein as it gets broken down.

Attempts to protect the body's protein tissues by feeding minimal doses of amino-acid supplements, as certain medically supervised weight-reducing regimes have recently proposed to do, may or may not be as effective at solving the problem of protein loss as they are intended to be: All indications from actual metabolic research seem to be that the body's first line of emergency glucose supply in starvation or underfeeding tends to be its own protein reserves, and this is true whether supplementary proteins are coming into the pipeline or not. Since the liver seems to find it easier to reconstitute glycogen from lean tissue than from fat, and since the brain must have glucose to the tune of 100 or 145 grams a day regardless of what the dieter is or is not eating in the meantime, the organism's first response to deprivation is to protect the brain's glucose supply by breaking down muscle tissue to get it. In the process, as it happens, rather large amounts of water are liberated and excreted by the kidneys, the lungs, and the skin—an effect that may show up almost immediately on the bathroom scales, with happy augurs for the dieter's morale. Only a confirmed spoilsport would want to insist at this juncture that such early weight losses involve relatively little (if any) loss of actual fat, as opposed to what is in fact a substantial deficit of water and, worse still, of much rather solid brawn.

Be that as it may, sooner or later the fat will start to come off too, and in the meantime the original weight loss will have brought its tonic effect to bear on the dieter's spirit, if not necessarily on his adipose tissue reserves. Eventually (that is, sometime within the first week of dieting) the brain will probably begin to accept fat derivatives called ketones as an acceptable substitute for glucose (although this happens more slowly and less predictably in fat people than in normal ones); for if it were to go on getting its emergency supplies from the skeletal muscles, death from starvation would be apt to occur in a matter of weeks, whereas in fact human beings can probably go some two or three months without food before death from total starvation ensues.

A word to the cautious. Death from starvation while dieting can and does happen, even in people who are, relatively speaking, still quite obese at the time they expire. In one recent case on record where death did result from total fasting, autopsy showed that the cause of death was inordinate wasting of the vital organs themselves, notably the heart: At the time of death the heart of the young woman in question had been reduced to less than half its normal size, and what was left of it was simply not sufficient to maintain life. Since nobody can predict how quickly or how efficiently a given individual's metabolism can be counted on to shift over from protein breakdown to fat breakdown (and since this shift may never occur in the very obese) total fasting will always carry some element of risk, even when it is carefully medically monitored (as it was in the case mentioned here) and bolstered with all the right amounts of vitamins and minerals to boot. Furthermore, the switchover is never complete; it has been estimated that a loss of one pound a day, even if it has been underway for some time, represents one half pound of fat and one half pound of lean tissue (i.e., muscle, organ tissue, and possibly even bone). In the truly obese the lean tissue loss is probably less important than it is in less seriously overweight people, since additional fat in the seriously obese is almost always accompanied by a concomitant amount of organ tissue that has accumulated to help service the fat—tissue which is in other words not going to be missed once the fat itself comes off. But in people who are only moderately overweight, the balance between fat and supporting lean tissue mass may be more critical, and the effects of acute starvation—medical or otherwise— may be much riskier in the long run.

Growing children and adolescents (up to and including young adults; males in certain ethnic groups—notably Scandinavians—do not stop growing altogether until they are well into their twenties) are at a special risk from this kind of all-or-nothing approach to dieting, although they may be among the most vocal and best-motivated candidates for it. The demand for new protein that actual physical growth makes on the maturing organism should rule out this kind of approach to weight loss for adolescents, children, and young adults. For not only will fasting tend to inhibit growth, but long-term derangements of functioning as well as organ structure can and do occur when young people still in their growing periods are starved or fast for any appreciable length of time. This is not to say that young people should not or cannot diet, but only that any diet suggested for them should make adequate allowance for protecting brain glucose supplies, and for forestalling lean tissue wastage as it does so. This means that some form of starch or sugar will have to be included in the regimen; to the extent that it isn't, the young dieter will be defeating his or her own purpose, and sacrificing lean tissue without making much of a dent on available fat reserves. The same caveat applies to invalids or any other group of people with especially high protein needs, like athletes, pregnant or nursing mothers, dancers, and stevedores.

In real life (that is, real life as it is lived in the urban middle-class north in the middle of the twentieth century) starvation is usually short-lived—say from dinner to breakfast; or, as in certain cultural and religious rituals, from dinner one night to dinner the next—and is only, metabolically speaking, the other side of the coin of normal feeding and fat synthesis itself. Somewhere between exclusive fat synthesis and exclusive fat breakdown, though, ordinary workaday, give-a-little, take-a-little metabolism is in fact going on, and this is a process that represents an orchestration of two major events—food intake (and subsequent nutrient uptake by the tissues) and actual energy output in the form of physical energy expended and debited from the system.

These factors vary from day to day and have to be calibrated to each other on some sort of relative short-term basis. Food is obviously only one half the story. The other half is activity, vital function, special effort, growth, or the kind of tissue destruction (and replacement) that takes place in disease. In an acute infection, for example, the body may use up to twice its normal daily budget of calories, even though the patient is flat on his back in bed and hardly able to raise his head from the pillow to eat or drink. Depending on age, sex, and general health, just the business of keeping the heart, brain, lungs, and other vital organs going can require anywhere from 1,000 to 2,000 calories per day, before you even begin to get up in the morning, put on a pair of slippers, and bend over to pick up the morning paper.

In the resting state, the muscles account for roughly 20 per cent of the total amount of oxygen being consumed by the body on a daily basis. In hard physical work, however, this proportion rises by a factor of 50 per cent until, in extreme exertion, the muscles are using practically all of the oxygen available to the body. Oxygen turnover of this sort and on this scale speeds up almost all metabolic processes accordingly (with the possible exceptions of brain activity and digestion) but the only immediate energy substrate for all this metabolic sound and fury is the relatively small amount of short-term glucose stored in the liver; the body brings this reserve into action at once, uses it up, and then goes into the red by acquiring an "oxygen debt" which will eventually have to be paid off by hyperventilation or deep panting after the exercise is over. The breathlessness we feel for example after a sudden sprint for a bus or a train is the pulmonary expression of the unpaid oxygen deficit. This debt may take quite some time to repay, and the resulting long-range gain (or loss!) from exercise, hours later, is one that is simply not taken into account in the various tables which list the caloric equivalents of so many minutes of brisk walking (350 calories an hour for an adult 150-pound male) or a ten-minute track sprint (150 calories). These values represent the actual number of calories burned while the activity is still going on; what they do not compute is the continuing halo effect of all that effort on the organism as it seeks to re-equilibrate the altered acid-base balance in the blood, pay off the oxygen debt incurred in the meantime, and wind its way back down to a normal resting state. Research suggests that this process, depending on the violence of the effort expended, can keep metabolism at abnormally high rates for a considerable length of time after the activity itself has stopped: H. T. Edwards and his colleagues showed in 1935 that after two hours of strenuous football workout, players' metabolic rates did not even begin to approach normal again for some 15 hours.

A third level of physiological payoff from the original muscular investment is that in order to get back to a biochemically normal state of equilibrium, oxygen-using metabolic pathways are put to work at the expense of anaerobic, oxygen-sparing pathways; and as oxygen is speeded to the cells to replenish cellular supplies, the richly oxygenated blood gives an overall metabolic boost to all the tissues it perfuses. The sense of heightened aliveness that results is one that will be familiar to athletes, housewives, and gardeners as the normal metabolic afterglow of a good job well done. The resulting lift is not just psychological; there are good biochemical reasons for it as well. Provided physical exertion is not carried to the point of total exhaustion, the biochemical pick-up involved in exercise is by way of being virtue's own reward. Without some sort of physical effort on a daily basis, dieting itself becomes (biochemically) arduous; without exercise the dieter will find the metabolic going all uphill as the body overcomes its own inertia to adjust from an oxygen-saving to an oxygen-using system.

The probability that moderate exercise acts as a kind of gyroscope or stabilizer on weight gain in people of normal weight with normal dietary food intakes is bolstered by studies like Jean Mayer's, which logged the total number of hours obese adolescent girls spent in physical effort as against the hours of activity of their normal-sized peers, and compared the caloric intakes of the two groups of girls to each other's. Motion pictures of the obese girls showed that even when they were actively engaged in formal sports they moved significantly less than nonobese girls did. Earlier, Mayer and M. L. Johnson had done a study in which they established that while obese girls actually ate somewhat less than normal girls did, they also spent much less time, on a daily basis, in activities like walking and sports, and much more time in sedentary pursuits like watching TV, than girls of normal weight did.

Other investigators have had similar findings. W. L. Bloom and M. F. Eidex compared six obese housewives with six lean ones and found that the obese housewives spent roughly one hour longer in bed each day than the lean ones did, and that, even once they were up and around, they put in a good 15 per cent less of their time on their feet than their lean controls. By the same token, R. J. Dorris and Albert J. Stunkard found that, averaged out over a one-week period, 15 obese women walked a total of about 2.1 miles a day as they went about their daily work routines, while 15 nonobese women matched with them for age, occupation, and social class logged more than double that amount for an average of 4.9 miles daily.

The stabilizing effects of exercise on appetite probably only operate within a rather narrow range, as Jean Mayer points out. The cautionary advice that exercise stimulates appetite (a familiar complaint of dieters, and one that is routinely invoked to explain their sedentary bent) may as it happens have some basis in fact—but only when the exercise in question is really on a very grand scale. A day's stint of woodcutting, haying, or logrolling does indeed rev up appetite to the point of caloric no return. But surprisingly, according to Mayer's studies of Indian bazaar workers, so does just sitting still. Mayer discovered a natural laboratory for energy output and food consumption habits in a group of Indian marketplace workers in Bengal. The bazaar workers in Mayer's study came from different walks of life and performed a wide range of different daily tasks; but they all ate in the same restaurants and had access to the same kind of foods. Mayer found that the biggest eaters in his busy bazaar were clumped at both ends of the activity spectrum; they were almost evenly divided between the most sedentary workers of all and the most active ones in the bazaar. "Nonwalking" clerks and coolies, at opposite ends of the work continuum in terms of the caloric cost of their days' efforts, were almost evenly matched for the total number of calories they consumed, although their respective energy outputs were some 2,000 calories apart. Mild forms of activity, on the other hand, seemed to favor a diet which, to judge by the weights of the workers in these categories (i.e., clerks who walked to and from work, mechanics, drivers, weavers), was almost perfectly calibrated to energy output: Workers in these jobs tended to eat just enough to bring them to the break-even point in the daily metabolic bookkeeping of food eaten and work expended.

Why the most sedentary workers should have consumed as much food as the most active ones remains something of a puzzle. The same sort of thing has been observed in animals, so the chances are that it is not psychogenic—or sociological—in origin. Sedentary supervisors and hardworking coolies eat remarkably similar food-stuffs in Mayer's West Bengal market place; since all workers were buying their meals at the same local outlets, social class cannot be invoked to explain the differences between their appetites or the kinds of food consumed, and the unmistakable conclusion is that it is exercise, and not food preferences, that accounts for the difference.

This experiment has not been replicated in an American factory or office building, but there is no reason to suppose the results would be any different in a Western urban setting than they were in an Indian bazaar. So chances are high that metabolic factors must be involved in this democratic paradox. One possible explanation is that decreased activity lowers circulation, and the decreased oxygenation of the tissues that results can have a depressing effect on overall metabolism—which the individual may then proceed to mis-interpret as actual hunger. In fact, such "hunger" is much more likely to be the physiological analogue of tissue starvation, and may get misread by the brain as hunger for food, rather than hunger for oxygen, which it actually is. This can be the beginning of a vicious cycle: The more the sedentary bazaar workers overeat, the more fat they deposit; the more fat they deposit, the more sluggish they begin to feel; and the more sluggish they feel, the more they resort to food as a way of raising basal metabolism and waking themselves up.

But there are still other, and probably less easily remedied, reasons for the sluggishness of the obese, and while these may be less common than the situation described above they can have just as aversive effects. In an outpatient clinic population of obese adolescents, J. Lawrence Angel, M. Stutts, and Jean Mayer found that their obese patients had significantly lower serum iron levels than a group of nonobese children matched to them for age, size, and social class. Under the circumstances, the authors reason, "this might signal a situation in which exercise would unconsciously be avoided"—as it is in all forms of anemia, where oxygen hunger makes any kind of physical effort uphill going and tends to foster an unenterprising, if not a downright sluggish, life-style.

"Better to be eaten to death with rust," said Falstaff, "than to be scoured by perpetual motion." The dictum is one that should earn at least a token amen from anyone who has spent the better part of his or her life carrying ten, twenty, fifty, or a hundred pounds of extra weight around with him wherever he goes about his daily tasks, and who cannot remember when he had much more than the modicum of energy on tap needed to move a human body from the armchair to the supermarket and back.

Given the bioenergetics of the situation, though, people with this problem would do well to go the extra mile—thereby interrupting the vicious cycle between inactivity, low tissue oxygenation, and overweight before the extra load incurred becomes so oppressive that just getting up out of the armchair demands a caloric outlay equal to riding a bicycle several yards uphill. Human hearts, bones, muscles, and connective tissues were not designed for inanition; and, especially for the constitutionally obese, it may in the long run be easier to regulate appetite at the far end of the equation (that is, at the output side) than to curb it at the near end, or the intake side. Both kinds of regulation require effort—one physical, the other psychological. But, for the truly obese, it is always an open question which of the two kinds of effort is really more strenuous—staying out of the kitchen and away from the supermarket in the first place, or setting off on a good brisk walk in the opposite direction after the fact. From a physiological point of view, in any case, it is no contest: Physical activity will prove to be the least arduous in the long run, even if it hurts the most at the start.

And yes, to take Falstaff up on his challenge—it is undoubtedly better to be scoured to death with perpetual motion in the long run than to be eaten to death with rust in the short.

8 Psychology: The Brain as a Digestive Organ

Although the fact of human obesity has a long and well-documented history (the Spartans once ostracized a man for being fat; and Socrates is supposed to have danced every morning to keep his figure within reasonable bounds), the existence of human hunger has an even longer one. Vicissitudes of climate, agriculture, and hunting have probably been a factor in all the great migrations—both human and animal—of prehistoric and modern times; and the politics of food supply and demand are at least as old as the dynastic Egyptians, whose control of the granaries gave them political carte blanche in the Nile Valley 4,000 years before the birth of Christ and determined Pharaonic succession for upward of at least two millennia thereafter.

Considering the pervasiveness and the very ancient history of human starvation and famine, the now widely accepted notion of oral greed as a form of infantile sexuality gone wrong may seem to be adding insult to injury; anyone who has gone without food for any considerable length of time can vouch for hunger itself as a drive perfectly capable of holding its own among other largely autonomous passions like thirst, sleepiness, lust, and the urge to evacuate. In all probability starving people can and do beg, borrow, and steal for food without any reference—conscious or otherwise—to sex or mother love. In a subtler sense, though, the psychoanalytic theorists have scored an important point; for it is undoubtedly true of hunger (as it has been said in another context of sex) that the most important digestive organ in the body is probably not the stomach but the brain.

In the psychoanalytic literature of the last thirty years obesity has traditionally been viewed as a form of infantile fixation at the earliest, and therefore by implication the "lowest," developmental level; put in its simplest terms, the obese patient has never really psychologically weaned himself from the memory of his mother's breast; the hunger that dogs him and may go on dogging him for the rest of his life refers back to infantile feeding conflicts, and the resulting obesity is assumed to speak for itself.

The assumption implicit in this point of view is that overeating represents an act of dependency gratification, indulged in well past the age at which we are all developmentally entitled to it. In the case of one fourteen-year-old described by analyst-pediatrician Hilde Bruch, the boy's mother would get down on her hands and knees as a matter of course during office visits to help him on and off with his shoes. This case sets the tone for much of the psychoanalytic literature on dependency behavior in the obese: Mothers like this one are presumably still re-enacting the rituals of the nursery years after their children have grown up and gone on to other things. Later on in adolescence, though, the same mothers may stand the problem on its head: As one of Bruch's young patients complained, "All the time she tells me, eat, eat, eat. And now she's angry that I'm too fat!"

Hilde Bruch is one of the towering figures in the field of obesity research; Bruch's many years as a practicing pediatrician before she took psychoanalytic training impressed her with the strong undercurrent of maternal domination and childish compliance that exists in the life history of the obese child. Other psychoanalytic thinkers on the subject have stressed the psychosexual components in adult obesities: fantasies of oral rape, impregnation, and general voracity loom large in these descriptions. Still others have reasoned their way backward from the "oral rage" of the obese to the depression that may result when this rage turns inward against the patient himself.

Regardless of what brings it on, depression has been a consistent occupational hazard of obesity—and vice versa—throughout much of recorded medical history. (Recovering from a serious episode of "melancholy," for example, when his earliest published work didn't receive the accolades he had anticipated, no less a witness than philosopher David Hume was startled to find himself getting inordinately fat, and, as he wrote to his physician in the summer of 1731, "there grew upon me a ravenous Appetite, [with] an Effect very unusual, which was to nourish me extremely, so that in six Weeks' time I past from one extreme to the other, and being before tall, lean, and rawboned, became on a sudden the most sturdy, robust, healthful-like Fellow you have seen."

The connection between obesity and depression is thus no modern invention. As with so many psychological syndromes, though, it is hard on the face of it to work out priorities of cause and effect: Do the obese get depressed because they are fat, or do they get fat because they are depressed? Any meaningful answer to this question will have to take account of the fact that, oddly enough, and despite the fact that the two conditions often go together, the obese have a suicide rate that is well below the national average; so if as a group fat people are more depressed than others in the general population, they would at least seem to have learned the right medicine to take for what ails them. Food in the last analysis constitutes the outstanding over-the-counter nostrum for depression in this and other affluent countries, despite its obvious side effects—not to mention the vicious circle which it manages to set in motion.

If food is the cheapest and most abundant mood-altering drug on the market, psychoanalysis is undoubtedly the scarcest and most highly priced. Psychoanalytic theory—what Philip Rieff has called the "negative community" in deference to its insurgent beginnings—may have started a revolution in twentieth-century thought, but has ended up as one of its dominating intellectual canons. To say that it has had less success in its own chosen arena (i.e., the therapy of mental disorders and dysfunctions) than in the intellectual market place of its day is not to devalue the insights that it has unquestionably brought into that market place. For even though Freudian psychoanalysis has not proved over the years to offer much in the way of certifiable clinical cures for many of the ailments it had once set out to deal with (phobias, schizophrenia, obesity, and sexual dysfunction among others), its organizing ideas have served as points of departure for other disciplines to apply and for other practitioners to test out. Freud's, Bruch's, and Deri's ground-breaking essays on the psychopathology of obesity strike the keynote for much subsequent research on the subject, and during the forties and fifties many psychologists raised in the Freudian tradition but trained in the experimental labs of empiricists like John Watson took it upon themselves to flesh out the Freudian canon and case reports with good hard empirical research findings.

Obesity soon came in for its fair share of this fact finding, with results that supported the psychoanalytic orthodoxies in some cases and refuted them in others. Uppermost in many workers' minds was the question, not so much whether the obese represented a psychologically disturbed population (it was simply taken for granted that they did), but rather just how disturbed the obese actually were, as compared both to nonobese people in general and to other disturbed people in particular. The answers were somewhat surprising, as it turned out, and might have given the psychoanalysts pause.

According to one recent English study, for example, among a group of 344 Londoners, 10 per cent of the men of normal weight and 40 per cent of the women of normal weight got high scores for personality disturbance, as opposed to 7 per cent of obese men and 33 per cent of obese women measured on the same protocol (the Cornell Medical Index in this case). Researcher R. F. Suczek used another instrument, the Minnesota Multiphasic Personality Inventory, and a projective test, the Thematic Apperception Test (TAT), to assess the personality characteristics of 100 obese women and got similar but somewhat more equivocal results. As a group, the women in Suczek's study were about 41 per cent above their ideal weights, and most of them had been obese for at least two years. What Suczek found to be the predominating personality configuration of his overweight subjects was not mental disturbance but almost the opposite—a kind of hypernormalcy and social proficiency that flies in the face of most psychological stereotypes of the obese. These women did not see themselves as weak, dependent, or depressed. On the contrary, the fatter they were the more socially competent and psychologically resourceful these women appeared to be, as if their very largeness disposed them to a sort of take-charge, earth-mother self-image as old as the Wife of Bath. Since Suczek's subjects had been recruited from a group of women taking part in a weight reduction program, it was easy to correlate their personality data with their diet and weight curves from the original survey; interestingly enough, as it turned out, the poor weight losers in the group had lower dominance scores than the successful weight losers did. The dominators in short seemed to be able to dominate everything in their milieu—including themselves and their own appetites, once they had turned their minds to the job.

Other unexpected and provocative insights emerged from this research. Compared to other groups of subjects, for example, the obese women's projective test responses tended to be rather flat and undramatic—even, to call a spade a spade, a little bit boring. This finding, which could hardly have been predicted from the mere fact of the obesity itself, closely echoes research done by B. Kotkov and B. Muranski, who studied the Rorschach responses of 81 obese women; their work was published in 1952 and they reported that obese women in their group tended to give constricted and extremely concrete word associations to the famous Rorschach inkblots. The authors noted that for some reason repression seemed to go deeper in obese women than in women of normal weight; on the inkblot tests Kotkov and Muranski's women tend to emerge with the same sort of personality profiles as out-and-out compulsive neurotics. Considering the impulsiveness that makes fat people overeat, and which ought by rights to be a major factor in any form of gluttony, this finding represents a paradox and a challenge: If the obese are so good at repressing things in general, why do they have so much trouble repressing the urge to eat?

And this was not an isolated finding; Mary E. Moore, Albert J. Stunkard, and L. B. Srole were to report much the same peculiarity some ten years later in their famous midtown Manhattan study in which a group of 1,660 New Yorkers were studied exhaustively by a team of psychiatrists and social scientists in the late 1950's. These authors admitted themselves to be baffled by the evidence and tried every way they knew to make good Freudian sense of the data. Obese subjects in Moore, Stunkard, and Srole's population were more "immature," more "rigid," and more "suspicious" than their nonobese neighbors and peers; and while the finding of immaturity in fat people did not strain the authors' conceptual framework much (after all, a return to the breast is not the average "mature" grown-up's psychological ambition in life), the other findings did. For why should obese people be any more rigid, everything else being equal, than other people of the same age, city, and social class?

The question is a tantalizing one, but one that current research has left unanswered. Some guesses may not be out of order; given the disesteem that attaches to fat people in this culture, a tendency to gain weight is one that the individual learns early on to deal with by a degree of self-control and self-browbeating that are not usually required of people in the population at large. Once mastered, this personality trait may spread to other areas of functioning that go well beyond the daily battle with appetite and food. It is not impossible, then, that the rigidity of the obese may be a sort of compensatory mechanism used to keep the rein on their own appetites and eating habits, and then unwittingly generalized to many other areas of the individual's personality as well.

To talk about the self-control of the obese is to invite skepticism, if not downright disbelief; after all, the theory goes, if fat people really could control their own feeding, how on earth did they ever manage to get so fat in the first place? This is a fair question, and one that is not as unanswerable as it seems. Recent research has shown that the obese are not in the normal course of events the constant, steady nibblers that the nonobese imagine them to be; on the contrary, we know now that in most cases weight gain has a cyclical, on-again, off-again pattern. In many cases people get fat by literal leaps and bounds, not by slow insidious increments—and then proceed to maintain the new, higher weight on caloric budgets that can be and often are well below the usual rations for normal-sized people of their age and sex. Physicians refer to these ups and downs as the active and passive phases of weight gain; in effect, though, the passive phase represents a plateau of sorts, with the metabolism having adjusted to its new inflationary caloric economy and the resulting obesity remaining stabilized at its own higher level, sometimes indefinitely and probably—at least from time to time—in the face of considerable and dogged self-denial.

The compulsiveness and rigidity that make their surprise appearances in the psychological test results of the obese may therefore represent a reaction to intermittent onslaughts of the ungovernable hunger that triggered the original eating binge (or binges), with the patient having learned over the years to exert a considerable amount of psychological counterpressure against his own impulses to gorge. If he or she tends to get a bit rigid and unbending in the process, the symptom may be nothing more or less than the psychological penalty entailed by wrestling with the devil of voracious appetite on and off for so many years, and with seesawing degrees of success and failure.

It is one of the problems of modern science that we measure only the things we have yardsticks for. Rightly or wrongly, psychological tests have been faulted for their tendency to measure not what is necessarily the most important or relevant part of a given problem, but only what the test itself is specifically designed to assay. I.Q. tests, for example, have been roundly criticized for measuring only what passes for quick-wittedness on the tester's own native ground; and the Rorschach and TAT could be similarly belabored. These tests are culture-bound. Their inventors were psychoanalytically oriented diagnosticians with a penchant for Freudian analogies, symbolism, and explanatory criteria; and one of the first fish to be caught in their nets is therefore not surprisingly their subjects' feelings and attitudes about the great psychoanalytic theme song of sex. Confusion about sex, size, and body image on the projective tests may therefore re-emerge on the analytic couch as confusion about gender and sexuality. Several authors have noted that the obese seem to be uneasier about their sex roles than other people are; others have challenged this view or stood it on its head.

Like most mammals, human beings as a species tend to run to large males and smaller females; the sheer physical bigness involved in obesity may therefore be enough to make a fat woman feel less feminine than her normal-sized sisters—if not much more masculine into the bargain too. This view is prevalent in clinical circles and should probably be reevaluated in the light of new thinking about hormonal effects on behavior, sexual and otherwise, and on anatomy itself. An interesting contribution to the problem of femininity and body size is one raised by the Dutch physician Frits deWaard, who believes that, although most estrogen is produced and distributed by the ovaries, there are also smaller, local estrogen factories in the body cells of any genetically female individual, which can and do add their share of female hormones to the body's total estrogen load. And the fact that large females have more and larger cells than smaller females do may be a factor in their over-all estrogen counts. If deWaard's hypothesis is correct, and estrogen levels are a function of total body size and not just of the hormonal exuberance of a given woman's particular pair of ovaries, then it would follow that large women are at least endocrinologically speaking more "feminine" than small women, on an absolute, if not a relative basis.

Reasons for the "unfemininity" of large women therefore probably have less to do with hormone counts and reproductive or erotic proclivities than they do with aesthetic ideals and cultural stereotypes about big men and little women, and their respective roles in the sexual marketplace. So in spite of the fact that the "unfemininity" of big women seems more of a social fact than a biological one, confusion or ambivalence about sex and sex role emerges, for whatever reason, as a common feature of obese women's projective test responses. (Unfortunately there seems to be no comparable data for men.) Despite findings like Shipman and Schwartz's, some two decades later, that fat women are sexier than thin ones, Suczek's study reported, among other things, that obese women tended to mention the sex of the characters on the TAT cards less frequently than a group of nonobese women did; and of those who did identify a figure on the cards as being specifically female (most TAT figures are deliberately somewhat hazy in this respect) half identified her as being a low-status person of some sort—i.e., a maid, a daughter, or a family dependent. Thus, although Suczek's obese subjects tended to see themselves as powerful, the fact remained that whenever femininity was mentioned on the TAT card as such, the female figure involved was placed at the wrong or masochistic end of the social power pole; women as a group were in other words seen as powerless even though the obese subject taking the test might actually see herself—at least on other tests—as a competent, take-charge person in her own right.

Other studies have had somewhat different results. A. Feiner, for example, is another investigator who was specifically interested in the femininity of the obese girls he studied; his research was based on a battery of projective test measurements and led him to conclude that the girls in his sample were more feminine on overt measures of femininity, but less so on covert ones. This was especially true in tests where the gender cues could be more easily disguised or camouflaged by the tester, as for example in figure drawings, a picture story test, and the MMPI (Minnesota Multiphasic Personality Inventory). The implication of work like Feiner's is that the femininity of the obese girls may just be a particular instance of their over-all propensity for social compliance: When they know they are being assessed for evidence of gender identification they make the responses they assume are going to be interpreted as socially "right"; but when the test itself offers no clues about what is really being tested, they drop the mask of compliant femininity and show themselves in their true and not so very feminine colors after all. The same tests showed the obese girls to be more dependent on their parents than nonobese girls and, in particular, to be more dependent on their mothers, and more aggressive toward their fathers, than other girls.

Findings like these corroborate Hilde Bruch's original conceptual model of the situation; but Bruch herself was charier of interpreting the results of a series of projective tests she personally administered to some of the obese children in her own practice. She concluded that the Rorschachs in her own sample were simply too diverse to say anything definite about, beyond drawing the very general conclusion that obese children seemed to have a striking preoccupation with body size and a concomitant confusion about it. In Bruch's obese sample there was a tendency for the symmetrical inkblots to be identified in terms of complementary sexing—man and woman, for example, and boy and girl—and not, as is usually the case with mirror-image Rorschach blots, as same-sexed twins or identical, unisex pairs. Thus, like Feiner's subjects but unlike Suczek's, Bruch's obese children have a Noah's ark vision of the world and see things and creatures in couples, two by two. Gender matters to them; and so, by implication, does sex itself.

The point is not an unimportant one; sex is a need state just like hunger and thirst, and it stands to reason that people who have had trouble with their impulses in one area of life may have trouble with them in another too. Ways of dealing with bodily needs can run the gamut from total repression to a raging voracity. William G. Shipman's fat sex-starved wives, reported earlier, were almost unanimous in their desire for more sex than whatever amount of it they were currently getting in their marriages; while normal and thin women in the same study were reasonably contented with their sexual lots. One of psychoanalyst M. B. Hecht's obese patients described herself as so sexually ravenous that she was capable of orgasm if and when her husband merely touched her; this patient was aware of the connection between her hunger for sex and her hunger for food, and drew the appropriate parallels. When she was sexually excited but not gratified she turned to food and ate voraciously. The "alimentary orgasm" that such people seem to be looking for sets the stage for their periodic eating binges, with disastrous consequences not only for their figures but sometimes for their gastrointestinal tracts as well. Some years ago the popular press covered the story of a Long Island girl whose last eating binge resulted in a ruptured stomach and fatal peritonitis. Physiologically of course the alimentary orgasm is a complete misnomer, since nothing in the consuming end of the digestive tract is remotely capable of anything like ogasm (and if it were might produce something far less pleasurable than anything the food addict had ever bargained for).

Elsewhere, on the other hand, the sexual appetites of obese women have gotten a less lurid but equally negative press; psychoanalyst George Reeve has described a classical case of female frigidity in a woman who had the happy faculty of "putting weight on and taking it off at the drop of a hat," as the bemused reporter puts it. "It was very easy to establish a correlation between her weight and the status of her love affairs," says Reeves of this 1940's college girl. "When a suitor became very interested and attentive she would eat huge quantities of food and candy. When a suitor became disgusted and left her she promptly lost weight." Intrigued with his patient's ability to don and doff layers of adipose tissues like a suit of armor, Reeve interpreted this pattern to mean that the young woman's weight gain kept her defended by a living wall of fat from any threatened sexual seduction; whenever the issue of sex arose in the normal course of a boy-girl relationship she would make herself as unpresentable as possible by puffing herself up like a species of pouter pigeon and frightening off the supposed predator with her sudden girth.

If this interpretation is correct it implies a level of self-awareness and self-manipulation that some investigators think may be seriously lacking in the obese. What Bruch classified as confusion about body size has been described by other reporters as downright self-delusion: Fat people do not necessarily even see themselves as being fat. Peter Wyden in *The Overweight Society* describes a Chicago advertising agency's study of obese people's attitudes toward overweight in which fat and thin women were given lists of fat and thin celebrities to scan and asked what it was that people on each list had in common. Fat women in the study were at a loss when it came to making the implicit distinction, but thin women applied the right yardstick and correctly pinpointed what it was that was different about people on the two lists. Obese women would seem, on the basis of this evidence, to be fat blind the same way some people are color blind; fatness simply does not seem to them to be a pertinent classificatory ticket to hang on one group of people over and against another. By implication this finding would seem to suggest that overweight women do not see themselves as others see them, and that they do not see other fat people that way either when all is said and done.

At apparent odds with this conclusion, though, are the data from a study conducted by L. Perry and B. Learnard, who discovered that in a group of 144 obese subjects, individual weights as reported by the subjects themselves were almost 100 per cent accurate—a somewhat higher rate than would be expected from the population at large, who are likely to have fewer occasions than the obese to get on and off their bathroom scales in the course of a week or a month, and may therefore be less up to date on their current weight than fat people are. Perry and Learnard's finding makes it clear that the obese are not kidding themselves in any fundamental (i.e., arithmetical) way about the subject of their own weight; most of these subjects know exactly what they weigh down to the last pound or fraction of a pound. At first glance this finding may seem not to jibe with the data reported above. But Perry and Learnard's data do not necessarily challenge the validity of those reported by Wyden from Chicago; for while fat people in both studies may know exactly what they weigh, it doesn't necessarily follow that they also see themselves as fat. The correlation, if there is one, may exist only in the eyes of the (thin) beholder. Stature, build, and well-cut clothing have a way of tricking the eye, and appearances can therefore be deceiving. Fat people are usually old hands at this particular kind of deception, what is more. The result may be, as reported by Wyden, that they have judiciously decided that obesity is a mere detail—and a misleading one at that.

Most of us, fat or thin, are not as able to inflate and deflate ourselves at will as Reeve's sex-shy college girl and, if we were, might find other than romantic reasons for doing so. But weight does go up and down in response to external cues, including psychosocial ones. And just as depression has traditionally been implicated in overeating, so has stress been viewed as a common emotional trigger to weight gain; fat college undergraduates in a classic study of the early 1950's were shown to gain weight during exam periods, while their thinner dormitory mates lost weight or broke even. Later studies of fat and thin business executives have pinned this relationship down and refined it; in an unpublished study by J. Maher, reported by researcher Stanley Schachter, it developed that fat executives in high-stress jobs gained no more weight than fat executives in low-stress jobs did: Occupational stress per se therefore is not what makes the fat get fatter. On the other hand, though, stress does play an interesting role in weight control by virtue of being exactly what it is that makes the thin get thinner: Maher's thin executives in stressful jobs did get thinner than their equally thin colleagues in more relaxing jobs. What this suggests is that stress may indeed be a factor—even the crucial factor—in weight gain or loss: but only in thin people, not in fat ones. If so, the psychoanalytic model will have to be revised, for Maher's data suggest that what may be critical in the overeating-obesity equation is not so much the overeating itself (thin people do this periodically too!) as the failure to actually *undereat* when the emotional heat is on, as skinny people apparently do, thereby redressing the balance in favor of the original weight set point.

(Ned Rorem, composer, diarist, and ectomorph, has left a mouth-watering description of a thin man on an eating binge that will serve to illustrate the point: A sudden yen for something sweet sends Rorem to the bakery one day for a lemon meringue pie, which he eats in blissful solitude—hastily hiding the remains of the feast like an "alcoholic with rum bottles" when a visitor puts in an unexpected appearance; the following day, with the mood still upon him, Rorem repeats "the process with Sutter's four pound devil's food cake, and the following day with twelve cream puffs.")

Fat people may take what solace they can from this confession of unembarrassed gluttony. But not much; the eating binges of the obese are at once more chronic, less reversible, and more metabolically consequential than those of the constitutionally thin. Thin people only overeat spasmodically; but fat people are always hungry, and cannot count on the natural ups and downs of their own appetites to redress the balance in favor of the status quo ante as thin people can and evidently constantly do. Hence the equivocal finding that the obese react to stress by overeating. In fact, as later studies on the eating behavior of the obese were eventually to make clear, the obese react less to inner cues like stress than to outer cues like availability of food, ease of access to it, and the general attractiveness of the food's presentation when it comes to actually sitting down to eat.

The thrust of findings like Maher's is away from the Freudian psychodynamics of overeating and obesity and into the relatively fresher pastures of psychobiology and behaviorism. Most researchers presently at work in the field would probably agree with this decision; for when it comes to the therapy of overeating and obesity, psychoanalysis has simply not done the job. Janet Wollersheim of the University of Illinois compared the weight losses of four groups of obese subjects undergoing psychological treatment regimes for weight control. The four groups represented different weight-loss strategies and different philosophies of appetite control, ranging from a social pressure approach like TOPS or Weight Watchers; a behavior therapy or operant conditioning approach; an "insight"-oriented, psychodynamically based program; and an untreated control group of people matched to those in the other three groups for age, social class, and degree of overweight. Those receiving the psychoanalytically based insight therapy had the lowest success rates of the total sample (with the single exception, that is, of the control group, which of course received no treatment at all). S. B. Penick, R. Filion, S. Fox, and Albert J. Stunkard had very similar results with a treatment-comparison study they ran at the University of Pennsylvania in 1969; the behavior-modification groups outperformed the psychoanalytically oriented groups by a factor of almost two to one. Controlled statistical studies of individual psychotherapy results are harder to come by than this, but there is no good reason to suppose that the analytic couch has produced any greater successes on a one-to-one basis than psychoanalytically oriented therapy has managed to produce in groups—nor have the analysts ever claimed so. Thus, while the whole field owes a considerable debt of gratitude to the analysts for focusing attention on the role played by the brain in obesity, as opposed to that played by the body itself, most recent research has nevertheless tended to lower its sights from the cerebral cortex (where presumably the human part of human nature presides over the psychoanalyzable part of the mind) to the pituitary and the hypothalamus—parts of the "old," basic mammalian brain where hunger and thirst take place and are processed in all their naked preverbal and pre-Freudian immediacy.

Before moving on into this scientifically newer but evolutionarily older and less verbal arena, though, it may be well to stop for a minute and attempt a summary of work to date that has had its taproots planted deep, for better or for worse, in traditional Freudian soil. What, in the last analysis, did the psychoanalytically oriented researchers actually find in the way of corroboration of the founder's theories—and how did these findings diverge from the predicted ones?

First, in answer to the question implicit in many of these studies as to how crazy the obese actually are, the only fair answer is: not very—and if anything, perhaps on the whole just a little less crazy than the population at large. More depressed, possibly, yes: but less overtly psychotic even so. More placid and socially compliant, yes; but less impulsive and less excitable under stress as well. Immature, yes; passive and dependent, no. One exception to this picture of low-keyed and even sanctimonious normalcy is in the area of sex: The psychoanalytic literature had painted a somewhat lurid picture of the sexual avidity of the obese (at least of obese women), but the research findings were mixed, and a fair summation at this stage of the game might be a guarded maybe.

A final conclusion would have to be that, in large measure, these studies cast serious doubts on many of the assumptions which had generated them: The obese did not look the same in the hard-nosed empirical studies as they did in the psychoanalytical case reports. What was missing from the case records, by and large, was the rock-bottom, preverbal mindlessness of hunger itself. Several decades and many research studies later, the only safe generalization that could therefore be made about fat people after putting them under the research microscope at so many different powers of magnification was that they were a universally, unfortunately, and constantly hungry lot.

For, emotion and psychopathology aside, the major universal mental aberration of the obese is of course excessive appetite. Impatience with untestable Freudian theories, and the increasing evidence that psychoanalysis and psychotherapy have shown dismal results in the actual treatment of obesity itself, have combined to stimulate a great deal of research into the everyday workings of feeding and appetite over the past decade. Psychiatrists Albert J. Stunkard and T. B. Van Itallie, and psychologists Stanley Schachter and Richard Nisbett, are some of the outstanding names in this line of research; and Schachter, if not the Grand Sachem of this group, is at least far and away the resident working tutelary genius. In his early work an interest in the physiological equivalents of emotions and other self-labeled feeling states, and the events inside the brain which presumably accompany them, led Schachter into the behavioristic aspects of hunger as a sort of test case for the whole mind-body problem in general. Much of his most recent research has dealt painstakingly, exclusively, and sometimes downright engagingly with the behavior of the obese as opposed to that of people with normal body weights; over the years in fact, a whole academic generation of Columbia graduate students in psychology has followed in his footsteps and helped to round out the solid accumulation of experimental and naturalistic evidence in which Schachter's career is grounded. This work has taken students and professor alike from the experimental lab to local Chinese restaurants and back again, in an attempt to spell out where, when, and how the feeding habits of the obese differ from those of other people—and to determine, if possible, why.

The body of that work revolves around the relationship between the demonstrable physiological need to eat and the self-reported (or self-revealed) impulse to do so. Why do some people eat when they are (physiologically) not hungry? What makes normal people eat when they are? To answer these questions, Schachter and his colleagues and graduate students set up a series of ingenious and revealing experiments that showed the obese to be largely out of sync with incoming data of their own senses. Schachter was intrigued by Hilde Bruch's remark that fat children seemed never to have learned the difference between their own hunger and various other feeling states like loneliness, anxiety, discomfort, etc. To test the accuracy of this insight, Schachter set out to provoke anxiety in his subjects under varying conditions, and then measured its effect on their feeding behavior. To do this, he fed obese and nonobese groups of college students two largish roast beef sandwiches to fill them up, and then got them to sample some designedly tasteless crackers on the pretext that they were being used as guinea pigs in a marketing research experiment. The other half of both obese and nonobese groups were told the same story, but were not prefed on roast beef sandwiches. Both groups were then deliberately alarmed, anxiety being laid on in the form of a mild but unexpected electric shock. ("You don't have a heart condition, do you?" the experimenter asks disingenuously—just in case the shock itself has not been sufficiently scary.)

Fear itself is thought to be a potent appetite suppressor, and in thin subjects—both those previously fed on roast beef sandwiches and those being tested on an empty stomach—this supposition is amply borne out. In fat subjects, however, the picture proved to be quite different. Neither fear nor a full stomach had any significant effect on the number of crackers fat students ate after being shocked. Not only did they eat just as many crackers when they were fearful as when they were relaxed, but they did not up their cracker consumption when they were relaxed either; they simply carried on as if whatever connects the sensation of fear to the sensation of appetite in their brains had been either absent or not in good working order at the time.

Since neither hunger contractions, fear, or a well-filled stomach seemed to have any major effect on an obese subject's willingness to go on eating tasteless crackers, Schachter began to wonder just what did influence the fat person's decision to eat, not to eat, or to go on eating once he had started; and he found that when he manipulated other parts of the eating situation a clearer picture began to emerge: Fat people eat when something in the outside world reminds them to, while normal-sized people eat only when their stomachs are empty and start to contract painfully with hunger.

Setting the hands of an experimental-room clock ahead by an hour or so has no effect on the nonobese subject's hunger pangs; this paragon's stomach tells him the correct dinner time, and he responds by eating whenever his usual mealtime rolls around. Under the same conditions, however, fat subjects are quite unaware that a hoax is being perpetrated on them and seem to feel hungry as soon as the doctored clock registers the erroneous dinner hour. The same general effect could be dependably produced by setting the clock back or ahead by an equal amount of time; the fat do not, properly speaking, feel hunger in the same way that other people do—if indeed they ever feel "hunger," in the classical sense of a painfully contracting stomach, at all. Cues to start eating (and possibly to stop eating as well) do not come to them from their own viscera but from events in the world they live in, or, at the very closest to home, from ideas and images touched off by events in that world—a picture of mouth-watering food in a magazine, for example; or the words of a recipe in a cookbook.

Taste itself proved to be a powerful regulator of food intake for the obese, less so for normals. One of Schachter's colleagues, Richard Nisbett, performed an experiment to test the gourmandism of fat, thin, and medium people respectively; just as predicted, when confronted (if that is the word) with expensive vanilla ice cream on the one hand and a somewhat inferior product judiciously adulterated with quinine on the other, obese subjects did eat more of the good ice cream than either normal or thin subjects did. For the bad ice cream, though, the prediction was not borne out. All subjects ate about the same amount of the doctored ice cream (although Schachter hazards the guess that "this may be due to the fact that Nisbett's bad ice cream really was pretty bad, and that many of the subjects simply ate the token spoonful or two requested by the experimental instruction . . . while most others ate only enough to satisfy themselves that the taste was quite as weird as they had first thought").

This clear effect of taste on appetite is one that should ring a bell with anyone who has ever had a weight problem or a sweet tooth of long standing. Satiety seems to be a point that is much harder to reach with delicious-tasting food than it does with so-so or awful fare; even the obese will tend to feel full when the food is sufficiently bad.

The same cannot be said when the food is good or superlative; it is a complaint of food addicts, obese and otherwise, that once they start eating they cannot bring themselves to stop. Nisbett ran an experiment in which obese and nonobese summer-school students were exposed to varying numbers of roast beef sandwiches while ostensibly being asked to fill out a bogus questionnaire. Before coming to the lab all subjects had been asked to forgo lunch, under the pretext of having to measure various physiological responses like EKG's and galvanic skin responses on an empty stomach. It was Nisbett's prediction, based on similar research with rats, that when brought face to face with a lone sandwich on a plate, and the promise of more as needed from a well-stocked refrigerator standing nearby, the unfed obese subjects would stop at one if there was only one sandwich on the plate, regardless of how hungry they really were, while the thin subjects would go and get as many extra ones from the refrigerator as hunger dictated and impulse and time allowed. With three sandwiches on the plate, on the other hand, obese subjects according to Nisbett's prediction should have gone on eating until there was nothing left on the plate—while thin subjects would stop somewhere toward the end of the second sandwich. The predictions were borne out handily. "Presented with three sandwiches," says Schachter in describing this experiment, "obese subjects eat far more than either normal or skinny subjects . . . Presented with only one sandwich, however, the obese eat just as little as do skinny subjects and significantly less than normal subjects."

Data like these raise interesting questions about the reasons for the behavior in question. Is it something in the personality of fat people that causes their distinctive behavior in feeding situations—a kind of exaggerated social punctilio, born of the desire to appear less greedy than the next person, for example, at least when there are onlookers present? Or is their behavior more instinctive and less socially determined than that? In an attempt to test these alternatives out, Nisbett decided to move his experiments developmentally back in time as far as he could go, and transferred the scene of his experiments from the psychology lab to the newborn nursery of a large urban hospital. Interestingly enough, fat newborn babies prove to be just as unwilling to go out of their way to work for their food as fat Columbia students did; in a study of the nursing behavior of two- to four-day-old infants, Nisbett and S. Gurwitz gave sweetened and unsweetened formula to fat and thin babies and found that the heavier babies consumed 28 per cent more of the sweetened formula than the unsweetened, while lighter babies— although they liked the sweetened formula better too—only consumed 8 per cent more of it. By the same token, though, like the summer-school students who could not be bothered to get up and get themselves a second sandwich, the heavier babies worked less hard than the lighter ones to get what formula was available when the nipple holes were made small so as to slow down the flow.

Nisbett and Gurwitz's experiments were carried out under carefully controlled conditions in hospital neonatal nurseries where none of the babies was much over four days old at the time of the study. The point is an important one because it seems to establish the fact that there are indeed feeding differences in babies which predate any possible mother-child social interaction and therefore cannot be laid to maternal attitudes, handling, or unconscious motives, as the Freudian model for eating disturbances in babies demands. Fat babies in other words already exhibit feeding behavior at birth that sets them apart from thin babies in a significant and striking fashion; and since the difference is of exactly the same kind, and goes in exactly the same direction, as similar behavioral differences between fat and nonfat adults, the hypothesis has to be seriously entertained that there is a strong biological component both in the babies' body compositions and in their feeding behavior as well. If this is true, the psychoanalytic argument that disturbed mothers are the real villains of the piece in infant overeating may have to be re-examined from the inside out. Or, as the authors put it, "the peculiarities are apparently present at birth, and it therefore becomes unparsimonious to assume that the peculiarities in the adult are due to parental treatment differences and other social factors." Parsimony in science has the same function to serve as frugality in a well-run household; where one idea can be shown to be explanatory with respect to a given body of facts, introducing a second idea to explain the same set of facts becomes wasteful and counterproductive. By this measure, to explain infant overeating on the basis of innate constitutional factors and adult overeating on the basis of purely social factors is improvident and unenlightening: One of the two explanations is superfluous and may probably be safely jettisoned. In some situations, the question of which hypothesis to adopt and which to jettison is a matter of personal preference, bias, or a toss of the coin; in the present case, though, if it comes to choosing one or the other hypothesis, Nisbett and Gurwitz's study would seem to weight the choice heavily in favor of the constitutional, as opposed to the social, explanation.

Schachter's and his students' and colleagues' experimental manipulations of hunger and satiety in obese and nonobese subjects have become classics in their own field, famous not only for the ingenuity they have brought to bear on the measurement of complex responses to simple cues, but for their penetrating insights into some of the finer distinctions between the reactions of obese and nonobese subjects to eating and food. As an experimental psychologist, Schachter has no axe to grind either for or against the psychoanalysts, on the one hand, or for or against the psychobiologists on the other. Schachter is not, in research parlance, a "rat man" (an animal psychologist) and neither is he a Freudian. For a dedicated experimental psychologist it must nevertheless be difficult to come to the study of mind-body problems in this day and age without the excess baggage of one or the other of these traditional academic biases, and Schachter's breezy and occasionally downright waggish approach to the subject of obesity is therefore like a breath of fresh air in the academic ivory tower.

As the evidence from his research mounted, furthermore, it became increasingly clear that by striking out into previously uncharted behaviorist waters Schachter had discovered a new continent of sorts; the feeding behavior of fat people was not, as it turned out, the only area of behavior in which they differed significantly from thin and normal people. The differences were wider-ranging than that, and each new experiment seemed to breed new hypotheses to be tested; in the end, some of these tests took the experimenters rather far afield of their original lines of inquiry, and extended the whole scope of the inquiry into areas to which no one had hitherto really expected it to apply.

The hyperemotionality of fat people, an article of faith with most neo-Freudians (and something which incidentally shows up with some regularity in the literature about other brain-lesioned obese animals as well), had received its first unexpected and fortuitous experimental corroborations from Schachter, R. Goldman, and A. Gordon's finding that obese subjects were easier to frighten with the threat of electric shock than nonobese subjects were. To follow through on this finding and tie it in with other indications of emotionality and distractibility in the obese, J. Rodin, D. Elman, and Schachter used tapes of materials that were highly disturbing emotionally and compared the reactions of obese and nonobese subjects to the tapes, as well as to more neutral ones. Afterwards, all subjects were asked to rate their own responses on an "uneasiness" scale of from 0 to 100. Not surprisingly, the obese subjects reported themselves to be much more severely affected by the emotional tapes than nonobese subjects did. This was of course as predicted and in and of itself caused no special revision in the accepted thinking about the emotionality of the obese.

To see whether they were reporting accurately on their own emotional reactions, however, Rodin hit upon a way of testing out objectively the subjective statements of what did and what did not constitute a distraction to fat people. While listening to tapes, subjects were given nominal make-work chores to do—one a routine proofreading job, the other a somewhat more intellectually challenging time-monitoring operation. Rodin theorized that if her subjects were indeed as distracted as they said they were by the unpleasant tapes, it would have to have some observable effect on the work they had been set to do while listening to them, and this effect—if any—could be used as an objective measure of their actual reaction to the tapes.

The idea paid off handsomely. As it turned out, the strong emotional reaction reported by the obese to the more troubling tapes could be clearly verified by their job performances: Fat people performed much worse at both kinds of jobs if they worked at them while they were listening to the upsetting tapes. When the taped material was nonemotional, though, they performed much the same as the nonobese. Emotionally charged subjects, in short, seem to pack a more powerful punch with obese subjects than with normal ones, and the effect is not just subjective or self-dramatizing: It can be objectively gauged, measured, and verified. Like brain-lesioned laboratory animals, obese human beings overreact to unpleasant stimuli; like psychoneurotics on the analyst's couch they "feel the pain."

All these things add up to a cluster of personality traits that of course have little or nothing to do with food itself. The emotional reactivity, work habits, and pain or anxiety tolerance of the obese are certainly not things that can easily be equated with hunger or feeding; and yet, like their voracity, the obese seem for better or for worse to have these personality traits in common too.

Why this should be so is one of the more absorbing questions of ongoing obesity research, and has brought the research itself to within target distance of new formulations of personality theory and ego psychology. Going on the assumption that the reaction fat people have to food is simply another variant of their reaction to any other exciting or intense stimulus, Rodin, P. Herman, and Schachter devised a series of tests of attentiveness, concentration, and quickness to react, and predicted that fat people would behave significantly differently on these tests than normals would. The results were as predicted. Fat subjects for example are slower than others to make a simple response to a single, uncomplicated stimulus; but when the stimulus is more complex they are significantly quicker on the uptake than normal people used as controls—another instance of the principle that the obese may be more difficult to arouse than the nonobese but that once something has really captured their attention they seem to get turned on higher and stay that way longer than other people do. The intellectual ramifications of this principle are not inconsiderable. In a test to measure people's ability to recall items on a list, fat people did significantly better than others, not only when the list contained food items, but even when it was composed entirely of words having no conceivable relation to food. Schachter and his group are not alone in reporting findings like these; a similar study of fat young women at an eastern girls' college came to roughly the same conclusions: Fat girls are simply better "rememberers" on tests of this sort than thin or normal girls are.

Similarly, the obese are significantly more alert to and cognizant of words flashed on a tachistoscope than normals are; it takes them less time to see, decipher, and make sense of words flashed very briefly on the screen than it does the nonobese, and as a group the obese are far more uniform in this ability than other people are, with less variation from trial to trial and from one individual to the next.

What do these findings add up to? Are fat people smarter than nonfat people are—is it true, for example, as I. P. Bronstein and his co-workers concluded in their 1942 studies of children, that obese subjects simply have higher I.Q.'s than other subjects do? And, if so, can we generalize from the intellectual status of fat children to that of fat adults?

One problem with this approach, of course, is that obese children are in fact physically and developmentally advanced for their years from birth to adolescence; so the possibility that their high I.Q.'s may be an artifact of their general physical precocity cannot easily be argued away. But Bronstein's findings were not unique; Hilde Bruch had had similar results testing the I.Q.'s of grade-school children too. Fat children were significantly brighter than nonfat controls, and Bruch voiced the opinion that the results would have been even stronger except for the fact that the best students in her group did not always put in an appearance at the scheduled testing sessions. In addition, many of these fatter children did not speak English at home, and might have done even better in the test situation if English had been their native tongue. Rodin, Herman, and Schachter never actually tested their subjects' I.Q.'s, and were in any case dealing with college students in whom the developmental factor should no longer count (the cut-off age on the Stanford-Binet test is 16 years; beyond that point age differences do not appear to affect intellectual achievement), but they concluded tentatively even so that the obese are better "information processors" than other people are—because they take in more information than their normal and skinny peers in the first place, code it more efficiently in the second, and store it more securely in the third.

With the idea of the obese as prodigies, we have come full circle from the popular Pickwickian stereotype of the fat man as simpleton. Whatever intellectual qualities the obese as a group may or may not possess, stupidity is apparently not one of them. And whatever intelligence itself may turn out to be (one rueful definition currently making the rounds of academic circles is that "intelligence is whatever is measured by the intelligence tests"), the obese seem more than able to hold their own against the population at large with respect to this elusive quality. Schachter and his co-workers have meanwhile chosen, no doubt wisely, not to open this particular Pandora's box; their publications are couched in the traditional academese of experimental psychology and the authors have been careful to keep their conclusions as low-keyed and value-free as possible.

In speaking of the "field-dependence" and "stimulus-binding" qualities of the obese, researchers in this area meanwhile are describing a kind of sensory susceptibility and receptivity that characterizes fat people the way tonal discrimination might be assumed to characterize musicians, or kinesthetic awareness to characterize tightrope walkers. The question that remains is why the obese should be better information gatherers and stimulus binders than other people are. Does their hunger for food generalize to their hunger for all other stimuli as well? Or does general response capacity receive some sort of over-all hormonal or neurological boost in the obese that tends to make them overreact to everything that catches their eye or their fancy—up to and including food itself?

The answer would seem to be yes. One straightforward test of this hypothesis is to substitute thirst for hunger in the experimental situation and see if the model still works. Interestingly, it does. Water has no taste, no sedative action, and is not fattening: If fat people prove to react to water as appetitively as they do to food, the chances are that what determines both reactions is not something unique about food itself. Provocatively enough, it turns out that water has the same effect on thirsty obese subjects as food has on hungry ones. Koslowski and Schachter found that fat subjects drank much more water than nonfat subjects when the cue (that is, the water) was arrestingly visible and prominent, but drank just about the same amount as other people did when the cue was visually duller and physically farther away.

This raises questions, like the question of I.Q., that Schachter and his co-workers have deliberately chosen not to pursue, on the grounds that it could lead them too far afield into the speculative limbo of brain neuroanatomy and the centuries-old mind-body debate. Other investigators have been and will be less chary of entering this no man's land, though, and it may not be presumptuous in the meantime to remember that food is the universal stimulus, the primordial turn-on throughout the animal kingdom: It is food that moves the slime-mold amoeba to aggregate, it is hunger that triggers locomotion in the paramecium, and it is food that is used as a reward in learning experiments, child rearing, business lunches, and wedding feasts. Feeding is the infant's first extroverted piece of behavior in the world he has just been born into, and it may well serve as a model for his responses to other situations throughout his lifetime too. It can therefore be no accident that how we as individuals perceive and react to food becomes a measure of how we respond to the rest of the world beyond our bodies as well; certainly the bulk of Schachter's work reflects the dawning empirical certainty that the obese respond differently to the world at large from the way skinny and normal people do, and that their fatness is probably just a special aspect of this difference—an effect of that difference, in other words, and not a cause of it.

Where and how the difference itself arises is still a puzzle, but the fact that it exists is no longer at issue. Bit by bit over the course of a decade, researchers in the behaviorism of obesity have begun to fill in the mosaic of the psychology of fat people, and the picture that is starting to take shape is clearly at variance with both literary and folkloric stereotypes on the one hand and classic psychoanalytic formulations on the other. Far from being the jolly easygoing slowpoke of the popular stereotype, or the greedy grown-up baby of the Freudian one, the image that begins to emerge from these new data is that of an affective powerhouse, slow to rouse initially but intensely reactive once aroused; emotionally susceptible and vulnerable, and capable of more than ordinary emotional intensity once moved; single-minded and hard to distract under ordinary circumstances, but highly distractible when the stimulus is emotionally unpleasant or otherwise negatively charged. In short, appearances are (as the obese would be the first to allow) deceiving. Contrary to tradition, literature, and folklore, it is the thin skin of the obese that distinguishes them from the nonobese; and not, as common sense would have it, the thickness of their fat.

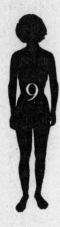

Psychobiology:
Fat Rats and
Starving Undergraduates

Excavating in the hills above Peking a little less than half a century ago, anthropologist Franz Weidenreich uncovered remains of one of the first communities of prehistoric cave dwellers in the human evolutionary line. The Choukoutien fraternity had inhabited this cave in an era of intense cold at the height of the Riss glaciation as long as 150,000 years ago, and had disputed tenancy of its home site with bears and saber-toothed tigers off and on for several millennia. The first indisputable evidence of the domestication of fire appears at Choukoutien: Peking man built hearths inside his caves and in all probability made use of the fires he kindled in them for cooking purposes.

Another archeological "first" at Choukoutien was human cannibalism. Peking man seems regularly to have smashed the skulls of his enemies and scooped out the contents through a hole in the occiput. Presumably he then ate their brains. This practice is not unheard-of in primitive cultures today, for that matter. The Foré of highland New Guinea have been ritually feasting on the gray matter of their relatives and enemies for as long as tribal memory stretches. Recently, however, the Foré appear to have gotten their medical if not their ethical comeuppance: A fatal central-nervous-system disease called kuru has been traced to a slow-acting virus that incubates in the brains of its victims, and the relentless transmission of the disease in Sepik-area warfare has been ascribed to the practice of ritual cannibalism—specifically, to the funerary ritual of eating the brains of one's fellow man.

This realization of the law of talion—man-made or natural—is almost Aesopian in its simplicity, but aside from drawing the obvious moral that crime doesn't pay, there are other important lessons to be learned from it. As the evidence of Choukoutien and kuru attest, man seems from earliest times to have localized the site of the soul somewhere in the recesses of the human brain. Long before Descartes pinpointed this spot to a tiny pea-shaped structure in the midbrain called the pineal body, our primitive ancestors were imbibing the accumulated nerve, wisdom, and soul of fellow and enemy tribesmen through holes in their braincases. Whatever the mind of man may be, and however it has been described over the eons by the various cultures that have tried to define it, there is common agreement about at least one thing: its whereabouts. By general consensus, the human mind lives in the brain, and sooner or later if we would like to know more about the mind than we do now, we are going to have to have recourse to the brain to study it.

The mammalian brain made zoological history in the Cenozoic by ballooning out and forward around its modest vertebrate underpinnings, as a simple bulb at the seeing and smelling end of the spinal column. To the old motoric and olfactory hindbrain of lower orders of vertebrates, evolving animals added larger and larger chunks of gray matter capable of processing wider and wider ranges of information, culminating in the fragile cybernetic wonder of the human neocortex. But this process has proceeded by a sort of accretion of new parts onto older ones; man therefore still shares important structural components of the old mammalian brain with creatures considerably less complicated than he is himself, and in very much the same form in which he first inherited them. So, while the human neocortex is much larger and more richly convoluted than its counterparts in other mammal species, the old brain below the human neocortex seems not to have changed very much, either in structure or in function, since its humbler mammalian beginnings; and scientists engaged in research on such basic physiological processes as hunger, temperature control, thirst, and sex have banked on the not unreasonable assumption that, in matters as primordial as these, the histories of mice and men are apt to be more or less interchangeable.

The histories of rats and men might be a more accurate summation. Man shares a long, exasperated, and star-crossed past with the genus *Rattus*, which arose at about the same time in zoological history as the first primates did, and which has probably always exploited much the same territorial resources and econiches as the ground-dwelling primates have—ourselves among them. Over the years, a kind of surly parasitism seems to have evolved between man and rat, flowering in the catastrophe of bubonic plague in premodern Europe, and culminating in the prolonged cold war that has held sway between the two species ever since—up to and including the standoff between the hybrid white rat and the working researcher in the laboratories of modern universities and medical schools today. The genus *Rattus* has meanwhile achieved a new econiche in human history; and laboratory rats are the unsung heroes of much of modern medical and psychological research of the past half century.

This latter-day alliance has turned out to be a useful one. Experiments with rats have monitored and measured an impressive array of mammalian behavioral puzzles, ranging from habit formation to feeding control and temper tantrums. To what extent findings about such matters can be extrapolated from data about rats and applied to human beings remains one of the open-ended issues of modern academic psychology. What moves a rat to learn his way in and out of a maze may not be quite the same thing as what moves a graduate student to learn how to administer an I.Q. test—and the resulting mental operations and cognitive engrams may not be even roughly comparable.

But in the context of mammalian brain-body feedback, this quibble seems less than earthshaking. Rats, like men, do control their blood salinity by drinking and their blood oxygen by breathing. They do respond to perceived threats in their environments by raising and lowering their blood pressure, and to perceived erotic overtures by raising their output of sex steroids. Like man, rats fight or take flight when threatened; like men, they can and do overeat when certain parts of their brains are destroyed by hemorrhage, tumor, or surgical interference.

The part of the brain at issue in all these behavioral maneuvers is the hypothalamus. The hypothalamus sits at the base of the two major hemispheres of the brain, sited slightly forward of the thalamus (from the Greek word for couch, so called because it forms a sort of cushion under the neocortex); and it controls feeding and satiety, body temperature, blood pressure, and sex—among other things—from its central position deep inside the brain. Research in the area of feeding and satiety, like that on obesity and overeating, has therefore tended in recent years to focus more and more closely on the hypothalamus. The main function of this organ in the body's over-all scheme of things seems to be to mediate between information from the viscera, blood, and skin, on the one hand, and information to and from other parts of the brain on the other—for example, the pituitary gland just below it, and the rhinencephalon just behind it. The pituitary is the body's so-called master gland; hormonal messages from the pituitary instruct other, specialized glands elsewhere in the body to manufacture their own special hormones on orders from the hypothalamus; while the rhinencephalon (or "olfactory" brain) is the part of the old mammalian hindbrain that controls instinct, smell, and feeling, and subsequently funnels sensory data to the hypothalamus to compute.

Together with the thalamus, the hypothalamus serves as a sorter for sensory input, on the one hand, and the hormonal and emotional output that must be conjured up to deal with it on the other. The hypothalamus is thus the brain's little black box, connecting our sensations to our feelings and our feelings to our hormones; the little "brain within a brain" that computes and orchestrates hunger, thirst, temperature, sex, and bodily comfort for us so that we are free to devote our conscious minds to other and presumably "higher" things.

As early as the second decade of the century, French pathologists doing autopsies on the brains of grossly obese subjects made the discovery that such people sometimes had measurable lesions or tumors in or near the hypothalamus at the time of their deaths. Implicit in this finding was the suggestion that something in the hypothalamus might be the factor that was responsible for regulating food intake and satiety, and that anything that interfered with this part of the brain might in turn lead to gross obesity if it went on long enough or was sufficiently widespread. American physiologists took up the challenge presented by this discovery, and in succeeding decades experiments with (live) laboratory animals elicited the fact that by making surgical incisions in the central section of the hypothalamus of such diverse animals as rats, mice, chickens, and a host of others—including, finally, even goats—it was possible to produce an animal so voracious that, as more than one worker has observed, it staggers over to the food hopper immediately after its operation and begins shoveling in food as if there were no tomorrow.

Eating as if life depended on every mouthful, such animals go through a postoperative stage of intensive feeding and expectably rapid weight gain to match. Then, several weeks later, the animal's weight tends to level off and food intake stabilizes at a point slightly higher than its preoperative level and somewhat higher than that of a normal, nonlesioned animal's. During both phases of this process, meanwhile, the animal behaves quite differently from his unlesioned littermates in ways that, oddly enough, have nothing very much to do with food itself.

The resulting psychological profile is not a particularly ingratiating one. The brain-lesioned rat is a snappish animal. He is picky and easily riled, and must be handled—sometimes almost literally—with kid gloves. If this cluster of personality traits has a familiar ring to it, it is not surprising; psychiatric and psychoanalytic case histories of obese patients are full of similar descriptions. And the resemblance is probably not as adventitious as it sounds; for although rats do not have human egos and human conscious (or even for that matter unconscious) minds, they do have similarly organized brains, and obese rats who overeat chronically may be as moody and irritable as human beings who do the same.

The laboratory rat is a convenient experimental animal: genetically standardized, easy to come by, cheap to feed, and quick to reproduce himself. Research on obese rats is therefore a reasonably uncomplicated undertaking. But for many years there were no comparable data on hypothalamically damaged human beings, and for obvious reasons the rat experiments could not be replicated on human subjects. Nevertheless, short of actually operating on human beings to induce surgical lesions in the hypothalamus—or implanting electrodes in their brains to get the same effect—Schachter and his group at Columbia set out to do what they could to match the animal obesity studies coming out of Harvard, Yale, and Rocke-feller universities, with research on human behavior that would ei-ther corroborate the animal data or refute them as the case might be. Their painstaking catalogue of studies on obese hypothalami-cally lesioned rats eventually paid handsome research dividends; it turned out that in almost every instance where such data exist or could be realistically duplicated by comparable experiments using obese human beings as subjects, the human studies upheld the ear-lier findings from studies of obese laboratory rats. Nobody, to hear Schachter tell it, was more surprised or intrigued by this outcome than he and his colleagues were.

Schachter's classic study of obese human beings' dependence on outside cues to stimulate appetite and induce feeding, in which he manipulated the hands of a laboratory clock backward and forward to simulate mealtimes, showed that obese humans were much more responsive to this kind of experimental flimflam than nonobese sub-jects were apt to be. The same thing was known to be true for brain-lesioned obese rats when light cues were juggled to simulate dark and daylight at odd and erroneous hours. Like the obese human beings, obese rats took their cues from the environment, real or doctored—and not from their own bellies, blood, or brains. They ate when darkness fell, regardless of real time and, presum-ably, of their own real circadian feeding schedules and actual ca-loric ups and downs. They were, in Schachter's phrase, "cue-dominated"—as opposed to the self-starting and self-dominating feeding habits of the nonobese.

Previous studies from the labs of various teams of investigators had shown that once past the first postoperative phase of gross overeating, hypothalamically lesioned obese rats ate very slightly more than control animals did on a day-to-day basis. They also ate fewer but larger meals. And when they did eat, they ate more rap-idly than normal animals did. Interestingly enough, all these obser-vations could be made with equal accuracy about obese human beings observed under experimental conditions too. Study for study, and variable for variable, obese human beings turned out to manifest the same differences vis-à-vis nonobese members of their own species as obese rats did vis-à-vis theirs.

And the parallels do not stop with caloric factors. For reasons that are still not clear, obese brain-lesioned rats will not work as hard to get food as nonobese rats will. The same peculiarity was to prove to be true of obese and nonobese newborn babies, and of obese and nonobese Columbia undergraduates too. By the same token, obese rats and obese humans will both eat more of a good-tasting food, even when their stomachs are full, than nonobese humans and lab rats will. On the other hand, though, the actual caloric load of a meal makes little impression on the appetites of obese humans (and obese rats) unless it happens to be ingested in liquid form. When food is eaten in solid form, both obese rats and obese humans (as opposed to normal individuals of both species) seem not to be able to assess the caloric measure of the food they have just eaten (or if they can do so, they do not act accordingly), while their assessment of liquid calories stays reasonably accurate. This is a finding which might incidentally turn out to have interesting—and helpful—consequences for dieters, if it proves to test out in larger populations than the ones sampled to date.

Taken all together, the major message from this impressive bill of particulars of rats and men is the fact that obese human beings and rats share striking similarities in areas that have nothing to do with food and feeding itself. Not only are their feeding habits distinctive, but both are also more emotional than normal individuals of their own species are; and both are significantly better at learning to avoid unpleasant stimuli (in the form of electric shocks) than their nonobese conspecifics are. The implications of such behavioral differences thus do not begin and end with the differences in their feeding habits but go way beyond the simple arithmetic of caloric intake and energy expenditure, and strike at the very roots of personality and character as well.

Aggression is one of the personality factors that affect feeding in species and classes as far away from each other on the Linnaean family tree as fish and mammals: Evolutionary taxonomy suggests that hunger and aggression have gone hand in hand throughout zoological history. José Delgado, who pioneered in electric stimulation of the brain in experiments at Yale Medical School during the fifties and sixties, found that he could turn affectionate, even-tempered cats into raging aggressors merely by stimulating a site at either side of the hypothalamus. The sites in question were close to—and possibly even coterminous with—sites normally known to be activated when the animal was in the process of feeding or stalking food. Milder nastiness (hissing and growling) could also be elicited by stimulating a somewhat more forward part of the same structure. This peculiarity of brain geography jibes well with observations about affect and obesity from other labs: It was becoming a commonplace of obesity research with hypothalamically lesioned animals that something or other apparently intrinsic to the syndrome of obesity itself seems to predispose obese animals to varying degrees of meanness, testiness, or outright rage.

If these were human beings, we might, like the Freudians, suppose that their rage was a cognitively determined one—triggered, say, by knowledge of the injustice of their fate, appetitive or otherwise, or at least of their inability to do anything much about it. Since rats lack the higher brain structures that are involved in such judgments, though, logic suggests that the source of their rage must be located much closer to the source of their hunger than "consciousness" is, and the fact that emotional reactions can be triggered by hypothalamic stimulation—as Delgado's work demonstrates—would seem to strengthen the case.

From Nature's point of view this arrangement is not an unreasonable one; hunger by itself is emotionally neutral and does not constitute a strong-enough impetus in and of itself for the unfed animal to commit predatory mayhem in an ecologically complicated world; some sort of even more intense emotion may be the catalyst that is needed to set the proper behavioral chain reaction in motion and carry it through to its logical (and biological) conclusion. In carnivores in particular, but to some extent in omnivores like man and rats as well, the requisite emotion may be something akin to anger. Anyone who has ever had dealings with an unfed, sulky child will appreciate the connection between crankiness and hunger—in human beings, at least. And presumably meat-eating animals are not moved to stalk and kill their prey by sheer pleasure in the chase or even by simple gluttony. As it turns out, something more sometimes proves to be necessary; and aggression may well turn out to be the emotional common denominator of food-seeking behaviors among animals who have to catch their dinners before they can actually make a meal of them. If so, evolutionary forces may sensibly have conspired to wire aggression and general irritability into the basic brain circuitry that governs appetite and feeding—especially in animals who routinely make their livings by predation.

In this respect, rats and man stand somewhere midway between the carnivores and the herbivores. We are neither as passive as the herbivores in getting our daily bread nor as active as the carnivores; but self-feeding in a human being normally requires at least some modicum of nonruminative, go-getting behavior. And the adrenal fight-or-flight hormones, epinephrine and norepinephrine, may be among the major biochemical signals for setting this biological enterprise in motion.

Evidence for the role of the adrenal hormones in turning both rage and hunger off and on comes from research in the brain chemistry of laboratory rats—and may even be generalizable to man. While epinephrine itself appears to be the hormonal "agent" or messenger for fear in the body, norepinephrine is the form of the hormone that seems to be highest in displays of rage and anger. Psychologists at Wyeth Laboratories in Pennsylvania have shown that there are definite receptor sites for norepinephrine in the part of the hypothalamus that governs satiety. When these sites—which actually consist of bundles of nerve endings—are biochemically treated so that they cannot pick up and "bind" a certain form of norepinephrine, laboratory animals so treated will go on gorging on their favorite foods long after they have actually had their fill. This fact would not be so interesting in and of itself, except for the additional fact that norepinephrine is apparently also simultaneously the body's chemical message carrier for rage (as Funkenstein had previously posited); and since the act of feeding in normal animals "binds" norepinephrine and removes it from the circulating blood, it may be that feeding not only neutralizes hunger but that it also neutralizes rage at one and the same time. Conversely, it may be that it is the high levels of unbound, free, norepinephrine circulating in the blood of unfed (or underfed) animals that causes them to be as cranky as they are—in the case of rats and humans—and as downright bloodthirsty as they are in the case of lions, tigers, and wolves.

The insight to be culled from experiments like these is not, however, that human beings are ratlike (or lionlike), or that rats and lions are humanoid; but only that, given a similar abnormality of body size and shape (obesity) and a similar cause for it (uncontrollable overeating)—the rats and humans in question should turn out to have so many other behavioral peculiarities in common too. And since we know what caused the rats to start overeating and get fat in the first place (i.e., a lesion in the ventromedial section of the hypothalamus, made to the experimenter's measure and put there deliberately to elicit the gluttonous behavior that ensues), the inference that obese human beings may have something awry in the same part of the hypothalamus is hard to keep from drawing too.

Research along these lines is clearly taking us close to the day when the connections between physique and behavior, and appetite and overweight, can be spelled out in some if not all of their enormous complexity and put to some good practical use in the control of obesity and other feeding disorders. So far, though, the work that has been done in this area has been tantalizing in its elusiveness, and has raised many more questions than it has had any immediate hopes of answering. For, contrary to popular ideas on the subject, feedback between the stomach (empty or full) and the brain (aroused or sated) is maddeningly inexact—especially in people with a weight problem, but even, to some extent, in those without.

Mouth, stomach, gut, and brain are all major way stations on the feedback shuttle between hunger and satiety; and to begin to get an idea of how things can go wrong with this system in obesity, we should probably aim for some reasonably clear-cut notion of the way things happen when everything is going right. Theoretically, the shuttle operates something like this: Hunger contractions in the stomach of the unfed animal get relayed to the hypothalamus through a major neural pathway (called the splanchnic nerve) that runs between the viscera and the head. The animal responds by locating food, grasping it, opening his mouth, and feeding. Sensations about the taste and texture, the liquidity or solidity and possibly the temperature of the food are relayed back to the hypothalamus through the trigeminal and gustatory nerves that run between the mouth and the brain; when these sensations are pleasurable or "right," the electrical activity in the feeding centers of the hypothalamus gets turned on "high," and the animal is given the go-ahead to keep feeding. Meanwhile, as he feeds, nutrients from his food pass into his digestive tract, gradually filling his stomach and passing on into his small intestine. Here they are picked up by the blood and sent around to the cells—including of course, among others, the cells in the brain.

Glucose is the fuel that the brain runs on, and special receptor cells for glucose in the lateral hypothalamus bind molecules of glucose now slowly beginning to circulate in the feeding animal's blood. When these special brain receptor cells receive their due share of glucose, their electrical activity increases, activating the cells that trigger satiety, on the one hand, and damping down on cells that trigger feeding on the other. This double-barreled message from the hypothalamus signals the animal that he has had enough to eat; whereupon the vagus nerve stops signaling the stomach to contract, and with the stomach no longer contracting and brain sugar receptors in the hypothalamus well saturated with glucose for the time being, feeding activity winds down and eventually comes to a stop. The animal feels fed and full; and, if all goes well, the feeding cycle will not repeat itself until available blood sugar is exhausted again sometime within the next few hours.

This is the model, however inexact it may be—and it is of course an ideal one at that. New research is constantly modifying it and fleshing it out; new ghosts in the machine are constantly rising up to obscure the basic outlines of the model as originally constructed. In the obese one or all of these ideal relays may get slightly out of kilter, go awry, or simply stop functioning altogether. Things can go wrong at any point in the circle—and do. Damage to the trigeminal nerve in rats and pigeons, for example, can close down the whole feeding mechanism in these animals from start to finish; conversely, pleasant sensations in the mouth and an overcharged or easily roused trigeminal nerve may keep animals (and people) feeding long after satiety actually sets in, with or without interference from somewhere farther down the line. Furthermore, incomplete feedback between the hypothalamus and the vagus nerve may keep the stomach contracting long after it is full; while an overresponsive splanchnic nerve can magnify the intensity of stomach contractions beyond all reason—regardless of whether the stomach was empty or full when the nerve originally began firing.

But even if all these neuronal relays are in good working order, getting glucose out of the food and into the brain glucose receptors where it belongs can be subject to all kinds of hormonal mishaps and various enzymatic ups and downs. Insulin and glucagon must be present in just the right amounts before glucose can reach receptor sites in the hypothalamus in the first place; too much insulin and the animal will go on feeding too long because glucose will be removed from the blood too fast to register in the satiety center in the appointed time; too little glucagon, and the circulating insulin will not be able to move what glucose there is out of the blood and into the cells themselves. Thyroxin gets into the picture by dictating the rate at which actual cell metabolism takes place during and after feeding: If metabolic reactions are going forward too fast, the satiety center may get activated too early in feeding for the animal to eat a fair-sized meal; if they are too slow the satiety center may get activated too late in the meal and the animal may go on feeding long after he is in fact "fed."

Any and all of these difficulties may be involved in the feeding and satiety miscalculation of the obese. One of the biggest surprises to emerge from early attempts to define physiological hunger was the fact that in certain important respects, the obese never do feel real hunger—at least not in the sense that normal people do. Albert J. Stunkard demonstrated this in an ingenious experiment that has become a classic in the field. He asked obese and nonobese volunteers to come to his laboratory early in the morning before they had had their breakfasts, and prevailed on them to swallow a gastric balloon which was set up to monitor their stomach contractions over a four-hour period. At regular intervals throughout the experiment subjects were asked whether they felt hungry or not; later, their answer at any given moment was matched to kymographic tracings of their own stomach contractions at the moment the question was asked. The results were startling. What emerged from this study was the finding that there was little if any relationship between stomach contractions as recorded in squiggles on the kymograph tracings of obese subjects and feelings of actual "hunger" as reported out loud to the experimenter by these same subjects themselves. Nonobese subjects, on the other hand, showed an almost perfect correspondence between kymograph tracings and "hunger" reports.

Obese people, in other words, do not seem to experience hunger when their stomachs are in fact contracting regularly, whereas nonobese patients do identify their own stomach contractions with the sensation of hunger regularly, effectively, and predictably. This means that either the obese do not feel their stomachs contracting when they are in fact doing so or, if they do feel the contractions, fail for some reason to identify the accompanying sensation with any specific desire to eat. The effect is not just an artifact of obese people's timidity about acknowledging their own appetites—since obese subjects were just as apt to report themselves hungry as nonobese subjects were, but these reports rarely jibed with the physical facts as recorded by the kymograph.

If the hunger that dogs some fat people and drives them to overeat on a chronic basis doesn't derive from sensations in their stomachs and viscera, just how do such people know when they are hungry, and why do they ever start eating—let alone overeating—in the first place? Increasingly, the answer to this question has tended to focus on the hypothalamus, and not on the belly itself.

In 1952 Neal Miller and associates of his at Yale, studying feeding and satiety in relation to the way rats learn certain tasks, discovered that while food injected directly into the animal's stomach worked as a perfectly adequate "reward" for lab rats in learning experiments, giving the same food by mouth was a much more potent reward than food delivered straight to the stomach. The implications of this finding were not immediately clear, and in order to find out more about them Miller began to implant electrodes into his laboratory animals' brains, and thereby monitor the consequences of their feeding behavior in terms of appetite, drive, and emotion.

Working with brain neurophysiologist José Delgado of the Yale Medical School, Miller confirmed the important discovery of pioneer brain researcher J. Olds that there is a certain site in the hypothalamus that, when electrically stimulated, acts as a pure pleasure center, uncontaminated by any baser drives or urges than that of pleasure itself. Animals stimulated in this part of their brain will press a lever in their cages over and over again to achieve the accompanying sensations; furthermore, they will press this bar in preference to one attached to a food hopper duly stocked with lab chow. And, as if to make matters even plainer, animals will press the pleasure bar in preference to the food and drink bars even when they have every reason to be hungry and thirsty, and presumably need food and drink much more acutely than they need a cheap nonspecific thrill. Delgado and Miller concluded that they had stumbled upon a new Atlantis in the brain: the pleasure center. In certain spots in the hypothalamus, electrical stimulation at that site caused rats to press the pleasure lever up to 5,000 times in one hour, and to go on doing so for hours at a time, to the point of virtual exhaustion. This behavior could be elicited altogether independently of feeding, drinking, or sexual arousal: The pleasure in other words was untrammeled by any instinctual content; it was an end in itself.

One of the implications of this line of research is that, whatever reasons the obese animal or person may have for overeating, pleasure as such, all by itself, need not necessarily be one of them. For just as the pleasure can exist without the feeding, it is not unreasonable to suppose that feeding can exist without pleasure too; and it is of course a common complaint of fat people that they can only bring themselves to quit eating when their stomachs are so distended that another mouthful would not only be unpleasurable but might be so positively unpleasurable as to be downright nauseating.

The question of pleasure is one that even the most enthusiastic of psychobiologists have been at pains to approach cautiously. Definitions are in order, but for definitions you need verbal consensus, and our pleasures are as notoriously hard to define and pin down as nuances of color, taste, and sensation. Does pleasure inhere in expectancy and anticipation—or does it have to reach a peak and then come to an end in order to merit the name? Is pleasure in eating, qualitatively and quantitatively, the same as sexual pleasure? Aesthetic ecstasy? Religious rapture? Is pleasure that goes on and on without peaking a pleasure—or a pain? Until recently, questions like these might have been considered philosophical, labyrinthine, or even downright windy; we are now beginning to find perfectly hard-nosed answers for them, and the answers turn out to be part and parcel of our understanding of the brain itself.

To find out whether the pleasurable component in eating is more tightly bound up with "hunger" or with "satiety," D. L. Margules in 1962 planted electrodes in the feeding centers of rats and then, after feeding the animals, delivered a mild electric current to the feeding centers to see if they could be turned back on again—to see, that is, if the animals could be induced to start eating again so soon after being fed—and well fed at that. Of the 46 animals Margules tested, only 28—or slightly more than half—could be induced to feed again in this way. But those that did start eating again showed an interesting difference from those who did not: The refeeders all proved to be animals who exhibited an extraordinarily high "self-stimulation" (or pleasure-seeking) score when put into a Skinner box with a self-reward lever and watched to see how many times they pressed the "thrill" lever when left to their own devices. There were notable differences among rats in this respect; and the refeeders were all measurably more pleasure-oriented, as it turned out, than their more ascetic, less food-cued littermates. On the other hand, though, their "hedonism" definitely affected their feeding behavior too; for although all the animals stimulated themselves with much more abandon as time passed and they grew genuinely hungrier, the refeeders led the pack in this respect: their bar pressing when they were hungry was much faster and more furious than that of the other rats.

It is clear from experiments like this that anticipating food is at least as great a source of pleasure as eating it is. But the pleasurable aspects of satiety are unfortunately much less clear. Meanwhile, work with brain-lesioned rats done by Jean Mayer and his colleagues at Harvard in the early fifties made it plain that it was not damage to the feeding centers of the hypothalamus that led lesioned animals to overeat, but damage to the satiety centers that did the trick. Mayer's brain-lesioned animals were not abnormal with respect to their appetites as such, in other words, but only with respect to whatever mechanism it is that is supposed to turn appetite *off* after the animal has received a calorically adequate supply of food. The resulting obesities in Mayer's lab animals were not the consequence of any unusual voraciousness on their parts, but of the animals' simply not knowing when to stop feeding. Like obese human beings, obese rats and mice seem not to know when they have had enough, and tend to rely on simple mechanical limits in the gut—if not outright nausea—to do the hypothalamus's work for them. Pleasure, in short, may be what turns feeding on; but it is something else again that turns it off. Nature has been careful to make sure that animals will feed when they are hungry by surrounding appetite with all kinds of cheap (and extraneous) cerebral thrills; but when it comes to satiety she has left matters to chemistry and common sense. The results can be unpredictable—and fattening in the extreme.

From his work with T. B. Van Itallie, Mayer eventually concluded that the hypothalamus contains sugar receptors especially designed to monitor the level of glucose in the circulating blood. Classical thinking on this subject had held that when glucose levels are low, the stomach will start contracting and the subject will acknowledge feeling hungry; when they are high, gastric contractions will cease and the subject will feel "fed." But where, when, and how did the organism become aware of the fact that there was new sugar in the system, and manage to take a reading of its own blood-glucose levels? Clearly, the sugar monitor was not in the stomach; if so, eating a piece of hard candy would be all that was ever needed to pacify hunger. Neither—by the same reasoning—was it in the mouth. This left the hypothalamus as the likely candidate for the site. Reasoning along these lines, Mayer coined the term "glucostat" for the mechanism that presumably turns appetite on and off in the hypothalamus. Like an ordinary house-furnace thermostat, this hypothetical monitor would tune up the feeding centers when blood-sugar supplies were low, and turn them off again when the subject had eaten and they were high.

In defense of this theory, Mayer designed an experiment to test the brain's specific propensity to bind sugar. The key to this puzzle proved to be—literally—golden. Working with Norman Marshall and Russell Barnett, Mayer discovered that parts of the hypothalamus could be destroyed by a chemical compound called gold thioglucose, which is composed of an atom of gold, an atom of sulphur, and a molecule of glucose. Gold was the lethal agent in this compound: Mice in whom a section of the hypothalamus had been destroyed by gold thioglucose became voracious and soon grew enormously fat. But the destructive action of the gold in gold thioglucose could only be counted on to do its damage when glucose itself was present; substituting other common forms of sugar (like sorbitol, or galactose) or fats (like glycerol and other fatty acids) for the original glucose molecule in the compound had no effect at all on the animal's hypothalamus, appetite, or weight. What seemed to be happening, according to Mayer, was that glucose exerted such a strong attraction on the satiety centers in the hypothalamus that any glucose in the vicinity of the organ would immediately be annexed by these centers—even at the expense of the cells themselves and of the integrity of the organ that contained them.

The lesson to be drawn from this phenomenon is not so much that gold is toxic to the hypothalamus (which of course it is) but that certain structures in the hypothalamus have such a strong affinity for glucose that they will pick it up and bind it even when it is indissolubly attached to a lethal atom of gold, and doing so therefore amounts to certain cellular death. The particular structures involved in this form of biochemical suicide are, on the evidence, those that tell the animal he has had enough to eat—in other words, the satiety centers. Mayer had thus effectively demonstrated in this experiment that, in the first place, there are indeed nerve-ending clusters that act as "satiety centers" in the hypothalamus; and that, in the second, these centers are specifically designed to bind glucose in any way, shape, or form they may happen to find it in—lethal or otherwise.

From observations like these, the inference is strong that the brain's ability to bind glucose must have something important—if not something downright decisive—to do with feeling satiated after a calorically nourishing meal.

Mayer's idea of a hypothalamic glucose monitor or "glucostat" is a convincing one, but it is not necessarily the only possibility. Hypotheses abound; the possibilities are almost as numerous—and puzzling—as the hypothalamus is complicated. Physiologist J. R. Brobeck had been doing research on appetite and hunger along the same general lines as Mayer's at Yale, but had arrived at very different conclusions about the mechanisms involved. Brobeck was interested in the fact that thermal factors seem to play a crucial part in an animal's decision to eat or not to eat according to the day, the climate, and the season, and noted that food intake seems to fluctuate with impressive predictability according to the weather or the temperature inside an animal's cage: When the environmental temperature is high, animals of widely varying species eat less than they do when it is low.

A wide-ranging and heterodox literature exists to back this observation up. As long ago as 1916 Anton Julius Carlson had measured the frequency of stomach contractions under various temperature conditions, and concluded that stomach motility increased impressively as the temperature dropped. The same phenomenon was noted in dogs by C. K. Sleeth and E. J. Van Liere in 1937; stomach-emptying time decreased significantly in animals who were exposed to a marked drop in temperature immediately after a feed. There thus seems to be some solid physiological evidence for the common impression that cold weather produces hearty appetites; our stomachs get the message that it is cold outside without any assistance from our conscious minds, and react accordingly. This effect has recently been pinpointed to a certain small area in the forward part of the hypothalamus: Rats who have been surgically lesioned in this area get their thermal and appetitive signals seriously crossed, and eat too much in a hot environment, too little in a cold one—suggesting that this part of the hypothalamus has the very specific function of calibrating hunger to temperature and sending the appropriate message on down the line to contractile tissues in the stomach itself.

This interesting addendum to the anatomy of the hypothalamus is not without consequences for farmers and livestock breeders and those sectors of the economy that supply them. Experts in England have recently established the fact that, depending on the price of feed (and fuel) in any given year, it may sometimes be cheaper to heat the barn over the winter months than to lay in more fodder over the same period. This economic cost-accounting reckoning makes good thermodynamic sense: In the process of burning food for fuel, body temperature rises by a slight but predictable amount (about one degree Fahrenheit for most mammals) within an hour or so of eating, and there is good reason to suppose that the resulting temperature change may register somewhere in the hypothalamus as a signal to the animal that it has had enough to eat. This finding was given added strength by E. R. Buskirk's observation that basal metabolic rates rise after a meal, until they reach a high point within about an hour after feeding, then gradually fall back to their normal set points again. Since it is basal metabolism that governs heat production in the body, and since the hypothalamus controls basal metabolism through its action on the pituitary, the meshing of these three variables—basal metabolic rates, heat regulation, and appetite—all in one organ seems to imply a functional, as well as a merely structural, relationship between them.

Other research along these lines was not long in coming. C. L. Hamilton put rats into refrigerated cages to see whether food intake would have any effect on the animals' attempts to keep themselves warm. The rats could press a switch to turn on heating lamps inside the cage. It soon became clear that animals who had had little or nothing to eat used the heating lamps much more often than those who had been put into the cages fully fed, proving not only that food intake predictably raises body temperature, as advertised, but that the animal is in some sense accurately aware of his own temperature deficit when he has not been fed—and may thus, presumably, "learn" to feed when there is no other means of raising body temperature at hand. (If so, rats and livestock would not be the only animals to respond to temperature in this way: The highest per capita food consumption ever recorded in the world is that of human beings on an Antarctic research expedition in 1967.)

A third possibility is one first proposed by Kennedy in 1953 and more recently put forward by J. F. Brock and J. D. L. Hansen in Sweden and G. R. Hervey in Great Britain, who have proposed that there may be some "lipostatic" mechanism operating in satiety as well as, or even possibly in lieu of, the hypothetical glucostat proposed by Jean Mayer. In the view of these authors, glucose receptors cannot account for the well-known ability of fats to satisfy hunger faster and more lastingly than sugars and carbohydrates do—or for the even more striking (and puzzling) fact that something in the brain does indeed seem to monitor the total amount of body fat an animal is programmed to carry—if not on a day-to-day basis, at least over a period of several weeks.

Evidence for this assumption comes from the fact that force-feeding animals, even for quite prolonged periods of time, usually does not result in a permanent weight gain: Once the animal is taken off tube feeding, body weight (at least in normal, nonobese animals) tends to revert to pre-experimental levels all by itself. The same thing probably holds true for normal, nonobese human beings too: Most people can safely overeat at parties, over the weekend, or on vacations without incurring any longstanding and irreversible degree of overweight. Something—a sort of inner gyroscope—can be counted on to do the right caloric arithmetic and bring them back down to normal weight within a few days or weeks of their original eating binge.

Ingenious but rather macabre experiments have been devised to prove the point. In 1959, physiologist G. R. Hervey con' ^ted experiments in the "parabiosis" of fat and thin laboratory rats and mice. Parabiosis is an operation that joins two animals together by a skin and blood vessel graft and thereby produces a kind of artificial Siamese twinning of two animals of the same genetic make-up, usually but not necessarily littermates; the animals share the same blood and lymph supply and are thus immediately responsive to hormonal and humoral messages from each other's body fluids. When two normal, nonobese animals are parabiosed in this way, each animal's body fat slowly dwindles to about half of its original fat level. This process can take anywhere from five to nine months, and it is hard to keep from drawing the conclusion that something in both animals' nervous systems is picking up the message that there is simply too much adipose tissue on hand for comfort, and that the excess will have to be jettisoned. Both animals can lose considerable amounts of weight in the process—sometimes amounting to 50 per cent and more of their normal fat reserves.

By the same token, if nonobese rats are parabiosed to grossly obese animals, the normal rats lose virtually all of their body fat stores, become emaciated, and eventually die of starvation in what appears to be an irresistible attempt by something in the central nervous systems to keep adipose tissue levels within tolerable "normal" limits. The process is automatic, unreasoned, and unrelenting; and the suspicion that something quite similar may exist in human beings has put the damper on plastic surgery to remove fat tissue surgically in cases of overwhelming obesity; nobody can be quite sure whether the remaining adipose tissue deposits might not compensate by automatically reverting to their sorry pre-operative highs.

In short, the existence of a "lipostat"—some long-term regulator in the brain, the blood, or the fat tissue itself that may be monitoring the total body complement of fat and keeping it up to the mark at regular (perhaps weekly or monthly) intervals—is a notion to be reckoned with, and one that cannot be dismissed out of hand.

Last but not least in the roster of tantalizing ideas about where and how hunger and satiety actually meet, match, and cross each other out is the suggestion of Mauricio Russek that the real testing ground for this action is in the liver. Russek's reasoning goes something like this: Injecting glucose directly into the abdomen is known to stop hunger pangs a great deal more quickly than injecting exactly the same dose into the skin or even into the blood itself. And injecting glucose into the portal vein (which is the major highway for blood entering the liver) produces an even stronger effect. Even more striking than the way glucose can appease hunger when it is injected into the portal vein, though, is the way in which amino acids—the building blocks of proteins—do the same job, and the rate at which they do it. Amino acids introduced into the portal vein are five times as effective as a calorically identical glucose load in turning off hunger and producing satiety in laboratory rats.

Russek posits an electrically potentiating model for the way this process might work. While animals are fasting, glucose is being mobilized from the liver and released into the bloodstream. But the glucose outflow from the liver is accompanied by an outflow of potassium ions from the cell's interior to the cell surface (a normal-enough state of affairs in the transportation of nutrients back and forth across the cell's walls). In losing potassium ions, however, the cell membrane is simultaneously being depolarized, hence "depotentiated," for further metabolic exchange; and it is the loss of the electrical charge at the cell's surface that causes that feeling of visceral uneasiness or stalemate, which the brain in turn reads as hunger. When Russek monitored his lab rats on a round-the-clock basis, he found that hunger pangs (or at least feeding behavior) peaked very close to the time when the electrical charge at the animals' liver-cell membranes became depotentiated. This suggests strongly that the two peaks are related to each other causally as well as chronologically, and that "hunger" begins when the electrical activity at the cell membrane leaves off.

The attractiveness of Russek's model is that it links two parts of the chain which have so far eluded connection. Glucose in Russek's model is only a sort of handy transport medium for the basic amino acids that constitute the real raw material of the human nutritional drama. We are, after all, made up of proteins at the level of our cells, our organs, and our blood; glucose is simply the form that the fuel takes as it runs through the pipeline. Glucose in other words is *in* the system without being *of* it: Russek's brainstorm provides the hook-up that has so far been missing between them.

And, what is perhaps even more important, Russek's model proposes at long last some really convincing explanation for the fact that people (at least nonobese people) unanimously experience hunger as a sensation somewhere in their guts, and satiety as an abdominal muchness. By the same token, it would also help explain why nausea, or anything seriously awry in the liver, tends to magnify the feeling of satiety to the point where feeding itself becomes unthinkable, if not downright impossible. At the same time, though, Russek's model does nothing to discredit Jean Mayer's theory of a glucostat in the hypothalamus, or Brobeck's theory of a thermostat in the brain, or Hervey's theory of a lipostat in the blood: It simply provides a link in the network that could hypothetically link all these systems together into a working, self-regulating whole.

Of course, it goes without saying that none of the brain-body servomechanisms enumerated here (lipostats, thermostats, glucostats, aminostats) need necessarily be mutually exclusive. And meanwhile, faced with so many different alternatives about the relationship between the brain and the belly in the state of hunger, a common-sense judgment might seem to suggest that there is merit in all of them. If Nature in her wisdom localized feeding and satiety, temperature and blood-pressure control, aggression, sex, and thirst in one small central and basal organ buried at the virtual dead center of the brain, a respectful guess would be that it was not done idly, and that all these functions may prove to be intimately interdependent once all the data are in. All may and probably do work together to achieve the organism's basic purpose—which is, logically enough, to keep the animal supplied with food and fuel as a means toward the end of staying alive and functioning.

But in the last analysis, if work like Hervey's, Brobeck's, Mayer's, and Russek's has any message for the obese, it is—as the Freudians were among the first to note—that the brain is the major arbiter of satiety and hunger in the long run. Whether one believes that that arbitration takes place in the neocortex—as the Freudians do—or in the hypothalamus—as the psychobiologists do—is pretty much a matter of training and point of view. But wherever in the head such feelings may originate, the basic mind-body connections obviously run both ways; and this means that understanding obesity should in the long run entail some understanding of its opposite number—emaciation—too.

Physiologically speaking, starvation and emaciation are the other sides of the coin of whatever it is that goes wrong in obesity; and here again, while the Freudians have staked a modest claim to understanding and cure, it is the psychobiologists who may prove in the long run to have the final say. If so, the crucial issue may revolve around the disease of *anorexia nervosa,* a syndrome in which patients appear to deliberately set out to starve themselves to within an inch of their lives. *Anorexia nervosa* patients are usually female, adolescent, and either mildly overweight or of just about normal weight when the disorder first sets in. In a brief for the psychogenic character of the disease, Hilde Bruch has pointed out that these patients tend to be perfectionistic, obedient, and super-achievers; losing weight may therefore be just one more way in which such a patient tries to achieve some wrong-headed version of physical "perfection" in a culture that overvalues leanness to the point of do or die. But the psychoanalytic explanation leaves important organic riddles unsolved. Psychobiologists for example point to the fact that as long ago as 1914 the English physician Simmonds had discovered evidence of recent hemorrhage in the pituitary gland of a woman who had died of cachexia (acute emaciation) following soon upon the birth of a child. This case has come to represent a model of sorts for the central mystery of the syndrome; all the elements of the (physiological) puzzle are there —emaciation, interrupted menstruation, midbrain insult—without any of the (psychological) elements of the *anorexia nervosa* syndrome as it would normally be described today.

While such clear-cut clinical findings have not been widely replicated (*anorexia nervosa* is by no means always fatal, and few cases ever end up on the autopsy table) they do crop up from time to time in the medical literature and must be dealt with by theorists on both sides of the issue. Furthermore, recent research tends to bolster the idea that there may be some fundamental midbrain disorder involved in the syndrome: Many anorectic patients show primary derangements not only of appetite but of temperature regulation, water metabolism, and daily steroid biorhythms as well—derangements that hang on even after the patient is eating regularly again and seems to have conquered the original phobia (if that is what it actually is) about being fat. These regulatory abnormalities have nothing to do with the physiological starvation process itself: Other victims of starvation do not manifest them, and neither do other psychiatric patients with phobias unrelated to calories. So, although it has been pretty much taken for granted by a whole generation of psychosomatically minded physicians that *anorexia nervosa* is a psychiatric syndrome, recent findings suggest that the matter is not quite so simple (or so complicated!) as the psychoanalytic theory supposes.

Self-starvation and regulatory disturbances are not the only hallmarks of this mysterious feeding disorder: other central-nervous-system indicators are present too. Certain *anorexia nervosa* patients for example are known to be peculiarly hyperactive and indefatigable. They pace the floor; they may literally walk around in circles (as one of Bruch's patients did) to work off energy, calories, and steam. Stunkard, like Bruch, has taken more than a passing interest in the syndrome; in a recent study he attached pedometers to the legs of anorectic patients to see just how hyperactive they actually were, and determined that they walked an average of 6.8 miles a day—almost twice as much, in other words, as normal women of the same age, social class, and life-style do. Symptom for symptom, therefore, the anorectic patient may have all the earmarks of someone who has overdosed on amphetamines; and whatever the intrinsic mistakes and oversights (or overreachings) of basic brain chemistry may turn out to be, these are among the clear indications that fundamental body regulatory systems are among the first things to go in *anorexia nervosa*, and that the metabolic mistakes involved are not secondary to the disease but part and parcel of its basic etiology.

Such a picture is of course almost diametrically opposed to the one seen in the real-life, unpremeditated, and unwilled starvation of human famine. Sub-Saharan refugees and German concentration-camp survivors set no pedometric records; in real starvation hyperactivity is the exception, not the rule, and people move around as little as is humanly possible in what is no doubt a sensible last-ditch attempt to preserve as much energy—and hence as much body tissue—as they can until the last possible moment of negotiable clinical time. Animals starved experimentally show a similar pattern: Up to the fourth day of fasting, starved rats exhibit abnormally heightened activity levels; but after this period inanition sets in and the animal moves less, then more and more slowly, and eventually not at all. The typical *anorexia nervosa* patient, on the other hand, never seems to reach this cutoff point; she (or in extremely rare cases he) is hyperactive and hyperreactive to the bitter end.

In one other important psychological respect, however, both kinds of subjects are very much alike: The anorectic patient proves to be, at least in a negative way, every bit as obsessed with the idea of food as the victims of true starvation are. And, just like victims of famine—though in a very different psychological and economic context of course—the *anorexia nervosa* patient thinks, dreams, and hallucinates food, even though she may go to extraordinary extremes to avoid eating it once it is actually there. (One of Bruch's patients, a woman in her early twenties, was so terrified of the quasi-occult power of food in her own icebox that she badgered her parents into shopping for staples three times a day, and then only in amounts just large enough to be consumed at one sitting—lest the siren song of the uneaten leftovers prove stronger than her own ability to resist them.)

But hunger makes even stranger bedfellows than these, and still another group with whom anorectic and starving subjects share their obsession (positive or negative as the case may be) with food are the bona-fide run-of-the-mill obese. For all three of these groups, food seems to have a coercive power all its own— something that operates quite independently of the subject's ethics, will power, or conscious mind. The *anorexia nervosa* patient fights back tooth and nail; the starving prison-camp inmate does what he can to hallucinate the taste and smell of food; while the run-of-the-mill obese citizen routinely gives in to the third sandwich on the plate; but otherwise the three kinds of responses are eerily similar.

From starved prison-camp inmates to refractory *anorexia nervosa* patients and obese laboratory rats and college students may seem a long way to go in cognitive time and space; but the incoming data warrant this considerable stretch of the scientific imagination, as work like Delgado's, Schachter's, and so many others had already amply demonstrated. Though the evidence to date may still be circumstantial, the connections clearly do exist: They can be described; they can be interrupted; the consequences of interrupting them can be measured and weighed.

The touchstone here is hunger, and the conclusion that anorectics and concentration-camp inmates are in fact physiologically famished, while hypothalamically lesioned obese rats are, metabolically speaking, just the opposite, is only marginally noteworthy; what counts is that from their own points of view, and from various relevant parameters in their blood, brains, and muscles, all these individuals are as effectively starving as if they had eaten their last meal several days ago and had no clear idea where or when they would be eating their next one—if at all.

But so, in all probability, and for a variety of good physiological reasons which are still by no means clearly understood, are the great armies of the unsung and underresearched human obese—sisters and brothers under the skin of Bruch's emaciated *anorexia nervosa* patients, Mayer's brain-lesioned rats, and starving refugees from the recent sub-Saharan drought. For the key to the psychology of plain, common garden-variety obesity—like the key to starvation itself—is hunger. Whatever the mental and physical antecedents of their condition may eventually prove to be, fat people get that way because they are hungry, and they stay that way because they are hungry too. And what is more, in view of an accumulating body of evidence from both animal and human experimental studies, the chances are beginning to seem considerable that the reason fat people are so hungry has less to do with their early mothering and other assorted vicissitudes of a troubled childhood than it does with the curious midbrain structure called the hypothalamus, which sits at the base of the thinking neocortex and tells the individual when to eat—and (if he is lucky) when to stop feeding and call it a day till the next time around.

Meanwhile, to the "Ventrem Omnipotentem" (or Almighty Belly) of Rabelais, modern science opposes the "Cerebrum Omnipotens" of Delgado, Mayer, and Bruch. The sixteenth century had taken a straightforward view of hyperphagia: Big bellies bespoke gargantuan appetites; gargantuan appetites demanded big feeds; big feeds incurred enormous bellies. The process could go full circle without even once tapping in on the thinking centers of the brain.

The twentieth century reversed this circuitry and stood the matter, more or less literally, on its head, so that, for the last three decades at least, fat people have been told that it is all in their minds.

But now, by the latest scientific reckoning, what was once supposed by the Freudians to be all in their minds is at present merely thought by the psychobiologists to be all in their heads. The difference is small but crucial; by moving the scene of the crime several inches downward—from the new brain to the old—scientists have changed the moral and psychological venue of the case, and in the process (or so it is to be hoped) uncoupled much of the guilt and self-loathing associated with overeating from the act of feeding itself.

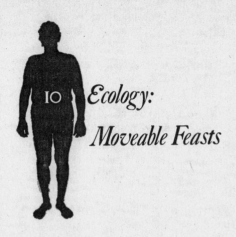

10 *Ecology:*
Moveable Feasts

To say that everybody talks about the weather but nobody does anything about it is to perpetuate a canard: Man's history as a cultural animal has largely been organized around the good and bad weather of his life—including changes from one to the other, escaping a change for the worse, and capitalizing on a change for the better. A vast chunk of human culture involves weather-related adaptations: Shelter, clothing, storage, planting, and harvesting are all responses to the vicissitudes of weather and climate. The man or hominid who built the first rock shelter was undoubtedly doing something about the weather, as was the human being who sewed the first fur cloak, sharpened the first tent pole, and fashioned the first clay water pot.

But technology is only half the story; the other half is physical adaptation. Climate affects our day-to-day physical machinery in ways that are still coming to light. A 1974 University of Pennsylvania study involving a total of 879 Philadelphians found that on days when the barometric pressure was high, a disproportionate number of people came to psychiatric clinics seeking help for depression, while on days of low barometric pressure admissions for alcoholism were higher than usual. Differences in barometric pressure are invisible, tasteless, odorless, and thermally imperceptible: and yet we are constantly receiving information about them even so, and, like the newest piece of meteorological hardware in the most sophisticated weather stations in the world, our bodies record these changes, "measure" them, and react accordingly. A 1965 World Meteorological Organization report found for example that work accidents of all kinds peak sharply—sometimes by a factor of as much as 20 per cent—on days when the air becomes heavily charged with unusually high numbers of positive or negative ions. Amputees and the chronically ill complain of pain twice as often on days of high atmospheric electricity as on other days. The ESP of everyday life outdoes thought transmission and table levitation and goes them one better; we are all old hands at it, whether we care to acknowledge the fact or not.

Other climatological factors are more visible to the naked eye but no less puzzling in their effects on our bodies and souls. Sunny days, for example, produce lower homicide statistics than cloudy ones do. In the same vein, a 1972 *American Heart Journal* report cautioned patients on the hazards of a change in the weather, or a move from one climate to another—or even a shift, within a given climate, from average to extremes of that season's prevailing weather. Illness and disability reduce the margin of homeostatic safety in living organisms, and extremes of the weather are no less noxious for sick people than extremes of emotion, exertion, or sensation. In Finland in 1972 a group of researchers studying 771 patients who had been victims of heart attacks in the recent past cautioned that deviations from the mean temperature for the season—regardless of whether the difference was good or bad (i.e., up or down from the norm)—resulted in an upswing of hospital admissions for heart attacks; while as early as 1926, Louis Wolff and Paul Dudley White of Boston had noted that in New England, at least, most heart attacks tended to occur in the winter months. Lest this finding be interpreted as just another argument against shoveling snow in the winter when the shoveler is not apt to be in good enough physical condition for any extreme exertion, studies have shown just the reverse pattern holding true in the south: in New Orleans and Dallas, for example, heart attacks occur most frequently in the summer months, when the living is easy and outdoor life is at a peak.

Change means stress, whether it is a change in the weather, the economic climate, or the social one, and even—as recent research seems to suggest—if the change itself is a change for the better, not the worse. According to Thomas Holmes of the University of Washington, for example, getting married is quantitatively only somewhat less stressful than getting divorced,—and moving from one house to another can be just as stressful if it constitutes a move up the social and neighborhood ladder as if it involves a move down. Walter Bradford Cannon's famous dictum that the body seeks to preserve its own status quo through all environmental alarums and diversions, and against all comers, seems borne out by work on stress and change; we are by nature physiological conservatives, and any change—whether for worse or better—is thus always registered as stress somewhere in our central nervous systems, and juggled with accordingly.

But how do we, as living organisms, deal with the after all predictable novelty of climatic stress? Going inside and shutting the door is a perfectly adequate way of shutting out the rain, storm, and snow; but exactly what is one to do about an excess of positive ions in the air or a lowered barometric pressure? Or, for that matter, against a sudden drop (or rise) in the season's mean temperature—especially in the absence of central heating, air conditioning, or an electric fan to bridge the gap? For most people, in most parts of the inhabited world and throughout most of human history, technology has never been sophisticated or affordable enough to ensure a dependable lifesaving interface between man and the elements; and adaptation—the ability to adjust physiologically, anatomically, and hormonally to environmental extremes of one sort or another—has always had to be invoked to make up the difference.

Man as a species was born into the midsummer Eden of Africa, the circum-Mediterranean, and subtropical Europe at the dawn of the last Ice Age, when tropical flora and fauna flourished along the Thames Valley in England, and no serious geographical or adaptive challenge existed to the species' slow northward spread. But about 80,000 years before the present era the picture began to change. The Gulf Stream from the Caribbean shifted toward Morocco, snow and ice built up around the poles, and the great Scandinavian glacier began to creep southward into the British Isles.

In the last 2 million years there has been a succession of greater and lesser Ice Ages, with warmer periods in between; but it is only during the last 50,000 years or so that the great vagaries of climate in the Northern Hemisphere have had much impact on our own species at all. Until then, man had simply not colonized the northern sections of the globe in great enough numbers to be put to the test, physiologically and technologically speaking, of true glacial living. But by roughly 60,000 years ago the ice sheet in northern Europe stretched all the way from Britain and parts of the North Sea eastward to Berlin, with a long finger jutting down from the Dnieper Valley in Russia, until at some places this southward extension reached to within 200 miles of the Black Sea. In western Europe, the Scandinavian glacier to the north and the Swiss glacier to the south held northern France, Belgium, Holland, and parts of Germany in a glacial pincer hold. By the height of the last glaciation, around 20,000 years ago, the ground in these parts of Europe was permanently frozen all year round, and the treeless horizon was much like that of the Arctic tundra today.

At this time, according to Karl Butzer, the University of Chicago paleogeographer whose comprehensive work on the subject is considered definitive, July mean temperatures were between 10° and 12° C., with annual mean temperatures of less than 2° below zero, and probably as much as 5° below zero in some locations. The Gulf Stream, which in our own times brings warm water from the Caribbean to the British Isles and points south, at that time dumped its currents at Morocco; in those days sea water off the coast of northern Spain was as cold as sea water off the coast of Greenland is now. Elsewhere—for example Czechoslovakia, Hungary, Romania, and European Russia below the 50th parallel, as well as most of Siberia—a somewhat more clement zone of birch forest (like those of Lapland and northernmost Russia today)—were covered by wind-driven dust or loess, and enjoyed (if that is the word) mean July temperatures of about 12° to 13° C. with a grand total of thirty to forty frost-free days a year—although midwinter temperatures were probably the same as those in the middle of the permafrost tundra of western Europe by and large.

The figures speak for themselves. People and animals living in climates like this had to evolve certain inborn biological defenses against the prevailing cold, and since human beings seem long ago to have lost the otherwise almost universal mammalian cold-climate adaptation of a thick coat of fur, insulation necessarily went under the skin in the form of fat. Fat is a first line of defense against cold in all vertebrates that are native to cold climates, including fish and birds as well as mammals; it is, in this sense at least, an evolutionarily older and more pervasive insulating mechanism than feathers or fur. Other cold-coping mechanisms are physiological rather than anatomical; they include shivering, which generates heat by putting muscles to work (exactly as if the shiverer were to start doing calisthenics or set off on a two-mile jog), and a good, quick-triggered vascular response—which lets the animal react to cold by constricting the small blood vessels in the skin, clamping down on the blood flow in and out of them, and shunting blood back to the internal organs where it is needed most.

Although we do not have very good evidence about the skin-fold thicknesses of our prehistoric forebears in glacial Europe, there is some historical evidence that our more immediate ancestors were a thoroughly cold-hardened lot; the bog men of the Danish early Iron Age—some of whose bodies have been dug up intact centuries after death or burial in the peat bogs of southern Denmark—apparently wore little else than short shoulder capes of animal skins. Corroborating evidence of a sort exists; a thousand-odd years later in the course of the Gallic wars Caesar noted that the "Germani" wore short skin garments to their hips, but otherwise went naked; and this is the way the Germani have been immortalized in Roman bas-reliefs of the period. Tacitus confirms the observation, describing the dress of the Germanic tribes as a shoulder cape pinned with a brooch; he adds that they were given to sitting around the hearth all day when not at war with nothing else on at all.

Tacitus and Caesar have nothing specific to say on the subject, but it is a safe bet that this sort of clothing would not provide much protection against the cold except in the presence of a healthy layer of subcutaneous fat, and an indomitable shivering and vascular response system. Both shivering and vasoconstriction are probably hormonally triggered: Humans and animals exposed to cold have been shown to have high levels of adrenal hormones, and the amount of such hormones mobilized seems to be directly proportional to the degree of cold. Recently, research has shown that in a group of young men in Norway, cortisol secretion was uniformly and significantly higher in winter and fall than it was in spring and summer. Other studies have shown that as adrenaline release goes up in response to cold, shivering in the same subjects tends to go down. It stands to reason therefore that people who can respond to cold with increased adrenal hormone output can probably conserve over-all energy expenditure in the process too, thereby saving calories and storing fat. The resulting body metabolism may make for a fatter, hence a more warmly insulated animal. Nature and evolution cannot have missed the point. Over eons, generations, and centuries, animals bred to withstand cold may have—perhaps even must have—developed the concomitant ability to pour out maximal amounts of adrenal hormones in response to exposure to cold.

In the process, the evolving physical format of the cold-adapted animal undoubtedly became shorter-legged and rounder-torsoed than the ancestral, warm-adapted prototype. For among the hormones secreted by the adrenal glands are small quantities of sex steroids, the estrogens and androgens; and when these hormones are activated early and for prolonged periods of time—as they may be in children exposed to intense cold throughout the early years of their life—their effect is to speed up sexual development, hurrying the onset of menstruation in girls and early sexual maturation in boys. One of the side effects of early maturation is a precocious closing of the growing ends of the long bones in the legs and arms, bones which seem to receive their developmental orders directly from the levels of sex steroids in the blood. (When adolescent girls, for example, are judged to be growing too fast and threatening to tower over their peers and contemporaries at maturity, estrogen is considered the treatment of choice, because it curbs bone growth and brings maturation to a climax months or years before the body was programmed to do so itself.) In cold-adapted animals, the adrenal glands and gonads seem to work hand in hand; Allen's famous zoological rule, that members of animal species in colder parts of their range have shorter legs, ears, tails, and noses than their more southerly cousins do, may work through some hormonal mechanisms like the ones posited here.

The resulting physical type is a historically and ethnically common one; many Asians and inland-dwelling Europeans are prototypical for the kind of short-leggedness and rotundity that generations of adaptation to cold are conducive to. These are the endomorphs and mesomorphs of the planet: stocky, fleshy, deep-chested and long-bodied specimens who probably owe their inherited physiques to the fact that small, inbred colonies of their remote progenitors once had to weather a few centuries or millennia of Ice Age winters in some isolated valley or geographical enclave where only the stockier members of each generation were able to survive and give birth to viable offspring—and where, even when the climate finally improved, geographic isolation still kept them breeding true to type.

It is perhaps only relatively recently (say from about 2500 B.C.) that man as a species has had both the technology and the climatological good luck to be able to migrate as freely as he pleased throughout Europe, the Mideast, and Asia. Until then small, isolated breeding groups were probably kept close to home by geographical happenstance, with the result that genes of the relative handful of our cold-adapted ancestors may have become copied and recopied out of all numerical proportion to their real usefulness in a postglacial world. In the steadily warming climate of postglacial Europe and China, for example, short legs, arms, toes, and fingers cannot have been as handy to the people who inherited them as they had once been to their severely cold-stressed forebears; but by then the genetic die had been cast, and since there was nothing particularly disadvantageous in that physique or those features either, the result was a certain prevalent body type whose phenocopies are still with us in rather substantial numbers today.

Interestingly enough, this sort of physique, although it in no way conforms to the current aesthetic ideal, is one that outbreeds many others: Short fat American army men marry younger and have more children than their taller and skinnier counterparts do, and endomorphic fathers seem to have larger families—though fewer sons—than the general population at large.

The cold-adapted physique is one that has well-documented prehistorical antecedents; the Venus figurines, some of which date back about 25,000 years, are a case in point. In recent research using frontal photographs of some of the better-known figurines, it was demonstrated that the more globular and least "leggy" of these statuettes were more apt to be found in sites which, by paleoecological determination, can be shown to have been among the colder areas of Europe at the height of the last glaciation; while the longer-legged and more gracile figurines tended to be found at the warmer and more meridional sites. This kind of distribution of physique by locale is still with us today, in spite of migration, famine, central heating, and various technological innovations like hot-water bottles, blankets, and stoves; and was even, as late as the sixteenth century, a well-known feature of certain southerly European populations, where the so-called vertical north of the Alps and Pyrenées bred a race of short-legged mountain folk who, according to historian Fernand Braudel, were held in some degree of contempt by the finer-boned lowlanders on whom they periodically descended to market their livestock in the fall of the year.

The continuing presence of mesomorphic and endomorphic physiques in sunny Italy and parts of mountainous Greece is understandable on this basis (and not, as popular wisdom would have it, on the basis of all the pasta such people are supposed to eat and the olive oil they sauce it with). Mean temperatures fall by a predictable amount for every few hundred feet of ascent as one climbs a mountain, and by the time you reach the tops of certain alpine peaks, you might for all ecological intents and purposes be living at the Arctic Circle.

Braudel, whose monumental work on southern Europe in the sixteenth century deals interestingly with the ecological causes and effects of the medieval and Renaissance Mediterranean world, even goes so far as to suggest that the mountainous uplands of southern Europe form the "poverty pocket of the Mediterranean world," and its "proletarian reserve." His data cast light on the social origins of the notable aesthetic edge that ectomorphs seem generally to have had over other body types in post-Christian painting and sculpture: Characteristically mountain folk were husky, raw-boned and low-slung. Winter in the mountains acted to speed shepherds downhill with their flocks against the oncoming cold; the immigrants were a rough lot, not much impressed with lowland civilities; and civilization itself, says Braudel, was thus primarily "an urban and lowland achievement."

The same relationship between mountain dwellers and lowlanders holds true in other parts of the world. Leo Africanus, a sixteenth-century Moorish traveler, was astonished by the "robust physique of the mountain folk of Mt. Megeza, while the plains dwellers were smaller men." Life in the oases exaggerated these distinctions; the oasis dwellers of northern Africa—"with a belly like Sancho Panza's"—were clearly made of softer stuff than the Bedouins who surrounded them. The oasis dwellers were the endomorphs of the desert.

People seem always to have guessed, in an intuitive way, that life-style and physique have more than a passing relationship to each other; whatever the hormonal and genetic means may be by which nature adjusts body size and build to life-style of a given group, the results are often visible, measurable, and striking. Climate is probably not the only factor that counts in this equation, but it is undoubtedly the basic one. Climate dictates food supply; climate determines what other animals and micro-organisms man will be sharing his natural resources with; climate determines the kinds of trees, rocks, and metals man will have at his disposal to build his shelters with, make his tools with, and fuel his hearth fires with.

Climate, moreover, can have a considerable role to play in the kind of diseases men are prey to, both from the human end of it (certain body types are more prone to certain diseases than others) and from the other end of the biotic spectrum as well (certain microbes and parasites can only flourish in a given climate, at a given latitude, and among a given flora and fauna). Before the discovery and widespread use of penicillin, pneumonia was one of the leading causes of death in northern Europe and the U.S.A., and there is evidence from animal studies that the pneumococcus itself is at its most lethal in animals whose body temperatures are one or two degrees below normal. The old wives' wisdom that chilling can put you to bed with a cold may thus be grounded in hard fact. Thermal factors like this could place a strong selective premium on the kind of body that is capable of maintaining adequate deep body temperatures under threat of intense cold.

But the effect need not be limited to the muscular and vascular systems of the animal in question either: Animal studies have shown that there is a definite difference between carnivores and herbivores with respect to the storage capacity of their livers and hence their ability to store fuel for the metabolic fire. Meat eaters can expand the fat and glycogen compartments of their livers almost instantaneously in reponse to high lipid intakes; grass eaters and other vegetarians cannot. It is anybody's guess whether the same distinction holds true between, say, Eskimos, whose diet consists almost entirely of protein and fat, and Asian Indians, whose diet is mostly vegetarian; but if it does, it might explain some of the more obvious differences in body build between the two groups, and other human "morphic" extremes.

Physique can thus have a considerable role to play in health and disease—not only in the sense that a "good" constitution acts as a kind of built-in actuarial warranty for the person lucky enough to get born with it, but in the narrower sense that certain physical types are just structurally more resistant to some ills the flesh is heir to than others are. During the nineteenth-century siege of tuberculosis that has been immortalized (and perhaps somewhat overdrawn) in so much of the literature and opera of the Romantic era, it was the long-legged, narrow-chested asthenic types who died of consumption in the flower of their youth, not the round-bodied, short-legged pyknics who were widely (and justly) considered to be at low risk from TB. As a matter of fact the serious overfeeding of children that has persisted down to the present day in the pediatric folk wisdom of many European and American subcultures may have its roots in this widely—and accurately—observed happenstance of differential adolescent morbidity.

Other upper respiratory diseases seem to have the same affinity for asthenics as TB once did. Remembering the pre-World War I death rates from pneumonia, and the terrible mortality statistics of the great influenza pandemic of 1918–1920, we may well get some idea of how body type and death from infectious disease can dovetail within a given population. One might even speculate that the increased mortality figures for heart disease in our own generation could be a direct consequence of this selective nightmare—by leaving the big-hearted, plethoric, round-bodied pyknics to their actuarial fate in the coronary units, after having previously winnowed out so many of the consumption-prone, "chesty" asthenics a scant half century earlier in the influenza wards. According to this line of reasoning, one of the reasons we may be seeing such high coronary death rates in the overweight adult population today is that nineteenth- and early-twentieth-century respiratory killers may already have taken such a toll of the asthenic types in our parents' and grandparents' generations that it has skewed the remaining population into the fat, pyknic quadrant of the present actuarial field.

But selection for a good pair of stout lungs (and the globular, short-legged physique that so often goes with them) must already have been strong in the days when people still lived in animal-skin tents and caves; anyone who has ever spent the night in a fire-warmed hut or igloo will realize that smoke inhalation and air pollution as such are not twentieth-century inventions. And when a recently exhumed Egyptian mummy was autopsied and found to have smoke-damaged lungs, the lesson became even clearer. Nowhere on earth has modern man ever been able to make do without fire for heat and cooking, and the farther north one goes the better the lungs must be designed to minimize the effects of smoke pollution. Living as they do in the so-called vertical north of high mountain ranges, highland dwellers even in mid-latitude countries tend to be co-adapted to cold, smoke-filled rooms, and oxygen scarcity. And the typical Alpine physique reflects this subtle patchwork of ecological imperatives.

Genetic designs for cold climate thus represent an integrated effort at co-adaptation, both to primary ecological infelicities (cold, seasonal starvation) and to their usual extenuating circumstances (crowded quarters, smoke, and disease). There is no need to belabor the fact that fat constitutes another basic biological strategy for dealing with cold. Anthropologist Carleton Coon has made the interesting point, however, that fat may be positively selected for only in those parts of the world where cold stress is seasonal or intermittent; in polar environments fat alone would not do the trick, and nothing short of fur outerwear and heated shelters can ever be equal to the task of keeping internal body temperatures up to the mark where midwinter temperatures regularly stand at 10°, 40°, or 140° F. below zero.

The fattest people in the world are therefore not found in regions of intense year-round cold, but rather in places where the summers are not quite warm enough for real creature comfort without a little assist from physique. Russell Newman's 1955 work on U.S. Army recruits bore this notion out; Newman recorded not only the absolute weights of his subjects but also their fat-to-lean ratio; he found that within the continental United States "men are fattest where the summers are coolest, and leanest where the summers are hottest." This of course is a somewhat different version of Newman and Munro's work showing that the *heaviest* army recruits came from birthplaces where the winters were coldest. Taken together, the two findings prove that weight and fat are not necessarily directly related, either in the body of an individual or in the ecological implications of his or her body composition.

In support of this kind of reasoning, it is interesting that Eskimos and other polar-dwelling peoples, although usually short and stocky, are not necessarily fat when compared to slightly more southerly peoples; and perhaps the same thinking can be invoked to explain the sometimes impressive adiposity of Hawaiians and Easter Islanders, who spend so much of their time in the water, and for whom fat may provide the aquatic margin of safety between the warmth of the tropical air on land and the more frigid sea-water temperatures that their semiaquatic fishermen's lives expose them to for several—and sometimes many—hours a day.

In this connection, racial variations—both in the amount of fat and in the way it is distributed over the body—are intriguing. Coon has compiled a schema representing most of what is known to date about fat distribution in twelve different ethnic groups; the results are enlightening and make good, though as yet only tentative, ecological sense. As far as chest, arm, and upper-body fat are concerned, the Polynesians are far and away the leaders in this dubious sweepstakes, with subscapular fat measurements up to 20 mm.; Europeans come next, with upper-torso and triceps measurements of between 10 and 15 mm., and waist, knee, and calf fat measurements of around 10 mm. Next fattest of the ethnic groups Coon had data for are the Alacaluf Indians who live in the cold year-round climate of Tierra del Fuego at the tip of the South American peninsula, making a precarious and frigid living as deep-sea fishermen, and who are notorious in the annals of anthropology for being able to withstand severe cold even when immobilized for hours at a time in unprotected fishing boats with nothing but a sort of loose cloak or blanket for body covering.

Vying in degree of adiposity with the Alacalufs are the Japanese—another island-bound and fishing people with subscapular, side, and abdominal fat measurements slightly larger than those of the Alacalufs, and only nominally lower than Europeans. Next in descending order of fatness come the Lapps, Australian aborigines, Arctic and Andean Indians, Chinese, Eskimos, Micronesians, and Bushmen. Since these figures were all culled from measurements of males, the famous steatopygia or fat buttocks and thighs of the

Bushmen females are not reflected in this profile—which does not include such measurements for any of the groups in question, but might be highly informative if it did.

Other interesting variations of fat patterning on the face and body in different ethnic groups come to light in these profiles. For example, Europeans, Lapps, and Indian and Eskimo groups all have high readings for cheek fat. Japanese data are incomplete on this score, but Chinese groups definitely score lower. The "apple-cheeked" physiognomy of northern European folk art is therefore no aesthetic exaggeration or aberration, but a certified morphological fact. Europeans are also interesting in that they have the fattest chins of any of the ethnic groups for whom such data exist, though what purpose a fat chin may serve in nature's scheme of things, and how to interpret this ethnic peculiarity, is anybody's guess. Alacalufs meanwhile are relatively lean in the sides and abdomen but have fat waists; like Europeans, on the other hand, Japanese people have fat backs, sides, and abdomens compared to other groups.

Another example of this sort of patchwork adaptation to cold is the fatty cheeks, feet, hands, and eyelids of certain Mongoloid peoples including the most northerly ones (i.e., Eskimos, Siberians, Manchurians, and Alaskan Indians) whose daily work exposes only these parts of their bodies to the Arctic temperature extremes from which the rest of their bodies are insulated by elaborate hooded and furred skin garments.

The general picture that emerges from such profiles—incomplete, inexact, and tantalizing as they may still be—is that a chilly life, especially if it is a watery or an insular one to boot, seems conducive to accumulating body fat, even where the living is far from easy, nutritionally speaking; while an intensely cold climate has the added effect of promoting a high degree of facial fat as well. Europeans seem to have the dubious distinction of measuring highest in all areas—but socioeconomic factors have to be taken into account as well as genetic ones in Europe, where standards of living are certainly higher than in aboriginal groups and undoubtedly higher than they are in all but a handful of Asian populations as well.

Cold is not of course the only thermal extreme that man and other animals are faced with over the course of a lifetime or a history; heat imposes its own biological stresses and strictures. Long legs and arms create increased body surfaces for sweat to evaporate from, and are characteristic features of many heat-adapted peoples and animals, including giraffes, camels, Bedouins, and Nilotic' blacks. So it is no accident that on a world-wide basis some of the longer-legged and skinnier peoples and animals of the world inhabit the warmer parts of the globe. From an ecological viewpoint, though, even more interesting adaptations to temperature can be surmised from the body types of people who live in areas where there is a strong shift from extreme heat to extreme cold in the space of a single day, thus calling for efficient cold- and heat-adaptive responses within the span of a 24-hour period. People indigenous to places where nighttime temperatures can be 30° to 40° lower than daytime highs sometimes show a combination of adaptive traits that mark a hodgepodge of anthropometric rules of thumb. The Papagos of Arizona and New Mexico may owe their thick and relatively fat torsos to the frigid night temperatures of their mesa homelands, while their long thin arms and legs represent an adaptive afterthought by way of accommodation to the hot arid days of their native climate. By the same token, the steatopygous Bushmen and Hottentots of Africa seem to have elaborated an even more interesting version of this major theme, by storing occasionally quite startling amounts of subcutaneous fat in their buttocks, while remaining lean—sometimes to the point of outright emaciation—above the waist and in the lower, distal portions of their extremities. The strategy may once have been widespread throughout Africa and not limited to rain-forest dwellers as it is now; American blacks, male and female, thin and fat, have more protuberant buttocks than American whites—a possible anthropometric hangover from the African past, and an interesting one considering that ethnically most American blacks trace their roots to West Africa rather than to the rain forest.

Oddly enough, moreover, although certain African groups can and do become quite fat (notably certain of the West African groups who live in a warm but very humid climate), their latter-day cousins in the twentieth-century United States seem to get less insulative effect from more fat than whites or Mongoloids with identical skin-fold thicknesses do. The pronounced obesity of some North American blacks may therefore represent a kind of thermal overkill: Since the fat they do deposit does not quite do the job of keeping body temperatures up to the mark in the cold winters of life in the Northern Hemisphere, they may tend to overshoot the mark and keep on storing more and more fat in an attempt to satisfy the hypothetical thermostat that calibrates fat to skin temperature in cold climates.

Cold, heat, and disease are among the major winnowing forces at work on human sizes and shapes, but other, subtler factors have also undoubtedly left their marks on our physiques, among them nutrition. Protein-poor ecosystems cannot support physical brawn in human populations on any major scale, and the small, slender body types may be at a distinct genetic advantage in regions where nutrition is poor. Essential amino acids from protein foods form part of the complex cellular underpinnings of all human tissues, including the antibodies and lymphocytes needed to fight infectious diseases, and it stands to reason that smaller bodies constitute less of a drain on available protein resources than larger ones do. It takes less protein to feed more people in marginal subsistence areas than it would take to feed large people under the same set of circumstances; in such places, reproduction is bound to favor smaller specimens over big ones over the long evolutionary run.

Another ecologically limiting factor in human nutrition is calcium. People can struggle along with varying kinds and amounts of vitamin and protein deficiencies, but children need calcium for bone growth, and adults need it for nerve-to-muscle impulse transmission—including those neuro-muscular relays which keep the heart beating on schedule, and therefore constitute the basic power grid of the body. A good source of calcium is milk and dairy products, and most northern Europeans and Asian Indians and certain African dairying tribes get all the calcium they need from cattle. But the vast majority of the world's peoples do not raise or own cows and cannot digest milk or milk products successfully once past the age of weaning (usually about 3 or 4 years old), and must therefore depend on other food and environmental sources for this basic mineral. While there is some evidence that in calcium-poor environments the human gut can adapt by extracting higher doses of calcium from relatively poor dietary sources, the idea has persisted that human beings in calcium-poor environments tend, like sheep and other livestock in such areas, to run to shorter and smaller-boned individuals than those from dairying lands or coastal, fishing areas, or regions where limestone is the native rock and drinking water is therefore rich in calcium.

On the other hand, sunlight itself is always a factor in this rather complicated ecological equation, and can never be left out of account when tallying the calcium needs of any given geographical group of people. In very sunny climates high doses of ultraviolet radiation can offset calcium deficiency, at least to some extent, by maximizing the amount of the mineral that gets taken up by the bones; Vitamin D, activated by sunlight working on the melanin in the skin, boosts the bones' ability to absorb calcium, and therefore in sunny climates there may be less need than in cloudy ones for dietary or background calcium sources. (Anthropologists have speculated that the reason children in wet, foggy, cloudy climates tend to stay blond until late adolescence is precisely because there is a selective advantage, in terms of bone growth, to being blond until the growing age stops; blond hair lets more ultraviolet rays penetrate to the scalp than dark hair does, and children whose hair does not turn dark until they have reached their full growth will thus make better use of whatever meager calcium they have access to than those with dark hair.)

As in all observations about the effects of ecology on body build, generalizations like this one are subject to a great range of caveats and outright disclaimers. Eskimos and Laplanders, for example, as J. S. Weiner has pointed out, both live in calcium-rich environments and have done so for unnumbered generations, but are nevertheless among the shortest peoples on earth. In this case, on the other hand, it might be wise to remember Bergmann's and Allen's rules, which state that animals in cold countries tend to be (a) bigger and (b) shorter-legged than their relatives in warmer climates. This does not mean that the principles of calcium economy and bone growth have suddenly stopped being operative when it comes to the Eskimos and Lapps, but only that we have not yet managed in these cases to master all the extenuating ifs, ands, and buts by which such simplistic scientific generalizations are normally, and maddeningly, surrounded and hemmed in.

While calcium-poor environments have been blamed for the small size of peasant peoples and agriculturists in many inland, non-dairying groups, other lines of reasoning suggest that the avail-

ability of iodine, a mineral necessary for proper thyroid functioning, growth, and intelligence may account for the general sturdiness
and presumed industriousness of islanders and other coastal-
dwelling peoples with access to fish and hence to a good, easily
renewable iodine supply (iodine is present in quantity in sea water).
There is of course no way to prove or disprove speculations like
these, and the same skepticism of necessity applies to another entic-
ing line of conjecture which holds that body build, as genetically
preprogrammed in any given local breeding group, will tend to be
governed by the kind of work that has to be done to make a living
in that particular kind of environment.

One of the most provocative publications in this general area was
an article written by anthropologist Alice Brues in 1959. In it,
Brues speculates that as long ago as the lower Paleolithic, work
requirements of forest dwellers as opposed to those of plains
dwellers were genetically molding whole populations toward one or
another of the popular physical stereotypes that Ernst Kretschmer
and W. H. Sheldon have made the basis of their morphological
studies of physique. In the plains and on the tundra, for example,
bagging the day's (or more likely the week's) big game supply was
a job for spearsmen, and depended on the hunter's ability to run
fast and to hurl a heavy spear or harpoon for a considerable distance through empty space. The resulting physique was thus a long-
legged, long-tendoned one with powerful shoulders and pectoral
muscles but slim hips—a build not unlike the ones we recognize in
skeletal reconstructions of Cro-Magnon man in the limestone-rich
Dordogne Valley of France, or in somewhat later cave paintings of
prehistoric hunters in northern Spain.

Gradually, though, as the Paleolithic climate improved and present-day temperate forests crept northward supplanting the scrub and
lichen flora of glacial Europe, there evolved a stockier, shorter-
armed kind of build, better adapted skeletally and muscularly to
hacking its way out of dense woodland and releasing an arrow from
a bow over relatively short distances. This newcomer made his living not as a big-game hunter with a tool kit full of harpoon points
and hafted spears, but as a trapper and an archer.

Brues speculates that the thrust needed for launching an arrow at
a target with due lethal propulsive force must have favored genetic
selection for short, massively muscled forearms—as opposed to the

long, loose-jointed and slender arms of successful long-distance spear throwers. Enter the mesomorph, who is of course still in demand today wherever brawn and cold resistance are at a premium. Life in the forest and a woodsman's ecosystem must have upped the selective advantage of this type considerably. Woodsmen live on small game which they either trap or shoot at relatively close quarters in forest undergrowth; they do not need to run fast or long, and can afford to sacrifice speed and leg length to the strong arm and well-braced thigh muscles of the "archer's" somatotype. We have been living in the temperate aftermath of the last Ice Age for the last 18,000 years or so, and it is no wonder that the colonists, sailors, and frontiersmen of our recent history were still well served by the short-armed and muscular physiques that once did so well by our Mesolithic ancestors.

But resourceful as mesomorphs may be in carving new paths through virgin wilderness, building new settlements in the middle of freshly cleared woodlands, and making a living by the sweat of their brows, they are nevertheless a protein-hungry lot and have not anatomically solved the problem of scarcity and famine. Once man has cleared his woods, built his enclaves, and settled in for the long hard agricultural pull, questions of reserves and storage become all-important, and it was at the point in human anatomical history when the species became agricultural and increasingly sedentary that the adaptive advantage of subcutaneous fat as a means of storing surpluses under the skin—and the face and figure to go with it—came into their own on a world-wide basis in both cold climates and warmer ones.

The Neolithic Revolution ushered in a new life-style for Europeans and Middle Easterners; with the end of the Ice Age man became less dependent on meat, fish, and fowl for his daily food needs, and more dependent on grains, legumes, and vegetables. The consequences were demographically dazzling: Agriculture could support many more human beings living at much closer quarters on an all-year-round basis than hunting and gathering had been able to do even in their best years, and human populations mushroomed accordingly. From an estimated 5 to 10 million people alive on the face of the earth at the start of the Neolithic Revolution, human population had increased by about 300,000,000 at the dawn of the present era, and has since risen exponentially and thus almost vertically to the present day—thanks to farming and the new technology that agriculture inspired and supported.

Malthus had seen the handwriting on the wall and drawn up the bill nearly two centuries ago, but until recently it was still possible to temporize. Then in 1972 world grain production fell by 4 per cent, putting an end to what had been a world-wide postwar trend of steadily rising food production. This dip in the horn of plenty triggered violent upsets in the economies of all the breadbasket nations of the world: Drought in Russia, China, and Australia created a vacuum for American wheat, corn, and soybeans to funnel into; and in America itself galloping food prices followed, with basic foodstuffs leading the list of inflationary items for which the country was to pay dearly, some months later, in the form of rising interest rates, recession, and unemployment. Between 1972 and 1974 the price of wheat had tripled on the world grain market. Ten years earlier, unplanted cropland and carry-over food surpluses in the world's granaries had accounted for better than three months' worth of food rations for every man, woman, and child on the planet. But by 1974 these stockpiles had fallen to slightly better than three weeks' worth of food; and famine in sub-Saharan Africa, Bengal, and the Punjab threatened to drain even these meager reserves toward the vanishing point.

The problem was—and is—as old as recorded human history. A granite tomb of early dynastic Egypt on an island in the Nile bears a chilling inscription to the ancient enemy, famine, that predates the earliest portions of the Old Testament. "I am mourning on my high throne," reads the legend of the Stele of Famine, "because the Nile flood in my time has not come for seven years. Light is the grain; there is a dearth of crops and all kinds of food. Each man has become a thief unto his neighbor."

Later, dynastic satraps would master the essential wisdom that by controlling the granaries in times of plenty and dispersing surpluses in times of famine they could effectively gain control of the rich agricultural Nile bottomland and reduce the peasantry to serfdom in the process. From the historical and ecological viewpoint, access to food has always represented the high road to survival; to control the granaries themselves, on the other hand, means to have arrived at the true confluence of political and economic power.

Foraging has had a place in human and infrahuman history from the dawn of time. Man's closest kin among the primates are all foragers, and some of the more primitive tribal groups alive today still practice the gut-level economics of hunt-as-you-go, culling that day's food supply as and where they find it, eating fruits and nuts in season and bagging the odd head of game as hunger and opportunity allow. This kind of life is of course only possible if and where the prevailing climate permits it; where there is a marked change in the kind and amount of food available from one season to the next such freewheeling provisioning becomes suicidal, and some more elaborate warehousing system must eventually be worked out.

Man is not the only animal to have been confronted with this problem: Other animals have faced it too and solved it in their own ways. The bee's hive is not just a nest and home base, but a carefully organized food warehouse; for mammals, the limits of territoriality have always been nutritional as well as defensive. The red fox may stash away the odd supply of rodents' corpses in winter in specially constructed corners of his burrow, while the European mole hoards upward of 1,000 earthworms in underground caches and tunnels radiating from its nest. Even the great felines of the Southern Hemisphere have been known to have their storage problems; when a leopard cannot eat its whole kill at one sitting, it drags what is left of the carcass up a tree for future consumption. And in colder regions, where food is generally more of a problem to begin with, cold storage is common practice: Polar animals like wolves, bears, and foxes may routinely bury part of their kills in the snow. Rodents all over the world are notorious food hoarders and collectors. Squirrels are legendary in this respect, and hamsters have been known to stash as much as 200 pounds of cereal seeds, peas, or potatoes away in special warehouses inside their territories—notwithstanding the well-known storage capacities of the expandable cheek pouches for which they are justly famous.

The ability to store food is thus part of the basic adaptive equipment of many mammalian species; animals who can make hay while the sun shines don't need to work quite so hard when it doesn't, and the saved time can be put to good use in territorial expansion or reproductive exuberance. The principle of food stock-piling is a widely utilized one, and it is no different in infrahuman species than it is in our own. It implies a seasonal rise and fall in the prevailing food supply and assumes the existence of ups and downs in luck and the weather. Food collecting and storage is not quite as fashionable in the tropics as it has of necessity become farther north (and south) of the equator; where the temperature and the weather do not change much from day to day or from one month to the next, neither does the surrounding vegetation or the surrounding game, and feeding and foraging will not vary much from one end of the year to the next. The proliferation of families, genera, and species and subspecies of plants, animals, and insects in the tropics reflects the climate's permissiveness. But as animals move ecologically farther from the equator into less clement econiches and less clement temperatures, their ranks thin out, there are fewer and less exotic variants of their species at large, and eventually, below a certain temperature, whole species may simply disappear from the geographical roster forever. Quality of life is determined by the quantity of flora and fauna left to enjoy it, and emigrants are therefore often made of sterner stuff than the parental stock left behind in the subtropical Garden of Eden. Man's northward journey from his ancestral tropical paradise imposed new strictures on his life-style and on the limits of his physical adaptability. Like other cold-adapted species he had to learn to survive the northern winters by storing food—and fat.

Perhaps mostly fat. Granaries and grain storage are only useful where there is a crop of some sort to be stored; where winter lasts ten months a year or more, there is no spring planting, no summer growing season to speak of, and no yearly harvest to bring in. In Pleistocene Europe at the height of the last glaciation the seasons were all but imperceptible, at least for horticultural purposes; life on the glacial uplands of western Europe was one long winter with a brief two or three months' slushy thaw in July and August to break the monotony. Storage was therefore not a real problem: There was no grain to be stored. Man lived on game—preying on the great reindeer herds, the woolly mammoth, aurochs, and bison of the glacial plain. The European Pleistocene hunter was for all intents and purposes a seasonal nomad, following the herds wherever their foraging and the weather took them. Thus in the long waits between kills there was only one sensible place to store extra provisions on a long-term basis, and that was on the individual's own body in the form of subcutaneous fat.

Man is not alone in this biological approach to the winter storage problem: Other cold-adapted animals had worked out the same general solution long before *Homo sapiens* began to colonize the colder reaches of the Pleistocene tundra and learned to winter over in it as the need arose. On a world-wide basis, cold has probably always represented a more stringent adaptive condition than heat. There are therefore far fewer cold-adapted animals than warm-adapted ones, and the only totally thermally cosmopolitan group of land mammals—besides man—are the bats and muridae (rats, mice, and small rodents like hamsters and moles).

Traditionally, animals not specifically adapted to harsh winter climates have had two major ecological choices: either to migrate south at the onset of cold weather, or to go to ground and hibernate. An animal's insulating capacity is determined by basic evolutionary factors like species characteristics and body size. The fur of an Arctic fox has roughly five times more insulating capacity than that of the tropical coati; pigs and seals gain roughly the same thermal protection from roughly the same thickness of adipose tissue, but seals have the added thermal margin of safety of a thick mantle of fur. Size, on the other hand, imposes thermal limits on the animal that have nothing to do with species traits like fur and fat: The smaller an animal is, the less over-all surface he has available to support a thick growth of fur. The Arctic hare is about as small as an animal can get, according to zoologist Laurence Irving, and still sport a thick-enough coat of fur to live through the Arctic winter in good condition.

Faced with this sort of conundrum, many small northern animals have taken the easy way out by simply curling themselves up in a ball and wintering over in a profound and almost unrousable sleep. Dormice, ground squirrels, hedgehogs, opossums, bats, hamsters, and marmots all hibernate in rigorous climates; other species hibernate under certain sets of circumstances but not under others, and there is even a sex factor in hibernation, with females of some species (California ground squirrels, for example, and polar bears) tending to go to ground in winter more regularly than males of the same species do.

Different animals have different thermal limits and requirements, and these seem to be inherited as part of the genetic package that sets one species apart from another taxonomically. Among lab animals, according to François Bourlière, the guinea pig is the least thermally resourceful animal, with critical lower-temperature limits of $-15°$ C., as compared to $-25°$ for the white rat and $-45°$ for the rabbit. Hibernating species operate within these limits too, but they do so on an annual basis and according to instinctual, unlearned protocols. In the dead of winter the hibernating hedgehog's and ground squirrel's body temperature drops to $6°$ C.; brain temperature, though, remains some two or three degrees higher, so that even in the depths of its annual cold storage the animal can still receive and react to incoming messages through its nervous system, rewarm itself to normal cruising temperatures if need be, and take appropriate action when the occasion warrants it. Meanwhile, heartbeat may have dwindled to one beat per minute, and in all important respects the animal may appear to be—to invoke the old phrase—as dead as a dormouse.

What triggers hibernation is one of the continuing mysteries of current zoological research, but theories abound. Nutrition and eating are closely implicated in the process; V. R. Young and R. S. Scrimshaw have shown in their work with human subjects that vastly lowered metabolic rates are normal responses to prolonged starvation—presumably because lowering metabolism lets the animal eke out existing glucose supplies for use by the brain for the longest possible amount of time. Heat output is therefore sacrificed to general conservation of tissue protein supplies after the first week of total fasting—though in this case the master plan is an economic one, and not a thermal one. Hibernating animals, like starving humans, probably follow the same general metabolic blueprint too.

The mechanisms for this metabolic slowdown are not too well understood, but hormones and seasonal variations in light and temperature and food supply undoubtedly play their part. Testosterone injections have been known to bring ground squirrels out of profound sleep in the middle of winter, for example. In some species (including our own) testosterone levels in males are highest in the fall and decline gradually until they reach their lowest annual levels in the month of May. (How this may affect the spring birth rates, and whether there is any biological master plan built into this annual hormonal variation, remains an open question, and an interesting one; if men are at their most virile and sexually active in the late summer and fall, births should tend to cluster 9 months later in May or June—which just happens, incidentally, to be a very favorable time for getting born in most temperate and northern regions, everything else being equal.)

Seasonal variations in amounts of other hormones have also been documented in the scientific literature. J. G. Bernstein found adrenocortical hormones to be higher in the winter than in the summer months, perhaps in response to cold stress; and the winter depression of certain Scandinavian and circumpolar groups has been attributed to seasonal variations in brain neurohormones, possibly triggered by the absence of sunlight and the effect this has on the pineal and the pituitary glands. In this case, as in a growing number of instances where the mind-body relays are either undocumented or obscure, science is being harder and harder put to assign causality to the chicken or the egg: does the depression trigger the brain chemistry changes or is it the other way around? There is as of this moment simply no way of knowing the answer to such questions.

Insulin is another hormone which appears to have a seasonal rhythmicity. R. Pannhorst and A. Rieger noted a definite increase of new diabetic cases in the winter months, especially among younger patients; and these data have been corroborated by W. F. Petersen's statistics on the onset of diabetes in children. Other researchers have shown that there is a decreased need for insulin therapy from April to October in most diabetics, corresponding to a seasonal amelioration in the patient's metabolic status; and according to E. S. Dillon and W. W. Dyer, the death rate from diabetes is definitely higher in winter than in summer. These data do not seem to be determined by seasonal variations in eating habits, but operate independently of nutritional factors and therefore seem to have their roots in some much subtler over-all endocrinological ebb and flow.

Our bodies seem to know the difference between summer and winter, or between night and day, even in a world full of the climatological red herrings of electric lights, central heating, and air-conditioned rooms and buses; but how we monitor these changes in the thermally and luminously homogenized environments we have created for ourselves in certain privileged portions of the world remains a mystery. On the evidence, taking gross experimental liberties with a hibernator's natural day-night cycles by leaving the lab lights on 24 hours a day, or even turning them off and on according to schedules that simulate summer hours in midwinter, or winter hours in midsummer, need not interfere with the animal's biological urge to hibernate at all. Zoologists E. T. Pengelley and K. C. Fisher kept ground squirrels in rooms where lights were left burning 24 hours a day and where a normal room temperature was maintained around the clock at all seasons of the year, and found that their animals went into hibernation on schedule regardless of these visual and thermal abnormalities. The mechanisms for these annual bioclocks remain puzzling and have come in for more than their fair share of scientific excitement lately; space scientists would like to know more about this natural version of suspended animation for its possible applications to long-distance space travel, but so far nature is keeping her secrets well.

Another group of researchers who would like to know more about hibernation are the obesity experts. The major way in which a hibernating animal prepares for winter is by gorging in the fall; dormice can double their weight within a period of a few weeks; the pregnant polar bear feasts heavily on seal blubber before digging her nest ten feet under the snow, not to re-emerge until spring, having dropped her cubs and sustained herself, and them, in the meantime on the fat stored on her body months earlier during the summer and fall. The ability to store fat is the physiological sine qua non of hibernators; without it the hibernating animal would have to rouse itself periodically and spend precious stored energy rewarming itself to feed.

In some parts of the world this is simply not a viable winter option. The animal's natural prey may be hibernating too; or if he is a vegetarian, his normal food supply may only be available in the summer and fall. In such cases the ability to store enormous quantities of body fat in season is the literal precondition for making it through the winter alive. Animals otherwise not known for their adiposity—unlike, say, pigs, seals, and polar bears—can thus gain up to twice their normal body weight in a matter of weeks; and the way they do it has fascinating parallels to the ways in which surgically brain-damaged rats studied by Schachter, Nachman, and P. Teitelbaum accomplish the same gastronomical feat.

N. Mrosovsky's work with dormice and ground squirrels has al-most uncanny resemblances to Teitelbaum's work with ven-tromedially lesioned laboratory rats. Mrosovsky's hibernators were placed in cages where they could only get a food pellet by pressing down a bar lever—a device not unlike an ordinary bubble-gum dispenser; and their behavior was compared to that of both normals and artificially lesioned obese rats as well. When Mrosovsky made things easy for his hibernating ground squirrels and dormice by loosening the leverage on the dispensing bar, the animals would gorge themselves on lab chow; but when he tightened up on the bar they reacted just as Teitelbaum's brain-lesioned obese rats (and Schachter's obese Columbia students) had done, by turning corre-spondingly lazy and unwilling to work very hard to get their food.

The hibernators, in other words, behaved to all intents and pur-poses exactly as if someone or something had deliberately set out to interfere with the satiety centers in the middle part of the hypo-thalamus by carving a specific lesion into it with a surgical in-strument, just as Teitelbaum had done to produce experimental obesity in his laboratory rats. The point to be made is that in the hibernators' case—as in the case of Schachter's obese college stu-dents—nobody had done any such thing. The resident surgeon in this case was nature, or the animal's genes, and the operation was a far subtler one than any that has ever been perpetrated on laboratory animals by man.

The outcome was of course vastly different too: Teitelbaum and Nachman's surgically lesioned rats could look forward to a lifetime of fussy and sluggish obesity; while Mrosovsky's hibernating dor-mice and ground squirrels could count on returning to their normal svelte proportions sometime on or about the onset of the vernal equinox. Once having eaten their fill (however lazily), the hiberna-tors would simply conveniently lower their body temperatures to some species-prescribed minimum, go into their annual doze, and spend the next six to eight months literally sleeping off the calories they had greedily cached in the fall.

This seasonal procedure is not without puzzles of its own: Hiber-nating species have in common with newborn mammals of many different species a special kind of adipose tissue called brown fat, which is not found in adults of the same species or of nonhibernators, and this is what they live off during their prolonged winter fast.

Brown fat is thermally as well as anatomically special. Heat from brown fat gets distributed throughout the body by way of the blood, and physiologists M. J. Dawkins and D. Hull estimate that in newborns fully one third of all cardiac output is channeled directly through this amazing tissue, which is conveniently located for that purpose around the neck and shoulders, over the breastbone, and (in human beings) some way down the length of the spine—thus putting it in close thermal proximity to most of the major organ systems of the body. Brown fat takes its name from the darkish color of its specially rich blood and mitochondrion supply, which presumably makes it much quicker to respond to hormonal signals in the blood than the white fat of grown-ups and nonhibernators. Not surprisingly, therefore, brown fat can produce energy and heat at a rate some 20 times higher than white fat cells can—a rate that rivals that of working heart muscle, incidentally, and goes it substantially better.

The environmental trigger for this cellular heat supply is cold. Newborn babies and hibernators have in common the rigors of a low ambient environmental temperature and relatively unresponsive nervous systems: Newborns cannot raise their body temperatures by shivering (a mechanism that does not mature, in human infants at least, until several weeks after birth), and many nonhuman newborn mammals are just as hairless and vascularly defenseless as man himself. It is standard operating procedure in many modern American hospitals, what's more, to give the baby a bath of some sort as soon as the umbilical cord is cut, and this can lower skin temperatures dramatically.

Brown fat has an active as well as a passive role to play in keeping the newborn animal (or the hibernating one) warm, and seems to be high on the list of the body's priorities when it comes to maintaining homeostasis. Rabbits kept unfed in a cold environment for 48 hours start borrowing glucose and free fatty acids from white adipose tissue to keep their brown fat cells supplied. The priority treatment implied in this process seems specifically related to brown fat's heating function: The order of the day for a newborn mammal is to safeguard the integrity of its operating temperature;

otherwise nothing else can proceed according to schedule—including nutrition, growth, and life itself.

In sum, brown fat is undoubtedly critical for survival in infants (recent research by R. L. Naeye at the University of Pittsburgh suggests that it may even have some role to play in the mechanisms of the infant crib-death syndrome, in which babies who seem to be in perfectly good health may be found dead in their cribs at the end of a nap or an uneventful night's sleep). But newborn animals soon learn other ways to keep warm; and as adults our own supply of brown fat has probably all but disappeared by the end of the first year of life—with at most some residual deposits still extant around the nape of the neck.

For man is not, after all, a hibernator. Unlike the dormouse and the ground squirrel, human beings do not curl up in the fetal position at the first sign of cold weather and sleep the winter away from equinox to equinox. Unlike the polar bear, female human beings do not hole up indoors at the onset of winter to gestate and bear their young. And unlike the hamster, man does not usually squirrel away 200 pounds of seeds and grains in some protected corner of his territory and retire from the world for the season's duration.

There are, however, certain parallels. For although man himself is not a hibernator, some of the animals he preyed on for many centuries of his own prehistory did go to ground in winter as a matter of course and according to their own species programs. Fat summers and lean winters were therefore in all probability our Paleolithic ancestors' lot. A considerable body of archaeological evidence bears this hypothesis out. The kitchen middens of European Paleolithic hunters prove the seasonal fluctuation of their game supply; certain sites can only have been inhabited till midwinter, because their garbage piles contained practically no shed antlers, proving that the sites were occupied only while the bucks still carried their antlers—which they only do until November or December in the normal course of events.

Reindeer may have been hunted all year round, with the hunters basing their winter campsites on the proximity of the herds; but small game like fowl and hare were not to be had for the asking in winter; and even in the case of larger game like reindeer or mammoth, winter in the tundra must have imposed strictures of its own, just as it does among circumpolar peoples today. It is in other words a fairly safe bet that the tundra dwellers' food supply was seriously curtailed in winter even if the reindeer herds held stable and suitable campsites could be found. For at the height of the Paleolithic, there was no nutritional alternative to game; except during the very brief summer months, man's only access to vegetable foods was through the animals he preyed on. Reindeer and other herbivores can scratch for mosses and lichens through the snow and thus subsist throughout the winter on this vegetable source, but man cannot digest lichens even if he wanted to or cared to dig them up out of the snow. Man stands at the pinnacle of the food chain in nature—especially in polar or tundra conditions; his vitamins and proteins come to him preprocessed through the bodies of the herbivores he kills and eats. And when this source of vital supplies runs short—as it does of necessity in winter in the Northern Hemisphere—man too must tighten his belt and learn to lie low until the return of good weather and fat flocks.

The result is hibernation of a kind, in fact if not in name. Physician and bioclimatologist Frederick Sargent has suggested that there is a vestigial mechanism operating to adjust man's metabolic juices to seasonal factors exactly as it does those of the true hibernators—and that this mechanism is still operating even in our climatologically homogenized environments today, long past any real need we may once have had for such a mechanism. There are for example measurable differences in the way we metabolize fats and carbohydrates from one season to the next. The spring and summer months (the "anaphase," in Sargent's terminology) are times of high carbohydrate consumption and low fat intake. Physiological fat turnover is lower in the summer than in the winter, and so are levels of the substance choline which helps to metabolize fats and keep them from building up dangerously in the liver. Conversely, fat turnover is higher in laboratory animals—and perhaps also in human beings, although experiments to prove it have not been done yet—in the winter "cataphase" from November to April. This phenomenon is particularly marked in hibernators, but the same effect is clearly present in nonhibernators too. Blood cholesterol for example is also known to be higher in both dogs and humans in the spring and summer than it is in the fall and winter months, and so are the ketone bodies which appear in blood and urine when fats are incompletely burned. Both these findings seem to suggest that man, like other cold-adapted animals, is more "fat-tolerant," or better at burning his own fat reserves, in the winter than in the summer months. The lowered activity of winter is thus offset by nature at least to some extent by the higher fat turnover of the hibernating season, and people who are at least moderately active in winter would therefore seem well advised to go on a diet in the first months of the year, before the summer fat-building season begins.

Carbohydrate metabolism also has its seasonal ups and downs. Adipose tissue carries less glycogen (a glucose precursor) in the winter than it does in the summer months. In 1920 Strouse reported that the blood sugar of healthy adults was higher in March than in July, and studies by other researchers have tended to bear this finding out. The phenomenon makes good sense: Food sources and nutritional carbohydrate supplies are bound to be higher in the spring and summer than in the colder months, and although this may not have had any direct effect on the metabolism of human tundra dwellers, it was bound to affect the tissues of the herbivores they preyed on. The seasonal increase in insulin production in the summer months seems well designed to deal with this ecological circumstance; and the fact that insulin output increases in diabetics too would seem to emphasize the adaptive, universal nature of the effect. Nature and our own metabolisms thus conspire to fatten us up in summer and fall, and diet us down in winter and spring, if we would only give them half a chance.

Granted that man is not a hibernating animal; but in his northernmost ranges he once shared his ecozone with numerous other animals who were. His cold-climate adaptations have therefore always been somewhat calibrated to theirs, and may always have included mechanisms for dealing with shortages brought on by the biograms of his hibernating neighbors in the animal kingdom. Thus, even though in the last 2,000 years or so human culture itself has relaxed many of the climate's most rigorous pressures for somatic and genetic adaptation to cold, it may be well-nigh impossible by now to draw sharp lines between our unmediated physiological responses to winter and our culturally and symbolically mediated responses to the dwindling of day length and the smell of snow in the air that winter ushers in. The American Thanksgiving ritual has given official and cultural sanction to annual autumnal gorging; and the midwinter solstice has long been a seasonal cue for feasting, especially in the northern reaches of the culture area that conveniently celebrates the birth of its major iconic hero in December.

In other words, in that part of his range that is widely populated by true hibernators, man may always have had to make adaptive arrangements for some sort of quasi-hibernation of his own. Until the forests spread north into western Europe and Russia so that nuts and cereal foods could be harvested in fall and stored against winter shortages, man in the colder reaches of his habitat must have had to store a substantial part of his winter food supply under his own skin in the form of subcutaneous fat if he had any hopes of surviving six-, seven-, or eight-month spans of regular seasonal famine. Under such conditions the man who (like the ground squirrel and the Arctic hare) could store the most fat in the autumn and mobilize it most efficiently throughout the long winter months of semistarvation would be bound to survive more winters than his thinner and metabolically more spendthrift neighbors would—and, other things being equal, would tend to outlive and outbreed them and go on to leave more of his genes to the next generation's gene pool when the time came, too.

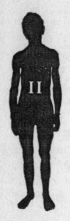

II   *Solutions:*
"Fasting as Fast
as We Can"

"No matter, since you are so steadfast and have us fast, let's fast as fast as we can and then breakfast in the name of famine."

—*Rabelais*

There are few vices to which people are less resigned than gluttony—probably because overeating is one failing that cannot be stamped out by simple swearing off. Hunger can only be curbed, not extirpated. We need food to stay alive, and the instinct that makes us go on eating is such close kin to the one that makes us go on breathing that we couldn't renounce it if we tried. Here, of course, the analogy bogs down: There is no such thing as too much breathing.

Too much eating is something else again. We can and do overeat, and whether we do so from actual starvation, hyperinsulinism, boredom, hypothyroidism, oxygen depletion, or brain damage does not in the end do anything to alter the basic causal sequence between too much food and too much fat—or the social and medical sanctions attending that sequence.

The medical consequences of overeating are easily rehearsed in the differential mortality statistics. Overweight people, both men and women, die significantly earlier and oftener of heart and artery disease, of kidney disease and strokes, of liver and gall-bladder cancer, of diabetes, appendicitis, and accidents than normal people do. Overweight men die significantly more often of hernia and intestinal obstruction; overweight women die significantly more often in childbirth than normal women do. But there are compensating factors. Fat women, according to a 1950 Metropolitan Life Insurance study, have significantly lower breast cancer rates than other women do. Fat people as a group have significantly lower TB and suicide rates, less schizophrenia, and only just about as much psychoneurosis as (or possibly a bit less than) other people do. Various studies of obese and normal city dwellers have shown obese subjects to be significantly more "stable" than the nonobese.

On the other hand, there is evidence that substantially large numbers of the obese tend to be divorced, separated, or widowed than the population at large, and since the mental health of unmarried people in this culture (especially men) tends to be poorer than that of the married majority, it follows that an unmarried individual's chances of being mentally ill do increase if he or she happens also to be obese. This probable side effect of obesity, though, is less a cause than an effect: In a culture that places a high value on thinness, overweight people constitute another disfavored minority group like the physically afflicted or certain ethnic outsiders; they are thus less likely to be chosen as sex, marriage, or occupational partners than more normal-looking people are, and the social consequences are heavy with psychological ones.

Jean Mayer in his informative and compassionate book on overweight has collected a series of vignettes about the social consequences of obesity that run the gamut from the edict of a Rhode Island judge who ordered a woman to reduce from 225 to 190 pounds (and gave her no more than ten weeks to do it in) to the party platform of a Danish reform group which included a proviso that fat people be taxed one hour's pay per month for every two pounds of overweight. In the same vein, a New York personnel placement professional recently ventured the guess that for every pound of overweight a man or woman carries, he or she stands to sacrifice roughly $1,000 a year in income.

It is understood on both sides of the issue that questions of social desirability and social status are involved, and while these questions cut across class lines it is a fact that the poor have more than their fair share of fat people and the rich have less. M. E. Moore, Albert J. Stunkard, and L. Srole's mid-Manhattan project established that while only 5 per cent of upper-socioeconomic-status women were overweight, fully 30 per cent of lower-class women were. That this difference is no mere accident of ethnicity or genes is attested to by the remarkable finding that among people who moved up the social ladder out of the class they were born into, only 12 per cent continued to be overweight. On the other hand, people who lose their original toeholds on the status ladder in the course of a lifetime tend to gain weight as they backslide. In England, J. T. Silverstone had similar findings, while in India—where food is still a scarcity item and hence a status symbol—the pattern was exactly reversed: K. N. Gour and M. C. Gupta in 1968 found that of a group of 68 obese patients, 60 were upper and middle class, and only 8 were lower and lower-middle class.

Considering the difficulties that actuaries and anthropometrists have always had in defining overweight, any excursion into the field of weight control on the part of judges, taste makers, and employers would seem presumptuous if it were not so commonplace. A flat belly seems to constitute all the credentials needed for this widely assumed badge of expertise, and the fat have rarely challenged the assumption; by and large the culture has taught them to take such treatment lying down.

But except to the moralizers, to whom the self-evidence of the proposition that people get fat because they eat too much knocks all other arguments overwhelmingly into a cocked hat, obesity is not as simple as it seems. For most of the chronically overweight, eating too much is only the last and possibly the least link in a long chain of causal connections between the food they eat and the flesh they end up carrying around. The preceding chapters have tried to bring some light to bear on some of the greater and lesser links in that chain, in hopes of taking the argument away from the moralizers and handing it back to the scientists to whom it so clearly belongs. Meanwhile, though, on the humble level of day-to-day living and common sense, we might as well concede the moralizers their point: Whatever the reasons for it may actually be, there is no way to get fat without eating too much food for the individual's own particular body to handle, and there is no way to get thin without eating less food than that same body needs to concoct more fat. A survivor's common sense suggests the obvious solution. For the overweight, it is always high time to go on a diet.

But what diet? There are so many of them. Magazines, books,

medical journals, newspaper columns, and hearsay abound with advice to the weight-lorn. Any living American who does not know by now the caloric value of an egg, an ounce of lean round steak, or a piece of bread (75, 50, and 75 respectively) cannot have had his ear to the ground of his own culture for the last few decades. We now know the caloric cost of a cup of breakfast cereal the way the Pilgrims knew the psalms or the way supermarket checkers know the prices of laundry detergents. Naming the caloric values of foods constitutes a new kind of American folk taxonomy, and it is common knowledge—disputed from time to time but never really revised—that to lose weight you are going to have to take in fewer calories in the form of food than you put out in the form of energy.

Books about obesity usually have two things in common: A list of the caloric costs of the most commonly eaten foodstuffs on the one hand, and some sort of magical formula for exploiting these lists to lose weight on the other. The present book offers neither: in the first case because calorie tables are widely available elsewhere, and in the second case because the research that has been done to date does not support the hopeful notion that there is any one all-or-nothing magical formula to achieve weight loss anyway.

Anyone who has had the patience to follow the arguments outlined and the research reviewed in the last ten chapters will probably be as convinced as the author was and is that the problem of obesity is too complex to yield its secret—or secrets—in one blinding Pasteurian breakthrough. We are conditioned to the "eureka reflex" by the fact that modern medicine won its first major stripes in the area of infectious diseases, where a single causal agent (whether a virus, bacterium, or some slightly larger organism) turned out to be responsible for a single well-defined disease. This single-agent model simply will not do for obesity, though, and we may have to relinquish our wishful assumption that it will. Heart and cancer research, incidentally, have had to yield to the same harsh empirical realities. It is in the nature of problem solving in medicine, and other fields too, that the easy jobs get done first—and to call the discovery of the immunizing action of the cowpox virus an easy job is not to belittle Jenner's achievement but to underline the challenge that faces investigators like Mayer, Stunkard, Brobeck, and Schachter. The list of these names is a clue to the multiplicity of fields that have overlapped in recent obesity research.

Mayer is a physiologist and a biochemist, Stunkard a psychiatrist, Brobeck a physiologist, and Schachter a research psychologist; but between them, they only barely begin to cover the field.

The same list catalogues the bewildering kind and number of proposed cures: There are as many therapeutic approaches to obesity as there are scientific disciplines involved in obesity research itself. How well all or any of them fullfills its clients' needs for solutions has become the focus of a small-scale research effort of its own. The scoreboard, at last count, was not brilliant—for any of them.

You would not in all probability be reading this book if you were not at least somewhat or sometimes interested in losing weight. And to the 40 or so per cent of the American population that is actually certifiably overweight the culture in its insistence on thinness has added half again as many citizens to the ranks of the potentially if not the violently weight-conscious. Many of us climb on the scales every morning with our hearts in our mouths; depending on where the needle stops fluttering we will sally forth that day in a good mood or a bad one. We are a nation of dieters and do not give up easily; what Frederick Exley has wistfully named "quitter's obesity" is probably a clinical rarity: It is in the nature of the dieter to try, try again.

The statistics, though, are not encouraging. In 1966 J. A. Glennon reviewed the available studies to that date and concluded that only 10 per cent of patients in scientifically conducted and statistically controlled clinical weight-reduction programs managed to maintain their original weight losses after one year; at two years this ratio had dwindled to 6 per cent. J. A. Strong estimated that only one eighth of any successfully treated population was apt to maintain its original loss, and A. R. Feinstein puts this rate at 1 to 2 per cent after a five-year time lapse. The biggest success rates reported for any groups were for male volunteers to an Anti-Coronary Club program in New York City, 71.7 per cent of whom had maintained substantial weight losses at four-year follow-up. The men enrolled in this program were a high-risk group in terms of age, life-style, and eating habits, and the aim of the program was a lot more complex than simple weight reduction; therefore, the results of the study probably reflect the life-and-death rationale attending the program itself, as well as a simple desire to lose weight.

Albert J. Stunkard, of the University of Pennsylvania, has done painstaking (and what can only be called unflinching) work in this field. Of eight studies involving a total of 1,368 patients, Stunkard found only one group with more than a 29 per cent success rate, success being interpreted as a weight loss of twenty or more pounds per subject. Stunkard's own patients at the Nutrition Clinic of New York Hospital fared no better. Of 97 patients enrolled in the clinic's program over a two-year period (most of them women), only 12 achieved a twenty-pound weight loss, and of these twelve, only six managed to keep the weight off for a full year after treatment. But at two-year follow-up this margin had been trimmed by two thirds: Only two of these six original losers were still slim at this time. Follow-up is the proof of the therapeutic pudding in weight loss: Charlotte Young of Cornell reported a 25.6 per cent success rate for a group of overweight patients treated in 1955, but ten years later the figure had receded to zero.

A word of caution is in order about informal studies reporting astronomical success rates. Such reports surface regularly. But few of them have been set up in advance specifically to test the statistical probability of any one outcome over and against another, and none of them volunteer any follow-up information. These studies appear regularly in the lay press but do not, for sound editorial reasons, find their way into the medical or nutrition journals; until they do, their authors' conclusions should be taken with a grain of salt. Stunkard, commenting on the results of thirty years' efforts in the field, concluded that the over-all results were miserable, and that the only generalization that could safely be made from the welter of data on age, sex, social class, and motivation of dieters was a simple one related to gender: to wit, that although relatively few men enroll in weight-reduction programs on a country-wide basis, when they do they are much more likely to lose weight and keep it off than women.

Notwithstanding the general gloom, dieters continue to go on dieting and researchers go on doing research, and a general review may still be in order. The eight reducing programs eventually selected for review by Stunkard and M. McLaren-Hume used a variety of methods to arrive at their results; basic to all of them, however, were re-educative efforts aimed at clearing up any misunderstanding about food and feeding their patients might have had, and regular clinic appointments to keep the dieters' morale up and the therapeutic pressure steady. In the late 1950's and early 1960's psychoanalytic theory caught up with dieting practice, and more serious attempts were made to introduce psychodynamic principles into the weight-loss programs, but without notable success. Consciousness raising of the obese became the therapeutic fashion in the late 1950's; group therapy, which had proved itself with delinquents, married partners, and unwed mothers, struck everybody concerned as a likely approach to the problem of obesity; hypnosis became another contender for this honor. Ten years later behavior therapy began to make a name for itself in the area of weight control. Remarkable results had been reported for it in the management of schizophrenia, phobias, and habit disorders; and obesity itself seemed a prime candidate for the so-called operant conditioning technique.

Given the known level of backsliding in weight control, followup is obviously crucial as a measure of success, and as of this writing none of these treatment modalities has been in effect long enough to determine how well graduates of the newer programs will prove to have held the line ten years, or even five years, after therapy. For the short term, however, one thing does seem to be clear: Where it has been systematically compared to other more conventional programs, behavior therapy can be demonstrated to outperform other popular approaches by an impressive margin.

Within behavior therapy itself, the techniques in service range all the way from "aversive therapy" to "operant conditioning." In the former, the patient is negatively conditioned to suppress the unwanted behavior; in the latter he is positively rewarded whenever he performs well. Radical aversive conditioning takes an opposite tack; patients are electrically shocked, or given emetics to take, whenever they own up to the thought of something good to eat. In the long run, aversive conditioning was found to be less effective in weight control than positive conditioning was already proving to be. T. Allyon reports a psychotic patient in a Canadian hospital whose compulsive gorging was effectively managed by simply (bodily) removing her from the hospital dining room whenever she displayed the undesirable behavior (that is, whenever she overate). After 14 months she had lost 60 pounds without any further therapeutic ado. The alternative form of operant conditioning depends on the principle of direct, positive reinforcement; this means that whenever the desirable behavior takes place the subject is immediately given some form of tangible reward. Working on this principle, J. L. Barnard brought a 407-pound female patient down to 337 pounds in seventeen weeks, reimbursing her for good behavior in a sort of clinical scrip redeemable for hospital privileges of various (inedible) kinds.

Anecdotes like these are rife in the medical literature, but must not be given more than their just due; life (and medicine) is miracle prone, and one or several isolated cases do not constitute proof of cure. Obese patients are notoriously individualistic in their response to therapy, and the only way to know whether the cure in question is some fluke of clinical luck or a genuine corrective is to do controlled studies of large groups of patients undergoing different kinds of treatment under exactly the same conditions and for exactly the same length of time, and compare the results statistically. Two such studies have been mentioned in an earlier chapter. In both of them behavior therapy came out ahead of competing treatment approaches—psychoanalytically oriented "insight" therapy for one, group pressure techniques for another, and re-educative approaches for a third. Although the groups studied were not large, the results of S. B. Penick, R. Filion, S. Fox, and A. J. Stunkard's study were impressive. More than twice as many patients in the behavior-modification group lost 30 to 40 pounds, and almost twice as many patients lost 20 pounds within the three-month treatment period, as patients in a group psychotherapy program did.

Hypnosis is another likely candidate for obesity treatment, and has reported some successes too. In a group of 525 randomly selected cases, consisting of subjects enrolled in a hypnotherapeutic weight-reduction program, Leo Wollman reported an average 30-pound weight loss over a three-month period. Subjects were men and women between the ages of twenty and forty, and were treated in groups of five, with the one-hour therapy sessions divided between trance experience and group therapy on a fifty-fifty basis. Wollman used aversive suggestion as well as positive, satiety-promoting suggestion. Other large-scale studies of the effectiveness of hypnosis are not on the books, so it is hard to know whether Wollman's results are unique or may turn out to apply to other similar populations too. As to how such results would fare in a countdown with behavior therapy, though, it should be said that hypnosis uses almost identical psychological mechanisms—i.e., aversive and operant conditioning—to produce the desired results, the difference being a matter of verbal technique on the one hand, and the level of consciousness at which the technique is put into operation on the other. If their results do indeed turn out to be similar, it would therefore come as no very great surprise.

Psychotherapy, behavior therapy, and group pressure therapies like TOPS and Weight Watchers all work on the principle of mind over matter; but there are other possibilities, and such is the concern with overweight in our culture that few of them have been left untried. Drugs used to treat obesity have ranged from hormones (thyroxin and estrogen head the list) to the amphetamines. But reputable physicians have remained unconvinced. Both thyroxin and amphetamines tend to be self-limiting because after a few weeks the body becomes habituated to them and demands larger and larger doses to maintain smaller and smaller effects. The more the medical community learns about the long-range effects of many hormones, meanwhile, the leerier doctors tend to become of them. Therapeutic estrogen has been implicated in breast and uterine cancer, and acute toxic reaction to thyroxin can constitute a clinical emergency of the first magnitude; growth hormone (including human chorionic gonadotrophin, which may be an active analogue of it) can have undesirable cosmetic effects on the face, hands, and feet if administered over any length of time.

This still leaves two interesting treatment possibilities based on the direct matter-over-matter approach (no will power needed). One is total starvation in a hospital setting; the other is intestinal-bypass surgery. Both solutions have had their defenders; both are radical procedures and carry a mortality risk that is probably only acceptable in cases where the gross amount of overweight is in the range of 100 to 200 per cent. Intestinal-bypass surgery attacks the problem at its source. In it, sections of the small intestine are simply tied off and the patient is put back into circulation with considerably less gut than he was born with—or may be able to make do with successfully in a normal postoperative life. Results can be dramatic in this operation, with weight losses of up to 100 pounds per year in spite of ad lib food intakes which may run to the same kind of caloric surpluses that got the patient into trouble before. Postoperative complications can be unpleasant, though, and may include diarrhea, abdominal pain, and a host of other trying gastrointestinal symptoms; and the surgery itself carries a 10 per cent risk of fatality (perhaps in part because only very obese patients are ever considered candidates for this approach, and they constitute a high-surgical-risk population to begin with).

Starvation, on the other hand, carries risks of its own. Even in the resting state the body uses 70 per cent of its incoming calories to service heart, brain, and viscera—and these tissues amount to 70 per cent by body weight over all. Total starvation not only deletes the calories needed for work and effort, but those that are needed just to keep the engine idling as well, and any deficit is therefore going to affect at least 70 per cent of nonactive (but nevertheless absolutely essential) body tissues along with active muscle. The game may be worth the candle to the dieter—but then again it may not. Reports of death as a result of medically supervised fasts are rare, but they do exist. E. S. Garnett and his co-workers described one such case in 1969: a young woman died after a 30-week fast in which she lost 58 kilos (127.6 pounds). Death occurred at the end of the fast, while the patient was beginning to eat normally again, and the autopsy report suggested that the patient had died of degenerative changes in the heart muscle itself. Still more recently, a 215-pound woman on a 500-calorie-a-day diet at a New Jersey diet clinic died of a heart attack after a four-day fast—presumably because of deficient blood minerals involved in maintaining the heart's electrical activity.

But these are extreme cases; careful attention to mineral intake might have averted the second tragedy, while nitrogen excretion tests might have warned physicians that too much lean tissue was being lost too fast in the first. By and large, short-term fasting in a hospital setting is probably no more dangerous than many other everyday, run-of-the-mill medical treatments are—and possibly somewhat less so than antibiotic therapy, X radiation, and simple surgery. The limiting factor, apart from mineral balance, is lean-tissue loss. In this respect, short-term fasting can be even more strenuous, relatively speaking, than long-term fasting; in 70 men who fasted for a ten-day period with a mean weight loss of 9.4 kilos (20.8 pounds), only 35.4 per cent of the recorded loss could be accounted for by fat; the rest, a whopping 64.6 per cent, consisted of lean tissue, including muscle, organ tissue, and bones. Ancel Keys's classic experiments on human starvation at the University of Minnesota in the course of the Second World War produced strikingly similar effects, even though his subjects merely fasted rather than being truly starved: Actual fat loss during the first three months was only on the order of 37 per cent of the over-all weight loss, and during the succeeding months it never increased to more than 70 per cent of the total tissue loss, suggesting that even in prolonged deprivation the body continues to break down its own protein reserves for energy, however nicely it may be burning fat in the meantime.

The point is an important one, because it means that in the long run it may pay the dieter to take in a certain carefully calculated number of calories a day rather than starve. M. F. Ball has noted that, paradoxically, in some patients on an 800-calorie-a-day diet, real fat loss was actually greater than it was on a regime of total fasting. This is because, with a bare minimum of nutrients coming into the system from time to time, the brain can still make do with holdover glucose supplies from that day's food intake, however meager, and the body's protein stores need not get called into action for emergency glucose deliveries to the brain. Fat will thus be burned for fuel, and lean tissue spared. A modicum of glucose, in other words, protects the body's protein reserves, and insures that energy needs will be met from adipose tissue instead of muscle. Recent approaches to this problem include the "supplemented fasts" now being touted in the popular press. The end itself is an enlightened one, but the means are still open to question: All indications are that in any prolonged fast the brain is still going to pull glucose by breaking down protein tissue, and a better way to preserve existing bone and muscle in the meantime might therefore be to provide a modicum of carbohydrate or glucose in the first place.

But the gist of all these efforts is that ways and means of losing weight do exist, short of full-scale psychoanalytic treatment on the one hand or major abdominal surgery on the other. To what extent the average middle-class, medium-fat and middling-determined citizen has or wants access to them is another question, though. Group therapy is not everyone's cup of tea, and some people are not capable of being hypnotized, even if they choose to be. Intestinal-bypass surgery is not a lightly undertaken procedure, and a medically monitored three- to six-month fast is probably no more realistic an option for most wage earners than a three- to six-month vacation with pay would be.

Still, the problem refuses to go away, and alternatives have been and will be found. The psychological and social costs of obesity are intolerable to many of the people who spend the better part of their lives paying them; and short of the more or less radical, more or less available weight-loss schemes described above, the long-suffering run-of-the-mill obese do have some realistic options in the matter of long-term, low-cost, no-fuss weight control.

But this is true only if they are willing to settle for something short of immediate and irreversible results. Knowledge is power, and to say that we do not really know what causes obesity, let alone how to cure it, does not mean that the bits and pieces of knowledge we do now have about obesity cannot be seamed together into a serviceable patchwork and put to good immediate use in day-to-day weight control. It is the premise of this book, however, that this is a lifetime, and not a one-shot, operation. If your constitution wants you to be fat it will take more than will power and the odd crash diet to keep you thin, and the sooner you face this fact the thinner you are apt to get and keep yourself. Dieting is not the answer; systematic, lifelong underfeeding is the gist of the medical handwriting on the wall. For the constitutionally obese, "proper" nutrition is overnutrition.

When it comes to weight loss or gain there are two ways of bringing mind to bear on matter; will power is one, information is another. The preceding chapters have been long on information, short on practical advice. In part this reflects the understandable caution of most workers in this line of research; obesity research has always been plagued by more than its fair share of charlatans and Panglosses. The truth is that there are no cures in sight, at least not at the moment, and serious investigators have run the risk of seeing their most judicious, limited, and prudently worded results logrolled into public panaceas without any regard for the medical or cultural consequences that might (and sometimes did) ensue. The high-fat diets of a decade or so ago came up against the heart-and-artery-disease statistics and eventually died a natural death; the no-carbohydrate diets are still with us, although the "meat eaters" will probably come to the same kind of grief on the bowel-cancer figures as the fat eaters did on the coronary tables. We have been oversold for so long on the notion that simple gluttony is what causes obesity that it has become second nature to assume simple asceticism is all that is needed to cure it. The facts are otherwise. Will power and liquid protein will not do the trick. For the long run, information, insight, and ingenuity are needed too.

Hunger is the dieter's ghost at the feast. Except in rare cases, there would have been no problem with weight gain to begin with unless the dieter's physiology and/or his psyche had not condemned him to a chronic nagging hunger that went to bed with him at night and woke up with him in the morning for the better part of his life. This kind of hunger is a problem that obviously is not going to go away with dieting. It is, on the other hand, probably not going to get all that much worse either; obese people have lived with hunger all their lives, and the additional hunger incurred by going on a diet is not going to be anything new to them either physiologically or psychologically speaking. The object in long-haul weight reduction is thus to learn to cheat that hunger as gracefully and as intelligently as one can.

Fat people are, to call a spade a spade, hungrier than other people are, and unless the feeling can be brought under control the battle is lost before it is joined. Three physiological subsystems are involved in hunger: the brain, the gut, and the endocrine system; and if hunger is to be manipulated in the dieter's favor he will have to be on the alert for ways to trick these three systems into complacency even when they are no more fed, full, or nourished than they were to begin with. The first line of defense against the false hunger of appetite is the brain—or that part of it that controls feeding and satiety in vertebrates, the hypothalamus. But how, where, and when can the ordinary fat person go about cheating his own hypothalamus into thinking that it has just been fed, when in fact it hasn't?

The answer lies in the structure of the hypothalamus itself and to some extent in its over-all neuroanatomical purpose. As the list of known regulatory systems originating in the hypothalamus grows, so grows the suspicion that its geographical placement is crucial to its function. The little black box that is the hypothalamus sits midway between the two major parts of the human central nervous system—the neocortex and the spine—and mediates all the sensory data that are constantly passing between them. Sexual responses as well as immunological ones have recently been added to the list of things that are thought to be organized and orchestrated in the hypothalamus; these are only the two latest additions to the catalogue as drawn. Hunger, satiety, circadian sleep-and-activity patterns, and temperature control had all been localized on the hypothalamus by earlier research. Included in this roster are some factors over which we have a modicum of control, as well as others over which we do not. Signals that we as dieters can inject into this cerebral black box include cues about body temperature, blood and tissue oxygen levels and, probably, tissue water saturation and glucose supplies. Research shows that all of these are factors which have some bearing on appetite itself.

Of these, perhaps the easiest to manipulate is heat. One way of persuading the brain that the body is being fed is to turn up body heat, whether by eating (or drinking) something hot or by deliberately setting out to raise skin temperature by putting on extra clothes and moving into a warm environment—or both. If J. R. Brobeck's theory of thermostatic appetite control is correct—and the whole prehistory of human physique suggests that it is—then the warmer you are the less apt you are to confuse real hunger pangs with other need states being monitored in the hypothalamus at the same time as the need for heat. Even in people with good regulatory feedback between the head and the viscera and skin, intense cold can interfere with these connections and throw them off. The human thermostat is—to judge from Brobeck's animal experiments—set to operate only within a thermal tolerance of roughly one degree Fahrenheit. Anything over this difference is apt to call for gross adjustment of body metabolism to right the balance. Severe cold stress raises thyroid and adrenal hormone levels; heat production goes into high gear and the animal starts to shiver and burn oxygen at a fast clip. This process may raise a hearty appetite, but if the animal starts feeding while all these things are going on, the effect of food on body temperature will just not be dramatic enough to signal the hypothalamus that food is coming in—unless the food itself is piping hot. Raising the temperature of the food itself thus raises the probability that the hypothalamus will perceive that it is being fed.

Interestingly enough in this connection, it should be pointed out that basal metabolic rates (and oxygen consumption) do not increase as much in obese people in response to cold as they do in people of normal size; this may be because the thick "electric blanket" of fat between the skin of a fat person and his own warm innards in some way short-circuits the lines between the individual's skin temperature and his brain's ability to monitor it correctly. Thus, especially in fat people, delivering heat to the viscera by way of hot food and hot drinks becomes a much more reliable (and faster) method of getting the message through to the brain than delivering it to the skin itself. And, last but not least, delivering the heat in liquid form constitutes express service. Liquids leave the stomach and reach the gut faster than solids and are therefore ready for action in the blood and hypothalamus well before any food that comes in solid form.

The night-feeding syndrome that plagues many obese people may be due in part at least to the same effect. Most people's temperatures show a rising circadian curve from noon till late evening, with temperatures peaking at or before midnight; but some people—and most species of hibernating animals—have a very different daily temperature curve, with high temperatures at noon and lows in the late afternoon or early evening. If the compulsive icebox raider turns out to have this kind of anomalous daily temperature curve it may manifest itself by sudden hunger pangs in the early evening. If so, drinking something hot and laying on an extra supply of blankets may help to keep him (or her) out of the kitchen and under the covers, where he or she is less apt to get fat. For people who have this problem, and for those who are seriously overweight, the thermal ante—both day and night—may have to be upped considerably, say within the fever range, before this bit of heat-regulating legerdemain can have any real effect on appetite. (At 104°F, as Brobeck has shown, all known mammals stop feeding, for better or for worse, until their temperatures come back down to within normal species-specific limits again.)

Another way to steal a march on the unfed hypothalamus is to persuade it that there is more oxygen in the tissues than may at any given moment actually be on its way to them. If the dieter has been leading a particularly sedentary life the lack of activity itself may be half the problem. Jean Mayer's study of Indian bazaar workers is a case in point. The least active workers in this sample actually ate as much as the most physically active ones did, in spite of the fact that they spent the greater part of the day sitting or standing in one place, and lived within very short walking distances of their work. Boredom and social factors may have explained part of this discrepancy between the calories the various workers took in and those they lost in exercise, but not all of it: Oxygen hunger may, in the brain, become misread as glucose lack, and the individual may think he is in the mood to eat when actually he is only so to speak gasping for air. If so, Mayer's bazaar clerks may have been the victims of an illusion many sedentary workers are prey to in countries all over the world. The best and fastest palliative for a raging appetite in these circumstances is to get up and go for a walk, do calisthenics or, in a pinch, simply fidget at one's desk. G. A. Rose and R. T. Williams found that even when sitting down, fidgeters can use up to 80 per cent more oxygen than more phlegmatic subjects do; and the resulting oxygen uptake in the tissues is felt first, most, and fastest in the brain. In the same vein, exercise physiologist Laurence Morehouse reports that Ph.D. qualifying-exam grades were significantly higher for fidgety students than for their more relaxed peers; this finding probably reflects brain glucose levels more nearly than it does the high I.Q. of fidgeters.

Americans tend to think of exercise as a planned extraneous element in their lives, something they are going to have to make time for, scheme for, and budget hard-earned money for. Most of us live in as automated a world as we can afford to, and one of the underlying shibboleths of American culture is that, at heart, nobody really wants to "work." From welfare chiseler to coupon clipper, the natural wisdom has it that we would all rather be off fishing or going to the movies. This assumption does both our bodies and our psyches wrong; man is a physical activist with a long evolutionary history of earth moving, trekking, portage, roof raising; and while the work patterns of industrial societies may satisfy most of his daily needs for camaraderie and money, as time goes on they seem to do less and less for his body's need for out-and-out physical action. Man was not originally designed for the inanition that modern technology has bequeathed him. But with a little forethought and consciousness raising we can all learn to steal a march of sorts on the entropic future that our supertechnologies seem to be condemning us to. Stairs still exist, even in skyscrapers; and in many buildings even if you live or work on the 35th floor, nobody can keep you from climbing to the third, fourth, or fifth floor and taking the elevator from there. By the same token, reversing the seemingly innate instinct of motorists to get as close to their destinations as possible, drivers may find it wise to park as far from their actual goals as they feasibly can, and walk the extra blocks to and fro (carrying as many heavy packages as they can stand to in the process!).

We have been brainwashed by efficiency experts into saving steps; what we need to do is reverse the process, and make steps for ourselves where none necessarily exist anymore. Housework and yard work make excellent exercise opportunities, especially those tasks that require a major displacement of the arms and upper torso. (Due to the force of gravity and the way major circulatory-system valves work, upper-body exercise is more calorically demanding than legwork is; housework is full of good object lessons in this principle.) The object of all these efforts is to get the blood moving—but not, as in so many organized sports, to get a real workout. The danger in exhaustion, for the dieter's purposes at least, is the mirror image of that involved in inactivity: to wit, that the brain will misjudge the signals and call for more food, rather than less effort, to compensate.

Fatigue, hunger, and cold are all monitored in the hypothalamus within a few hypersensitive millimeters of each other, and in the midbrain or regulatory obesities all incoming signals seem to get coded into the same message—that message being hunger. For those of us who suffer from this confusion, a lifetime of conscious self-monitoring and self-regulation is in order. The pseudohunger of people who react to cold with ravening appetites can probably be appeased with a hot drink (preferably something salty instead of something sweet and milky, since salt appears to enhance our perception of warmth while calcium attenuates it). By the same token, the raging hunger that can follow strenuous exercise or physical exhaustion may yield to rest and a glass of something noncaloric, if given half a chance. In both cases the hunger itself is no less real than if it were caused by an actual caloric deficit; the hypothalamus will reliably—but erroneously—respond by sending out the message that it is time to eat. This kind of hypothalamus is hard to live with and will have to be trained to distinguish the finer points.

Speculation has raged for decades about the origins of this kind of central-nervous-system derailment of appetite, with psychiatrists holding out for an emotional explanation and the physiologists for a hypothalamic one. But in the end it makes very little difference whether the hypothalamus got that way because the individual is neurotic, congenitally gluttonous, brain-damaged, or just plain unlucky. The net result is an incompetent appetite-regulating device, and the only cure is a conscious self-regulation to take the place of the automatic regulation the individual no longer enjoys, with the patient's own neocortex taking over where his confused and confounding midbrain leaves off.

One of the worst side effects of hypothalamic fuzziness like that described here is not knowing when to stop feeding. Satisfaction of appetite is still very poorly understood; the feedback loops between hunger and satiety are simply not as dramatic and full-blown as they are in anoxia, in sex, or in thirst. We all seem to know when to take a deep breath, when we have had an orgasm, and when we have had enough to drink to quench thirst. Knowing when we have had enough to eat is something else again; it seems to depend on orchestration of a huge complex of messages between our viscera, our blood, and our brains. In the regulatory obesities any or all of these message relays seem to get short-circuited: Uncontrollable overeating represents a breakdown of communications in one or all of these feedback circuits, and the only place in the circuit that the dieter can assert any degree of control at all is at the point of input itself. By juggling the actual amount of food he takes in against the number of calories he eats, he can, if he is clever, vigilant, and persistent, manage to cheat his own hypothalamus into thinking that there are more nutrients in the pipeline at any given moment than there are actually calories in the bloodstream at that time.

One way of doing this is to exploit what we know about the time it takes the various different food components to pass through the gullet and out into the blood. After water and minerals, sugars are the first nutrients to get digested and pass through the walls of the small intestine into the bloodstream for use by the cells. Starch and cellulose come next. The ideal meal plan for someone with an ungovernable appetite is therefore to start out the meal with something sweet and follow it with a salad; then get down to basics. Of the three major foodstuffs, proteins and fats take the longest to leave the stomach and are last to be absorbed through the intestinal walls; in some cases this process may take as long as six hours. Since neither proteins nor fats are therefore going to be present in the bloodstream within the first half hour of eating anyway, the person who has trouble knowing when to stop should leave these nutrients till last. Meat, cheese, butter, and eggs eaten at the end of the meal will enter the bloodstream at a stately enough pace to carry the dieter through many hours of fasting till the next meal, while keeping energy levels and body temperatures high enough to head off the false hunger of anoxia and cold.

The meal plan suggested here is of course almost a complete inversion of the normal one, which probably made good sense in an era when the need was to ingest as much food and store as much fat as appetite permitted at one fell swoop. But affluence and the modern food industry have reversed the ecological premises on which the old meal plan was based, and it is probably high time that the usual rituals were overhauled and adjusted accordingly.

Other ways to beat the system exist, but they are less immediately self-explanatory. Although there is good evidence from animal studies that frequent small feeds seem to exert a dampening effect on fat deposition, there is other evidence that starved tissues are less fat- and insulin-responsive than fed ones are. George Cahill conducted animal studies in which tracer dyes attached to foods were monitored isotopically to see where in the body's tissues the ingested fats actually ended up. His research showed that in animals who have recently eaten something, dietary fat bypasses the lean tissues and goes straight to the adipose tissue cells for storage, while in animals who have gone without food for several hours or longer, the newly ingested fats went directly to the liver and muscles, presumably for emergency use in ongoing metabolism. G. Hollifield found the same sort of pattern, this time with glucose as opposed to fats; in an unfed animal, adipose tissue has more trouble making fat from sugar substrates than it does in an animal who has recently been fed. This surprising clinical finding may explain why, at the end of a long diet, people's weights may stay stable for a few days even though caloric intake goes up sharply and exceeds immediate caloric needs; something in the newly thin animal seems to be resistant to renewed fattening. But whether this resistance is enough to offset the appetite-dampening effects of small, frequent meals noticed by other investigators and widely ballyhooed in the popular press has never been tested.

For the short term, however, the message from Cahill's and Hollifield's research would seem to be that, if you must go on an eating binge, be sure to cut way back on your calories a day or so before you plan to do so. Dieters who have trouble keeping their appetites in check at parties, weddings, and gala dinners usually try to salvage the situation by morning-after abstinence; but studies like the two reported above suggest that just the opposite strategy may be indicated: Partygoers should prediet rather than postdiet. The message is that, if you must overeat, do it on an empty stomach. (Of course, to the well-motivated dieter, a little morning-after abstention is not going to seem amiss either.)

So far most, if not all, of the artful dodges in this master plan have been addressed to the problem of how not to feel too hungry, too soon, or for too long; they are based on the premise that the hypothalamus is the place in the brain where we feel hunger and is therefore the organ to be reckoned with (and deceived) when we do. There are other, more primitive ways to feel fed—and one of them is simply to eat a lot of nonfattening foods. This may not necessarily damp down the fires of hunger—in fact, if there is any inadequacy in the midbrain it probably won't—but it may make the dieter feel so full that even where brain satiety can't begin to operate, bloat or nausea will. The point is particularly crucial for endomorphs. Autopsy findings confirmed Sheldon's surmise that endomorphs were apt to average significantly longer and larger intestines than mesomorphs or ectomorphs do, and whatever feedback relays may exist between the viscera and the brain, it stands to reason that it will therefore take more time and more food to trigger them in endomorphs than it will in members of the other two groups. Cellulose, accordingly, is the endomorph's best friend. To fill the gut as close to capacity as possible, and with as little caloric load as is feasible into the bargain, should be one of the endomorph's major nutritional aims in life. Salads and vegetables help; so do soups and those cereals that soak up a respectable amount of water or milk when they are cooked. And the hotter the food the better; hot foods leave the stomach and enter the gut more quickly than others and will thus send back signals to the brain faster than cold foods will—quite apart from any effect they may concurrently have on body heat and on the various thermal factors involved in appetite.

Water and other liquids in the body, incidentally, play a puzzling but ungainsayable role both in satiety and in fat mobilization as well: Francesco Grande of the University of Minnesota found that the water content of the body had a very significant effect on the amount of weight that was lost on a diet. When water and other liquids as well as calories were withheld from dieters, actual fat loss (as measured by densitometry) was substantially less than it was when dieters received the same number of calories but were allowed to drink water ad lib. This effect was especially strong during the first few days of a diet, with the difference amounting to some 500 calories per day. The advice to drink plenty of water while you are on a diet is therefore well taken—not only because it tends to make you feel full, but also because whatever works to preserve fat stores in the body seems closely calibrated to whatever it is that also conserves water. Schachter's review of the similarities between obese rats and obese human beings evinced a similar effect: In both cases animals tended to take in fewer calories when the calories were presented in liquid form than when they were presented in solid form.

Diets for mesomorphs present a special case; the high protein content of the dieter's own body probably demands a special attention to carbohydrate intake in order to spur complete fat breakdown and prevent metabolism from taking the path of least resistance through its own muscle stores to get glycogen and glucose for the brain. Fat burns best and fastest in the presence of carbohydrates, and the mesomorph's own lean tissue is at risk when there is no starch or sugar coming into the system to provide fuel for burning the fat. There may also be a sex difference here, with male dieters more concerned about maintaining their lean tissue stores than females are and rightly so; there may even conceivably be women who would go into the business of dieting away muscle tissue with their eyes wide open and full speed ahead. Just such a diet made news in publishing circles a few years ago. Practitioners of this sort of diet should be advised, however, that the lean tissue they stand to lose may not all be in their legs and biceps where it shows: The heart is a muscle too, and the viscera and blood vessels contain their fair share of essential protein tissues, none of them expendable, least of all to healthy, active mesomorphs.

Diets for ectomorphs? The very idea seems a little misbegotten, because ectomorphs rarely get fat, and when they do, the problem is usually local, temporary, unimpressive, and easily brought under control. Of all the basic somatotypes, ectomorphs are probably the only ones who can afford to take the classical medical advice—that is, to cut out sugars and starches and go easy on everything else— that is so randomly and optimistically promulgated by most diet doctors for most dieters. This regimen has never been known to do much for the seriously obese and may not do much for ectomorphs either, depending on how fat they are; but if anyone can lose weight on such a regimen ectomorphs can, and the only wonder is that it should ever have come to that with them in the first place.

Other ways to cheat either the brain or the body of their natural proclivity to help the obese make fat are less well researched and should be investigated further before they are added to the dieter's everyday bag of tricks. David Green's finding that it takes manganese to make fat while it takes magnesium to burn it might or might not be used to the dieter's advantage—if and when a test could be arranged without upsetting the body's natural mineral balance. As of now the data simply do not exist. These are therefore not questions for do-it-yourself dieters to decide, and such matters can only be definitively settled in the laboratory. Conceivably, a diet low in manganese and high in magnesium could be devised and clinically tested in human subjects to see whether it would have any measurable effect on the rate at which people gain or lose weight; but juggling the amounts of the body's trace minerals is not an undertaking for amateurs, and is suggested here not as a solution to a problem but as an area in which obesity research might someday begin to pay off.

Another study along these lines might look at the effect of salt and potassium balance on the ability of adipose tissue cells to take up glucose and convert it to fat. Normally, the balance between these two complementary body minerals is maintained by means of the so-called sodium-potassium pump at the outside surface of the cell. Inside the cell there are more potassium ions than sodium ions; but in the fluid outside the cells sodium ions are in the ascendancy, and in order for nutrients to get into the cell itself, potassium ions have to get shifted from inside of the cell to the cell surface to let them in. A sudden ion shift like this may cause the body to re-equilibrate its salt and water stores. Recently, biochemists B. Jeanrenaud and A. E. Renold of the Geneva Biochemical Institute found that when potassium levels inside the cell and at the cell membrane are artificially lowered (which allows sodium to pass over the membrane and get into the cell itself) over-all metabolic activity inside the cell goes up strikingly—and at the same time, what is even more interesting from the dieter's point of view, the cell in question becomes much less sensitive to insulin than it would normally be. Since insulin acts as one of the major inducements for cells to take up glucose and store fat, any over-all decrease in potassium in the body may therefore act to slow down the rate at which fat can be synthesized from blood-sugar substrates, and thus in the long run may prove to be one of the most useful minerals in the dieter's periodic table of elements.

These manipulations are of course not advisable for people with low blood pressure or any kind of mineral imbalances, and are mentioned with the usual strong caveat that they not be undertaken without the advice of a physician. And even so the dieter may not be safe, for the same caveat always applies, on a somewhat grander scale, to any of the medically approved but hastily researched dieting regimes which sweep the public imagination at intervals and attract their predictable armies of acolytes and casualties. Like everything else of any importance in a given era's cultural inventory, medical panaceas have a life history of their own, full of ups and downs, reverses, fashions, and eclipses—and obesity cures are no exception. William Banting, author of the first low-carbohydrate diet, seems to have been the first in what was to become a long line of messianic dietmongers, each with some final message to impart and truth to deliver; but he was not and will not be the last.

Banting's high-fat, high-protein, and low-carbohydrate diet has the virtue of starting matters off with a considerable and impressive body-water loss in the first days or week of the diet. We now know, however, that this kind of first-week loss, or beginner's luck, represents an unacceptable lean tissue loss with little if any concomitant wasting of actual fat. Most dieters—and their doctors—would find this a high price to pay for those first moments of rapture on the bathroom scale. Moreover, Banting was writing in a time and place (the late nineteenth century) when the advice to eat lots of fat was not so easily taken as it is now. Latter-day Americans and northern Europeans probably eat far too much fat for their own good to begin with, and while the data about fats and coronary and arterial disease are by no means conclusive at this point in medical history, there is increasing reason to suspect that a high fat and protein diet is largely responsible for unacceptably high colorectal and breast cancer rates in the more affluent, fat-eating countries of the world; and no responsible physician would want to ignore the implications of these findings, however tentative they may be. Meanwhile, it is well to remember that only 5 to 15 per cent of ingested fats go to work immediately in the cells themselves; the rest go to the adipose tissue for storage or into the arteries themselves, with even more sinister effects.

While the classical view used to be that fats cannot be used for fuel in the muscles and other organs without first going into storage in the fat cells and thence being processed into free fatty acids for uptake by the lean-tissue cells, newly discovered ways of charting the pathways taken by various foodstuffs (by injecting marked tracer doses of them into the blood and seeing just where they do in fact end up one, two, or twelve hours after injection) prove that a small proportion of ingested fats does actually go straight to the (nonadipose) cells. This rate may be even higher when the diet itself is abnormally high in fats; but the obverse of this equation is that less fat will then be drawn from storage to make up the cellular deficit. The advantage of the low- (or no-) carbohydrate, high-fat, and high-protein diets is therefore almost exactly the opposite of the one their originators have suggested: Stored fat is not released from storage more easily and efficiently than it is in other regimes, as claimed; what these diets do achieve, though, is to lower the rate at which new fat can be formed. They do this, however, at the expense of considerable loss of lean tissue. Is the lean-tissue loss involved in this transaction worth it? A little nutritional arithmetic would seem to suggest that it's not. By slowly depleting the body's lean-tissue stockpiles, all you are ultimately going to achieve is a lower basal metabolic rate; at the end of the diet you will therefore be using far fewer calories a day to maintain your own (diminished) tissue mass than you were before, and if you now decide to return to anything resembling a normal caloric intake for your height, age, and sex, you will gain weight at a much faster rate than normal because of the lowered metabolic baseline you are now operating from. This unhappy side effect of a low-carbohydrate diet probably accounts for the rapid swingback to previous weights that so many dieters experience when they go back to eating normally. With less lean tissue to fuel and refuel than it had before, the body no longer needs anything like a normal daily allotment of calories, and just eating the officially sanctioned daily regime spells an automatic gain in weight.

Everything that has been said about the zero- and low-carbohydrate diets can be said about starvation diets too, only more so. In the long run any such scheme is self-limiting and self-defeating; and for people constitutionally (or even just psychologically) programmed to get fat, it goes without saying that it is the long run that counts. Anybody can lose five to ten pounds of body weight on a short-term basis. Most fat people are experts at this; they have lost and regained the same five or ten pounds with boring regularity over the course of years. What counts is losing weight for good, and for this you need more than simple will power, self-loathing, and the short-term recklessness of the crash dieter—all of which the obese seem normally to have in good supply.

To lose weight for good the person constitutionally disposed to overweight needs time—the rest of his or her life, to be exact. Of all the bits and pieces of misinformation and false prophecy that surround the issue of obesity, the worst offender is the idea of diet itself. To people genetically programmed to obesity there is no such thing as a successful diet. Obesity itself is a physical disposition, not a passing indisposition; because it is not an indisposition it does not have a "cure" and does not invite "therapy." What it does need is a carefully cultivated and lifelong attention to the caloric value of incoming food and the energy value of outgoing effort. Like Europeans in the tropics, fat people in the modern urban hothouse are immigrants to a paradisical ecosystem that they are not properly genetically adapted to, and they must learn to make do in their new environment accordingly or pay the price in chronic overweight.

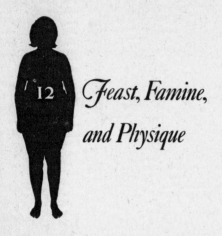

12 Feast, Famine, and Physique

We are what we eat, or so the saying has it. The biochemical implications of this maxim are fairly obvious; the social and historical ones are less so. In zoology, whole ways of categorizing animals have classically devolved from their feeding habits: The terms herbivore, carnivore, frugivore, and omnivore speak to the ecological and behavioral distances between those animals that graze for a living, those that hunt for a living, those that eat fruit for a living, and those who do a little of all three.

The distinctions are not arbitrary. Grazing animals, for example, share certain anatomical peculiarities like hooves and horns which are unknown to carnivores and frugivores and which, moreover, have nothing to do with their basic alimentary apparatuses at all. How an animal feeds and what he feeds on (and whether he is in turn fed on) can affect much more than his digestion: Such things can affect his means of locomotion, his angle of vision and hearing, his sense of smell, and his whole life-style into the bargain. If there is such a thing as "national character" there is no doubt also such a thing as zoological character. Cows do not just seem to be phlegmatic and "ruminative"; they actually are so. Cats owe their "cattiness" to the style of domestication that is their stock in trade.

How we eat, what we eat, when and how much we eat are questions that have resonances throughout all the other major areas of our lives; our feeding habits are as much a part of our unique personal signatures, both as individuals and as a species, as our faces, our voices, and our handwriting.

The history of human food-getting behavior reads like a history of human hegemony itself. We are the first primates and perhaps the last to have raised the sport of hunting to the level of a fine art complete with artifacts and learned to make a living at it in the process. In terms of feeding behavior, the basic primate blueprint is anything but a meat-eating one. Our simian ancestors were foragers and frugivores, and enjoyed the occasional meat meal only when they literally fell over it in the course of the day's real foraging action. Termites, birds' eggs, and carrion may have been fair game for some if not all of our simian and anthropoid cousins; but it is not until humanlike creatures arrived on the scene that hunting became a serious food-getting option for any of the major primate groups.

When it did so, something new had been uncontestably added to the sociobiology of feeding. As a carnivorous primate, man drew on two ancient traditions: To the spirit of teamwork that rules the food-getting strategies of carnivorous pack animals and killer felines, man has added the hierarchical genius of monkeys and apes. Meat eaters in the wild tend to be teammates and partners in crime; they need each other for success in the kill. Cooperation is thus the order of their day. This applies not only to animals like wolves and dogs that travel together in packs, but even to the large jungle cats as well. Wolves hunt in pairs when they are on the trail of animals that make easy marks, like sheep or caribou; but when they are on the scent of larger and more formidable animals like moose, the hunting party can swell to ten or more. Lions are more reclusive in their hunting habits than this, but while they may take on an individual gazelle singlehandedly, when they are tracking larger prey they may and often do enlist the cooperation of all the adults in the pride. Furthermore, like wolves and wild dogs, the big jungle cats may very well share out their food with other members of the pride, if only because the day's kill can be too much for one animal to make a meal of all alone. The logic of the food chain demands cooperation in the hunt and distribution of the kill in many groups of carnivores; as a result, an expedient "altruism" is one of the socio-biological earmarks of the killer carnivores.

Monkeys and apes have a very different approach to feeding. It is by and large a much more self-centered one—among foragers it is every man for himself, or, when there is a particularly choice tidbit to be had, or a sudden windfall to be apportioned, leaders first. The acting male potentate of a baboon or monkey troop does not share food with other members of his group; on the contrary, he stakes out a position for himself in the most lucrative corner of the day's feeding station and may even pre-empt a less dominant animal's grazing rights if he feels so inclined. In this situation it is rank order and dominance that carry the day. Decisions about who gets what to eat are made on the basis of size, status, and sex. Mutual give and take is not a big item of food-getting behavior in the primate repertoire.

Human reading, misreading, and rereading of these two basic food-getting strategies—the bloodthirsty team spirit of the carnivores on the one hand; the feudal highhandedness of the primates on the other—resulted for all practical purposes in a biogram unlike any that had been seen in the mammalian world until man arrived on the scene to invent it. In this startling new synthesis of two old traditions, it took the executive genius of the older men and the brawn and bravado of the younger ones to concert the day's hunt, just as it had done among the carnivores. Women and children, on the other hand, were left to themselves to forage in season just as their most remote primate ancestors had traditionally gone about it, and, if they were lucky or sexually or sentimentally favored, they could usually count on a reasonable handout of high-quality protein food from the men at the end of the day's hunt. In all probability it was therefore from very early on that typical male-female divisions of labor got established in the basic human way of doing things. When this happened the men lined up on the side of the carnivores in the mammalian family tree, while the women took their model from the frugivores.

Human marriage and work rhythms put down firm social roots in this new sociobiological soil. And so, no doubt, did the male bonding infrastructure from which so many of our political institutions—tribal, local, and international—have since evolved. Food and food getting are, however, only the beginnings of a longstanding economic deal between the individual and his group, or between one sex and another, one generation and the next. Social life itself begins at the breast, where the model for food sharing among mammals is that first unasked, instinctive, and essentially one-way distribution relay from mother to newborn child. Parental largesse is our first lesson in the dynamics of hunger and repletion. It is also surely one of our first lessons in comfort, company, pleasure and pain.

Armies travel on their bellies, according to the nineteenth-century punster; but the same thing can be said with equal justice for communities and nations as well. An assured food supply is the first order of the day not only for individuals, for families, and for cities, but for national governments as well. The "deal" between a citizen and his country is basically an economic one; how well this deal gets implemented, however, depends on a multiplicity of things, among which food resources and weather are neither last nor least. For even with all the technological resources of a modern industrial society, the breadbasket countries of the world still hold high cards: Fuel oil does not fill men's bellies; computers do not conjure up bread out of the thin air of data banks.

But food production, no matter how cleverly organized along cooperative-carnivorous lines, nor how finickingly distributed along hierarchic-primate ones, depends in the last analysis on growing conditions; and growing conditions depend first, last, and always on the weather. And in agriculture, technology ("mere technology," as certain environmentalists have learned to say) is not now and has never been a match for things as basic as the sun, the winds, and the rain. Man once knew this lesson in his bones; he has recently had to relearn it from the pages of his daily newspapers. By and large the famines that struck Bengal and sub-Saharan Africa in the early 1970's were treated by journalists as footnotes to the political history of the third world. In fact, an equally accurate view of the matter might well have been the exact reverse. In the long run it is probably just as fair to view our political systems as footnotes to our climates and our food production systems as it is to look at things the other way around. Since well before the beginning of the modern era, for example, the meat-eating north has tended to lord it over the grain-eating south. Western enterprise has generally been fueled by western plenty: It is hard to be enterprising (or even to stay alive) on less than 1,000 calories a day, especially if few or any of those calories are coming in in the form of animal proteins like meat, milk, fish, and eggs.

But Western man has increasingly paid the price of his rich granaries, fat bank accounts, and expanding gross national product, with relentlessly expanding waistlines to match. A fat carnivore may seem like a contradiction in terms: Animals who hunt for a living must ordinarily keep in racing trim. In this respect Western man seems to have outgrown the usual anatomical strictures implicit in the hunter's biogram. We do our hunting on the telephone now, from behind the ambush of a desktop, safe from the rigors of the weather and the actual chase. We do our foraging in shopping centers with our babies safely basketed in supermarket carts. Our climates are all indoor ones, equable and man-made. In what was once a hunter's rugged northern paradise, we have grown fatter and fatter with ecological impunity.

Or so it would seem, give or take a few squiggles in the mortality tables. Men evolving in climates which are benign enough to provide surplus food without being quite so benign as to produce unmanageable surpluses of population at one and the same time seem generally to have had it all their own way with history. The delicate equilibrium between climatic plenty and climatic rigor, between feast and famine, between hot and cold, is one that must be maintained if a species or a people is to prosper. Such an equilibrium, however, depends in the last analysis on the ingenuity with which each individual can manage to mediate his own metabolic needs in a constantly shifting ecological scene. Economic success as a civilization rests ultimately on the adaptive success of the individuals who foster it. And adaptation and adaptability in turn depend on genetic versatility.

The ability to gain and lose weight as the temperature rises and falls, or as granaries wax and wane, is one that has been meticulously bred into the genes of populations living between the climatic extremes of the so-called temperate zones. These zones are in a sense misnamed; their mild mean annual temperatures represent an average extrapolated from two highly divergent and thermally stressful extremes. Temperate-zone dwellers must be able to react with reasonable thermal and economic efficiency to both sets of extremes; and the fact that they can do so depends upon many things, not the least of which is their ability to accumulate fat. We may rail at our tendency, individual or collective, to gain weight; but temperate-zone populations owed their survival to this ability in the pre-industrial past, and if present trends in population, food production, and climate continue as they appear to be going, may well turn out to do so in the future too.

We live at present in an apparently cooling world. The trend is not universal (Australia, Antarctica, and parts of the southern Pacific seem to be exempt), but it is measurable and widespread. The growing season in England, for example, dwindled by a full two weeks between 1950 and 1975, and surface water temperatures in the North Atlantic have been dropping steadily throughout the same period. By the same token, between 1950 and 1972, there has been an 8 percent drop in the amount of autumn sunshine hitting forty-eight American states. Even so, when the mild winters that the Northern Hemisphere has enjoyed with minor ups and downs (and major complacency) over the last fifty years were rudely interrupted in late 1976 by record cold, citizens of an oil-fired and gas-driven world had sudden intimations of mortality. In the city of Buffalo six people stranded in cars during a January blizzard died of exposure to cold; so did two elderly men in an unheated New York City residence hotel. To a generation of Americans raised in the hothouse of thermostatically regulated central heating, the climatologists' persistent warnings of harsh winters ahead had fallen on deaf ears; it took the winter of 1976–77 to remind them of the killer colds our ancestors had once had to survive with grinding regularity.

The suddenness of it all is not without climatological precedent. Ninety thousand years ago a similar cold wave cooled Europe and parts of North America from temperate to glacial conditions within the course of a single century. Man or his manlike forebears left stranded by this change in the weather learned to live with it within the scope of at most three or four generations; his descendants in northern Europe, Russia, and China would otherwise not be alive to tell the tale today.

The story of their survival is one of the most impressive miracles of human adaptation so far recorded. Technology (fire, refinements of hunting skills, new inventions in architecture and home heating) must of course have played its part. But no innovation could have accomplished the whole job without an underlay of human biological ingenuity to build upon. To a large extent, that ingenuity involved coping mechanisms in our ability to mediate the stresses of extreme cold. And, to a considerable extent, such mechanisms themselves involved our ability to acquire and store surplus energy in the form of fat.

Human survival in Paleolithic Europe required the species to turn on the dime of its own adaptability and adjust from torrid to frigid weather, and from relative feast to virtual famine, within the course of a bare hundred years. We once did so with relative impunity and even a modicum of success; and that we may soon be asked to do so again does not now seem to be altogether beyond the realm of historical possibility. If the predicted cooling trend materializes, we may be in for another rude awakening not unlike the one suffered by our remote ancestors at the beginning of the Würm glaciation some 90,000 years ago. And if dwindling energy resources continue to dog us in the immediate future as they have done in the recent past, we may be forced to draw on the same biological coping mechanisms that man did then.

For despite the great arsenal of our technological inventions, despite all the refinements of our basic primate and carnivorous food-sharing relays, at the cutting edge of human hunger it has, historically, always been every man, every hamlet, or at most every nation for itself. And in a rapidly cooling world with its growing season and growing lands relentlessly whittled down by the encroachment of Arctic cold, the ability to put down and maintain fat may yet turn out to be at just as high a premium in the species' future as it must have been in the species' past.

We are the victims of ancestral circumstances. For many of us these circumstances were glacial, and therefore thermally and nutritionally decisive. Our ancestors rose to the evolutionary challenge by genetic instructions for more and better adipose tissue formation; we have inherited this solution in the form of excessive body fat. But every culture, if not every age, has its own idea of what constitutes an excess; and what may have been too much of a good thing in one time and place may turn out to be a niggardly bare sufficiency in another. In a changing climate and a possibly changing ecosystem, meanwhile, the case against fat and fatness has not been proved.

Bibliography

INTRODUCTION

Burnright, R. G., and Marden, P. G. "Social Correlates of Weight in an Aging Population." In Petersen, William, ed. *Readings in Population.* New York, 1972.

Malina, R. M. *Growth, Maturation, and Performance of Negro and White Elementary School Children.* Doctoral Dissertation, University of Pennsylvania, 1968.

Neel, James V., and Schull, William J. *Human Heredity.* Chicago, 1954.

Society of Actuaries. *Build and Blood Pressure Study.* Washington, D.C., 1959.

U.S. Public Health Service. *Obesity and Health* (Publication No. 1485). Washington, D.C., 1966.

1 GEOGRAPHY

Allen, J. A. "The Influence of Physical Conditions in the Genesis of Species." *Radical Review,* 1877.

Bergmann, Carl. "Über die Verhältnisse der Wärmeökonomie der Thiere zu ihrer Grösse." *Göttingen Studien,* 1847.

Coon, Carleton Stevens; Garn, Stanley; and Birdsell, J. *Races: A Study of the Problem of Race Formation in Man.* Springfield, Ill., 1950.

Eveleth, Phyllis. "The Effects of Climate on Growth." *Annals of the New York Academy of Sciences,* Vol. 110, 1963.

Hamill, Peter, and Johnston, Francis. "Height and Weight of Children 6–11." National Center for Health Statistics, Series 11, Vol. 104, 1973. "Height and Weight of Youth 12–17." National Center for Health Statistics, Series 11, Vol. 124, 1974.

Lindegard, Bengt, et al. "Male Sex Characters in Relation to Body Build, Endocrine Activity, and Personality." Lunds Universitets. Arsskrift NF Ard. 2, Bd. 52, No. 10, Lund, Sweden, 1956.

Millis, J. "The Effect of Equatorial Climate on Birth Weight and Subsequent Weight of Infants." *Journal of Tropical Pediatrics,* Vol. 3, No. 3, 1957.

Newman, Russell W., and Munro, Ella. "The Relation of Climate and Body Size in U.S. Males." *American Journal of Physical Anthropology,* Vol. 13, 1955.

Rensch, B. "Some Problems of Geographical Variations and Species Formation." *Proceedings of the Linnaean Society of London,* Vol. 149, 1936–37.

Roberts, D. F. "Body Weight, Race, and Climate." *American Journal of Physical Anthropology,* Vol. 11, 1953.

Schreider, Eugène. "Geographical Distribution of Body Weight/Body Surface Ratio." *Nature,* Vol. 165, 1950.

Sheldon, William Herbert; Stevens, Stanley Smith; and Tucker, William Boose. *The Varieties of Human Physique.* New York, 1940.

2 GENETICS

Angel, J. Lawrence. "Constitution in Female Obesity." *American Journal of Physical Anthropology,* Vol. 7, 1949.

Bjürulf, Per. "Obesity and Disease." In Brožek, J., ed. *Human Body Composition.* Oxford, 1965.

Darwin, Charles. *On the Origin of Species.* 1859.

Demole, M. J. "Dietetic Implications of Current Pathophysiological Concepts in Obesity." In Vague, J., ed. *Physiopathology of Adipose Tissue.* Amsterdam, 1969.

Dubos, René Jules. *Man Adapting.* New Haven, Conn., 1971.

Garn, Stanley. "Types and Distribution of Hair in Man." Abstract. *Annals of the New York Academy of Sciences,* Vol. 53, 1951.

Hanley, T. "The Aetiology of Obesity." In Baird, Ian M., and Howard, Alan N., eds. *Obesity: Medical and Scientific Aspects.* Edinburgh, 1969.

Hooton, Earnest Albert. *Handbook of Body Types in the U.S. Army.* Cambridge, Mass., 1951.

Hunt, E. E. "Hunger and Satiety in Health and Disease." *Advances in Psychosomatic Medicine,* Vol. 7, 1972.

Miller, D. S., and Mumford, P. "Gluttony: Thermogenesis in Overeating

Man." *American Journal of Clinical Nutrition,* Vol. 20, No. 11, 1967.

Nadal, P., et al. "Le Club des + 100 Kilos." *La Presse Médicale* (Paris), December 1, 1954.

Newman, Horatio Hackett; Freeman, Frank N.; and Holzinger, Karl J. *Twins: A Study of Heredity and Environment.* Chicago, 1927.

Newman, R. W. "Skin-Fold Measurements in Young American Males." *Human Biology,* Vol. 28, 1956.

Osborne, Richard H., and De George, Frances V. *Genetic Basis of Morphological Variation.* Cambridge, Mass., 1959.

Reynolds, E. L. "The Appearance of Adult Patterns of Body Hair in Man." *Annals of the New York Academy of Sciences,* Vol. 53, 1951.

Seltzer, Carl C. "Genetics and Obesity." In Vague, J., ed., *op. cit.*

Seltzer, Carl C., and Mayer, Jean. "Who Are the Obese?" *Journal of the American Medical Association,* Vol. 189, 1964.

Sims, E., et al. "Experimental Obesity in Man." In Vague, J., ed., *op. cit.*

Widdowson, E. M. "A Study of Individual Children's Diets." *Special Report: Series of Medical Research Council,* No. 257. London, 1947.

Withers, R. F. "Problems in the Genetics of Human Obesity." *Eugenics Review,* Vol. 56, No. 2, 1964.

3   WOMEN

Collinder, Björn. *The Lapps.* New York, 1949.

Ford, C. S., and Beach, F. A. *Patterns of Sexual Behavior.* New York, 1948.

Hunt, E. E. "The Developmental Genetics of Man." In Falkner, F., ed. *Human Development.* Philadelphia, 1966.

Klaatsch, Hermann. *The Evolution and Progress of Mankind.* Philadelphia, 1923.

Morris, Desmond. *The Naked Ape.* New York, 1967.

Shipman, William, and Schwartz, L. Unpublished (Michael Reese Hospital).

Singh, Devandra, and Sikes, S. "Role of Past Experience on Food-Motivated Behavior of Obese Humans." *Journal of Comparative and Physiological Psychology,* Vol. 86, March 1974.

Vallois, Henri. "Vital Statistics in Prehistoric Populations as Determined from Archaeological Data." In *The Application of Quantitative Methods in Archaeology.* Viking Fund Publications in Anthropology, No. 28, 1960.

Washburn, Sherwood L., and de Vore, Irven. "Baboon Ecology and Human Behavior." *African Ecology and Human Evolution.* Chicago, 1963.

4 PREGNANCY

Frisch, R., and MacArthur, J. "Menstrual Cycles: Fatness as a Determinant of Minimum Weight for Height Necessary for Their Maintenance or Onset." *Science,* Vol. 185, 1974.

Frisch, R., and Revelle, R. "Variation in Body Weights and the Age of the Adolescent Growth Spurt Among Latin American and Asian Populations in Relation to Caloric Supplies." *Human Biology,* Vol. 41, 1969.

Hytten, F., and Leitch, E. *The Physiology of Human Pregnancy.* Oxford, 1971.

Keys, Ancel, and Brožek, J. *The Biology of Human Starvation.* Minneapolis, Minn., 1950.

Oakley, Ann. *Woman's Work: A History of the Housewife.* New York, 1975.

Thomson, A.; Billewicz, W.; and MacGregor, I. "Body Weight Changes During Pregnancy and Lactation in Rural African Women." *Journal of Obstetrics and Gynaecology of the British Commonwealth,* Vol. 73, 1966.

Venkatchalam, P.; Shankar, K.; and Gopalan, C. "Changes in Body Weight and Body Composition During Pregnancy." *Indian Journal of Medical Research,* Vol. 48, 1960.

5 SOMATOTYPE

Bridges, P. K., et al. "Relationships Between Some Psychological Assessments, Body Build, and Stress." *Journal of Neurosurgical Psychiatry,* October 1973.

Child, Irvin. "The Relationship of Somatotype to Self-Rating on Sheldon's Temperamental Traits." *Journal of Personality,* Vol. 18, 1950.

Damon, A. "Some Host Factors in Disease: Sex, Race, Ethnic Group, and Body Form." *Journal of the National Medical Association,* Vol. 54, July 1962.

Damon, A., and MacFarland, R. A. "Physique of Bus and Truck Drivers." *American Journal of Physical Anthropology,* Vol. 13, 1955.

Garn, Stanley M., and Gertler, Menard M. "An Association Between Work and Physique in an Industrial Group." *American Journal of Physical Anthropology,* Vol. 8, 1950.

Hooton, Earnest Albert. "What Is an American?" *American Journal of Physical Anthropology,* Vol. 21, 1936.

Karvonen, M. J. "Physiological and Anthropological Studies on Participants in Lumber Competitions." *International Conference on Sport and Health,* State Office for Sport and Youth Work, Oslo, Norway, 1952.

Kretschmer, Ernst. *Körperbau und Charakter.* Heidelberg, 1948.

Lindegård, Bengt, et al. "Male Sex Characters in Relation to Body Build,

Endocrine Activity, and Personality." Lunds Universitets. Arsskrift NF Ard. 2, Bd. 52, No. 10. Lund, Sweden, 1956.

Naccarati, P. "The Morphologic Aspect of Intelligence." *Archives of Psychology*, Vol. 45, 1921.

Parnell, Richard William. *Behaviour and Physique*. London, 1958.

Schori, T. R., and Thomas, C. B. "Rorschach Factors and Somatotype." *Journal of Clinical Psychology*, Vol. 29, October 1973.

Sheldon, William Herbert; Dupertuis, C. Wesley; and McDermott, Eugene. *Atlas of Men*. New York, 1954.

Sheldon, William Herbert, and Stevens, Stanley Smith. *The Varieties of Temperament*. New York, 1942.

Sheldon, William Herbert; Stevens, Stanley Smith; and Tucker, William Boose. *The Varieties of Human Physique*. New York, 1940.

Tanner, J. M. "Physique and Function, Disease, and Behavior." In Harrison, G. A.; Weiner, J. S.; Tanner, J. M.; and Barnicot, N. A., eds. *Human Biology: An Introduction to Human Evolution, Variation, and Growth*. Oxford, 1964.

6 HORMONES

Ax, A. Cited in Funkenstein, D. H. "The Physiology of Fear and Anger." *Scientific American*, May 1955.

Best, C. H., and Campbell, James. "Anterior Pituitary Extracts and Liver Fat." *Journal of Physiology*, Vol. 86, 1936.

Bonner, John T. "Hormones in Social Amoebae and Mammals." *Scientific American*, Vol. 220, June 1969.

Bragdon, J. H., and Gordon, R. S. "Tissue Distribution of C^{14} After Injection of Labeled Fats." *Journal of Clinical Investigation*, Vol. 37, 1958.

Chalmers, T. M.; Kekwick, A.; and Pawan, G. L. "Fat Mobilizing Hormone in Human Urine." *American Journal of Clinical Nutrition*, Vol. 8, 1960.

Cleghorn, R., et al. "Psychophysiology of Lipid Mobilization." *Canadian Psychiatric Association Journal*, Vol. 12, 1967.

Elmadjian, A. Cited in Lischke, P. "The Psychobiology of Aggression." In Selg, Herbert, ed. *The Making of Human Aggression*. New York, 1975.

Heald, Felix. "Biochemical Aspects of Juvenile Obesity." *The Practitioner*, Vol. 206, February 1971.

Laron, Zvi. Abstract. *Acta Endocrinologica*, Supplement 100, 1965.

Meier, Albert. In Eleftheriou, B., ed. *Hormonal Correlates of Behavior*, Vol. II. New York, 1975.

Roth, J., et al. "Secretion of Human Growth Hormone: Physiologic and

Experimental Modification." *Metabolism,* Vol. 12, July 1963.

Rudman, D., and Seidman, F. "Lipemia in the Rabbit Following Injection of Pituitary Extract." *Proceedings of the Society of Experimental Biology and Medicine,* Vol. 99, 1958.

Schäfer, H. Cited in Best, C. H., and Campbell, James, *op. cit.*

Stevenson, J. A.; Box, B. M.; and Szlavko, A. J. "A Fat-Mobilizing and Anorectic Substance in the Urine of Fasting Rats." *Proceedings of the Society for Experimental Biology and Medicine,* Vol. 115, February 1964.

Stunkard, Albert J. "Glucose and Gastric Hunger in a Brain-Damaged Man." *American Journal of Clinical Nutrition,* Vol. 5, 1957.

Trygstad, O. Cited in Laron, Zvi, *op. cit.*

7 PHYSIOLOGY

Angel, J. Lawrence; Stutts, M.; and Mayer, Jean. In Mayer, Jean. *Obesity: Causes, Cost, and Control.* Englewood Cliffs, N.J., 1968.

Bloom, W. L., and Eidex, M. F. "Inactivity as a Major Factor in Adult Obesity." *Metabolism,* Vol. 16, August 1967.

Brady, Roscoe. "The Lipid Storage Diseases: New Concepts and Control." *Annals of Internal Medicine,* Vol. 82, February 1975.

Brobeck, J. R. "Food and Temperature." *Recent Progress in Hormone Research,* Vol. 16, 1960.

Cahill, George J. "Adipose Tissue Metabolism." In Rodahl, Kare, ed., *Fat as a Tissue.* New York, 1964.

Cheek, D. B. Symposium on Human Development, Temple University Medical School (unpublished), 1969.

Coon, Carleton Stevens. *The Living Races of Man.* New York, 1965.

Damon, A. and MacFarland, R. A. "Physique of Bus and Truck Drivers." *American Journal of Physical Anthropology,* Vol. 13, 1955.

Dorris, R. J., and Stunkard, Albert J. "Physiological Activity Performance and Attitudes of a Group of Obese Women." *American Journal of the Medical Sciences,* Vol. 233, 1957.

Edwards, H. T. "The Energy Requirements in Strenuous Muscular Exercise." *New England Journal of Medicine,* Vol. 213, 1935.

Galton, D. "An Enzyme Defect in a Group of Obese Patients." *British Medical Journal,* Vol. 2, 1966.

Green, David. "The Metabolism of Fats." *Scientific American,* January 1954.

Hausberger, Franz K. "Neurogenic Factors in Obesity." In Rodahl, Kåre, ed., *op cit.*

Hetenyi, M. Cited in Bruch, Hilde. *The Importance of Overweight.* New York, 1957.

Hirsch, Jules, and Knittle, Jerome L. "Nutrition and Cell Development: Cellularity of Obese and Nonobese Human Adipose Tissue." *Federation Proceedings,* Vol. 29, No. 4, 1970.

Johnson, Mary Louise; Burke, Bertha S.; and Mayer, Jean. "Relative Importance of Inactivity and Overeating in Energy Balance of Obese High School Girls." *American Journal of Clinical Nutrition,* Vol. 4, 1956.

Jones, Frederick Wood. *Man's Place Among the Mammals.* New York, 1929.

Keys, Ancel, and Brožek, J. *The Biology of Human Starvation.* Minneapolis, Minn., 1950.

Kreider, M. B. "Pathologic Effects of Extreme Cold." In Licht, S., ed. *Medical Climatology.* New Haven, Conn., 1964.

Maxwell, Nicole. *Witch Doctor's Apprentice.* New York, 1961.

Mayer, Jean. "Obesity." *Annual Review of Medicine,* Vol. 14, 1963.

Mayer, Jean. *Obesity: Causes, Cost, and Control.* Englewood Cliffs, N.J., 1968.

Monod, Jacques. *Chance and Necessity.* New York, 1971.

Riczak, M. A. "An Epinephrine-Sensitive Lipolytic Activity in Adipose Tissue." *Journal of Biological Chemistry,* Vol. 236, 1961.

Rolly, F. *Deutsche medizinische Wissenschrift,* Vol. 47, 1921.

Wassermann, Friedrich. "The Concept of the Fat Organ." In Rodahl, Kåre, ed., *op. cit.*

Winegrad, Albert I. "Adipose Tissue in Diabetes." In Rodahl, Kåre, *ibid.*

8 PSYCHOLOGY

Bronstein, I. P., et al. "Obesity in Childhood: Psychological Studies." *American Journal of the Diseases of Childhood,* Vol. 63, 1942.

Bruch, Hilde. *Eating Disorders: Obesity, Anorexia Nervosa, and the Person Within.* New York, 1973.

deWaard, Frits. Cited in Kushner, R. *Breast Cancer.* New York, 1975.

Fareni, J. "Do Fat People Like to Be Fat?" Cited in Wyden, Peter. *The Overweight Society.* New York, 1965.

Feiner, A. "Parental Figures and Sexual Identity of Adolescent Females." *American Journal of Digestive Diseases,* Vol. 21, 1954.

Hecht, M. B. "Obesity in Women." *Psychiatric Quarterly,* Vol. 29, 1955.

Hume, D. Cited in Bruch, Hilde, *op. cit.*

Kotkov, B., and Muranski, B. "Rorschachs of Obese Women." *Journal of Clinical Psychology,* Vol. 8, 1952.

Maher, J. Cited in Schachter, Stanley. "Some Extraordinary Facts About Obese Humans and Rats." *The American Psychologist,* Vol. 26, 1971.

Moore, Mary E.; Stunkard, Albert J.; and Srole, Leo B. "Obesity, Social

Class, and Mental Illness." *Journal of the American Medical Association,* Vol. 181, September 15, 1962.

Nisbett, Richard. "Determinants of Food Intake in Human Obesity." *Science,* Vol. 159, 1968.

Nisbett, Richard, and Gurwitz, S. "Weight, Sex, and the Eating Behavior of Human Newborns." *Journal of Comparative and Physiological Psychology,* Vol. 73, 1970.

Penick, S. B.; Filion, R.; Fox, S.; and Stunkard, Albert J. "Behavior Modification Treatment of Obesity." Paper presented at the Annual Meeting of the American Psychosomatic Society, Washington, D.C., March 1970.

Perry, L., and Learnard, B. Communication in *Journal of the American Medical Association,* Vol. 183, March 2, 1963.

Reeve, George. "Psychological Factors in Obesity." *American Journal of Orthopsychiatry,* Vol. 12, 1942.

Rodin, Judith; Elman, D.; and Schachter, Stanley. "Emotionality and Obesity." In Schachter, Stanley, and Rodin, Judith. *Obese Humans and Rats.* Potomac, Md., 1974.

Rodin, Judith; Herman, P; and Schachter, Stanley. "Obesity and Various Tests of External Sensitivity." In Schachter, Stanley, and Rodin, Judith, *ibid.*

Rorem, Ned. *The Final Diary, 1961–1972.* New York, 1974.

Schachter, Stanley. "Field Dependence, Drinking, and Urination." In Schachter, Stanley. *Emotion, Obesity, and Crime.* New York, 1971.

Schachter, Stanley; Goldman, R.; and Gordon, A. "Effects of Fear, Food Deprivation, and Obesity on Eating." *Journal of Personality and Social Psychology,* Vol. 10, 1968.

Schachter, Stanley, and Rodin, Judith. *Obese Humans and Rats.* Potomac, Md., 1974.

Shipman, William G., and Schwartz, L. Unpublished (Michael Reese Hospital).

Silverstone, J. T. "Psychological Factors in Obesity." In Baird, Ian M., and Howard, Alan M., eds. *Obesity: Medical and Scientific Aspects.* Edinburgh, 1969.

Suczek, R. F. "The Personality of Obese Women." *American Journal of Clinical Nutrition,* Vol. 5, 1957.

Wollersheim, Janet. "Effectiveness of Group Therapy Based Upon Learning Principles in the Treatment of Overweight Women." *Journal of Abnormal Psychology,* Vol. 76, 1970.

9 PSYCHOBIOLOGY

Blinder, B. J.; Freeman, D.; and Stunkard, Albert J. "Behavior Therapy of Anorexia Nervosa." *American Journal of Psychiatry,* Vol. 126, 1970.

Brobeck, J. R. "Food and Temperature." *Recent Progress in Hormone Research,* Vol. 16, 1960.

Brock, J. F., and Hansen, J. D. L. "Body Composition and Appraisal of Nutrition." In Brożek, J., ed. *Human Body Composition.* Oxford, 1965.

Bruch, Hilde. *Eating Disorders; Obesity, Anorexia Nervosa, and the Person Within.* New York, 1973.

Buskirk, E. R., and Thompson, R. H. "Metabolic Response to Cold Air in Men and Women in Relation to Total Body-Fat Content." *Journal of Applied Physiology,* Vol. 18, No. 3, 1963.

Carlson, Anton Julius. *The Control of Hunger in Health and Disease.* Chicago, 1916.

Delgado, José. *Physical Control of the Mind.* New York, 1969.

Funkenstein, D. H. "The Physiology of Fear and Anger." *Scientific American,* May 1955.

Hamilton, C. L. "Interactions of Food Intake and Temperature Regulation in the Rat." *Journal of Comparative and Physiological Psychology,* Vol. 56, June 1963.

Hervey, G. R. "The Problem of Energy Balance in the Light of Control Theory." In Mogenson, G. J., ed. *Neural Integration of Physiological Mechanisms and Behavior.* Toronto, 1975.

Margules, D. L. "Alpha-Adrenergic Receptors in the Hypothalamus for the Suppression of Feeding Behavior by Satiety." *Journal of Physiological and Comparative Psychology,* Vol. 73, No. 1, 1970.

Margules, D. L., and Olds, J. "Identical 'Feeding' and 'Rewarding' Systems in the Lateral Hypothalamus of Rats." *Science,* Vol. 135, February 2, 1962.

Mayer, Jean. *Obesity: Causes, Cost, and Control.* Englewood Cliffs, N.J., 1968.

Mayer, Jean, and Van Itallie, T. B. Cited in Mayer, Jean, *ibid.*

Mayer, Jean, et al. Cited in Mayer, Jean, *ibid.*

Miller, Neal E.; Bailey, C. J.; and Stevenson, J. A. F. "Decreased 'Hunger' but Increased Food Intake Resulting from Hypothalamic Lesions." *Science,* Vol. 112, 1950.

Miller, Neal E., and Delgado, José. Cited in Delgado, José, *op. cit.*

Russek, M. In Mogenson, G. J., ed., *op. cit.*

Schachter, Stanley, and Rodin, Judith. *Obese Humans and Rats.* Potomac, Md., 1974.

Sleeth, C. K., and Van Liere, E. J. "The Effect of Environmental Temperature on the Emptying Time of the Stomach." *American Journal of Physiology,* Vol. 118, 1937.

Stunkard, Albert J. "Glucose and Gastric Hunger in a Brain-Damaged Man." *American Journal of Clinical Nutrition,* Vol. 5, 1957.

10 ECOLOGY

Alland, Alexander, Jr. "Medical Anthropology and the Study of Biological and Cultural Adaptation." *American Anthropologist,* Vol. 68, February 1966.

Bernstein, J. G. "The Effect of Thermal Environment on the Morphology of the Thyroid and Adrenal Cortical Glands in the Albino Rat." *Endocrinology,* Vol. 28, 1941.

Bourlière, François. *The Natural History of Mammals.* New York, 1956.

Braudel, Fernand. *The Mediterranean.* New York, 1975.

Brues, Alice. "The Spearman and the Archer." *American Anthropologist,* Vol. 61, 1959.

Butzer, Karl. *Environment and Archaeology.* Chicago, 1968.

Caesar, Julius. *The Gallic Wars.*

Cannon, Walter Bradford. *The Wisdom of the Body.* New York, 1932.

Coon, Carleton Stevens. *The Living Races of Man.* New York, 1965.

Dawkins, M. J., and Hull, D. "The Production of Heat by Fat." *Scientific American,* Vol. 213, August 1965.

Dillon, E. S., and Dyer, W. W. "Factors Influencing the Prognosis of Diabetic Coma." *Annals of Internal Medicine,* Vol. 11, 1937–38.

Harrison, G. A.; Weiner, J. S.; Tanner, J. M.; and Barnicot, N. A., eds. *Human Biology: An Introduction to Human Evolution, Variation, and Growth.* Oxford, 1964.

Holmes, Thomas H., and Masuda, M. "Psychosomatic Syndrome." *Psychology Today,* Vol. 5, April 1972.

Irving, Laurence. "Adaptations to Cold." *Scientific American,* October 1971.

Mrosovsky, N. "The Adjustable Brain of Hibernators." *Scientific American,* Vol. 218, March 1968.

Naeye, R. L.; Freeman, R. K.; and Blanc, W. A. "Nutrition, Sex, and Fetal Lung Maturation." *Pediatric Research,* Vol. 8, March 1974.

Newman, Russell W. "Skin-Fold Measurements in Young American Males." *Human Biology,* Vol. 28, 1956.

Pannhorst, R., and Rieger, A. "Manifestierung des Diabetes und Jahreszeit." *S. Klinische Medizin,* Vol. 134, 1938.

Pengelley, E. T., and Fisher, K. C. "The Effect of Temperature and Photoperiod on the Yearly Hibernating Behavior of Captive Golden-Mantled Ground Squirrels." *Canadian Journal of Zoology,* Vol. 41, No. 6, 1963.

Petersen, W. F. "The Patient and the Weather." *Organic Disease,* Part II. Vol. 4, Ann Arbor, Mich., 1937.

Sargent, F. "Season and the Metabolism of Fat and Carbohydrate: A Study of Vestigial Physiology." *Recent Studies in Bioclimatology.* Champaign, Ill., 1954.

Tacitus, Cornelius. *The Complete Works.* Cambridge, Mass., 1925.

Teitelbaum, P. "Sensory Control of Hypothalamic Hyperphagia." *Journal of Comparative and Physiological Psychology,* Vol. 48, 1955.

Young, V. R., and Scrimshaw, R. S. "The Physiology of Starvation." *Scientific American,* October 1971.

11 SOLUTIONS

Allyon, T. "Intensive Treatment of Psychotic Behavior by Stimulus Satiation and Food Reinforcement." *Behavior Research and Therapy,* Vol. 1, 1963.

Ball, E. G., and Jungas, R. L. "On the Action of Hormones Which Accelerate the Rate of Oxygen Consumption and Fatty Acid Release in Rat Adipose Tissue in Vitro." *Proceedings of the National Academy of Sciences of the United States of America,* Vol. 47, 1961.

Ball, M. F., et al. "Comparative Effects of Caloric Restriction and Total Starvation on Body Composition in Obesity." *Annals of Internal Medicine,* Vol. 67, July 1967.

Barnard, J. L. "Rapid Treatment of Gross Obesity by Operant Techniques." *Psychological Reports,* Vol. 23, 1968.

Benoit, F. L., et al. "Changes in Body Composition During Weight Reduction in Obesity." *Annals of Internal Medicine,* Vol. 63, 1965.

Brobeck, J. R. "Food and Temperature." *Recent Progress in Hormone Research,* Vol. 16, 1960.

Cahill, George, Jr. "Adipose Tissue Metabolism." In Rodahl, Kare, ed. *Fat as a Tissue.* New York, 1964.

Feinstein, A. R. "The Problem of Treatment in Obesity." *General Practitioner,* Vol. 23, May 1961.

Garnett, E. S., et al. "Gross Fragmentation of Cardiac Myofibrils After Therapeutic Starvation for Obesity." *Lancet,* Vol. 1, 1969.

Glennon, J. A. "Weight Reduction—an Enigma." *Archives of Internal Medicine,* Vol. 118, July 1966.

Gour, K. N., and Gupta, M. C. "Social Aspects of Overweight and Obesity." *Journal of the Association of Physicians of India.* Vol. 16, 1968.

Grande, Francesco. "Comment." *Annals of the New York Academy of Sciences,* Vol. 110, 1963.

Green, David. "The Metabolism of Fats." *Scientific American,* January 1954.

Hollifield, G. "Influence of Food Intake and Physical Exercise on Adipose Tissue Metabolism." In Vague, J., ed. *Physiopathology of Adipose Tissue.* Amsterdam, 1969.

Jeanrenaud, B., and Renold, A. E. "Effects of Hormones on Adipose Tissue Lipogenesis." In Vague, J., ed., *ibid.*

Keys, Ancel, and Brožek, J. *The Biology of Human Starvation.* Minneapolis, Minn., 1950.

Mayer, Jean. *Overweight: Causes, Cost, and Control.* Englewood Cliffs, N.J., 1968.

Mayer, Jean; Roy, P.; and Mitra, K. P. "Relation Between Caloric Intake, Body Weight, and Physical Work: Studies in an Industrial Male Population in West Bengal." *American Journal of Clinical Nutrition,* Vol. 4, 1956.

Moore, Mary E.; Stunkard, Albert J.; and Srole, Leo B. "Obesity, Social Class, and Mental Illness." *Journal of the American Medical Association,* Vol. 181, September 15, 1962.

Morehouse, Laurence, and Gross, Leonard. *Total Fitness in Thirty Minutes a Week.* New York, 1975.

Mrosovsky, N. *Hibernation and the Hypothalamus.* Boston, 1971.

Penick, S. B.; Filion, R.; Fox, S.; and Stunkard, Albert J. "Behavior Modification Treatment of Obesity." Paper presented at the Annual Meeting of the American Psychosomatic Society, Washington, D.C., March 1970.

Rose, G. A., and Williams, R. T. "Metabolic Studies on Large and Small Eaters." *British Journal of Nutrition,* Vol. 15, 1961.

Silverstone, J. T. "Psychosocial Aspects of Obesity." *Proceedings of the Royal Society of Medicine,* Vol. 61, 1967.

Strong, J. A. *Diseases of Metabolism.* Philadelphia, 1964.

Stunkard, Albert J., and McLaren-Hume, M. "The Results of Treatment for Obesity." *Archives of Internal Medicine,* Vol. 103, 1959.

Wollman, Leo. "Hypnosis in Weight Control." *American Journal of Clinical Hypnosis,* Vol. 4, No. 3, 1962.

Young, Charlotte. Cited in Wyden, P. *The Overweight Society.* New York, 1965.

12 FEAST, FAMINE, AND PHYSIQUE

Bates, Marston. "Food-Getting Behavior." In Roe, A., and Simpson, G. G., eds. *Behavior and Evolution.* New Haven, Conn., 1958.

Schneider, S. H. *The Genesis Strategy.* New York, 1976.

Wahl, E. W., and Bryson, R. A. "Recent Changes in Atlantic Surface Temperatures." *Nature,* Vol. 254, 1975.

Washburn, Sherwood L., and Avis, V. "Evolution of Human Behavior." In Roe, A., and Simpson, G. G., eds., *op. cit.*

Wilson, Edward. *Sociobiology: The New Synthesis.* Cambridge, Mass., 1975.

Index

Catalog

If you are interested in a list of fine Paperback
books, covering a wide range of subjects
and interests, send your name and address,
requesting your free catalog, to:

McGraw-Hill Paperbacks
1221 Avenue of Americas
New York, N.Y. 10020